MINORITIES, MEDICINE AND HEALTH

RACIAL MINORITIES, MEDICINE AND HEALTH

B. Singh Bolaria
Rosemary Bolaria

Fernwood Publishing
Halifax, Nova Scotia

and

Social Research Unit
Department of Sociology
University of Saskatchewan
Saskatoon, Saskatchewan

Copyright © 1994	Social Research Unit
Department of Sociology
University of Saskatchewan
Saskatoon, Saskatchewan

All rights reserved. No part of this book may be reproduced or transmitted in any form by any means without permission in writing by the publisher, except for a reviewer who may quote brief passages in a review.

A publication of Fernwood Publishing

Fernwood Publishing
P.O. Box 9409
Station A
Halifax, Nova Scotia
B3K 5S3

Printed and bound in Canada

Second Printing

Canadian Cataloguing in Publication Data

Main entry under title: Racial minorities, medicine and health

Co-published by Social Research Unit of the University of Saskatchewan

Based on presentations made at a conference held at the University of Saskatchewan in June 1992

Includes bibliographical references.

ISBN 1-895686-41-5

1. Minorities — Medical care — Congresses.
2. Minorities — Health and hygiene — Sociological aspects — Congresses.
I. Bolaria, B. Singh, 1936- II. Bolaria, Rosemary.
III. University of Saskatchewan. Department of Sociology. Social Research Unit.

RA563.M56R32 1994   362.1 08 693   C94-950150-6

Contents

Contributors *xi*

Acknowledgments *xiii*

Introduction 1

PART 1: Racial and Socioeconomic Dimensions of Health and Illness

1. Social Status and Health Status: 9
   Does Money Buy Health?
   David I. Hay

2. Poverty, Homelessness and Health 53
   Valerie Tarasuk

3. Lifestyles, Material Deprivation and Health 67
   B. Singh Bolaria

4. Inequality and Differential Health Risks of 85
   Environmental Degradation
   B. Singh Bolaria and Rosemary Bolaria

5. Globalization of Environmental and 99
   Industrial Health Hazards
   B. Singh Bolaria and Rosemary Bolaria

6. Different Cultures or Unequal Life Chances: 113
   A Comparative Analysis of Race and Health
   Li Zong and Peter S. Li

PART 2: Immigrants, Race, Gender and Health

7. Mortality Differences Between the Canadian Born 127
   and Foreign Born in Canada, 1985-1987
   Frank Trovato

8. Immigrant Status and Health Status: 149
   Women and Racial Minority Immigrant Workers
   B. Singh Bolaria and Rosemary Bolaria

9. Health Status and Illness Patterns 169
   Among Asian Adolescents in Scotland
   Manfusa Shams

10. Hindu Asian Indian Women, Multiculturalism 189
    and Reproductive Technologies
    Vanaja Dhruvarajan

11. Racial and Ethnic Dimensions of Aging: 201
    Implications for Health Care Services
    K. Victor Ujimoto

12. Service Providers' Perceptions of 225
    Immigrant Well-Being and Implications
    for Health Promotion and Delivery
    Alexander M. Ervin

PART 3: Health Status and Health Care of Aboriginal Peoples

13. Colonization, Self-Determination and the 247
    Health of Canada's First Nations Peoples
    Terry Wotherspoon

14. Health Promotion and Indian Communities: 269
    Social Support or Social Disorganization
    James S. Frideres

15. Sick to Death: The Health of Aboriginal 297
    People in Australia and Canada
    Carol Reid

16. The Health of Aboriginal People in Saskatchewan: 313
    Recent Trends and Policy Implications
    Alan B. Anderson

17. Cultural and Socio-Economic Factors 323
    in the Delivery of Health Care Services
    to Aboriginal Peoples
    James B. Waldram

PART 4: Research Issues and Ethics

18. Problems and Limitations in the 341
    Study of Immigrant Mortality
    Frank Trovato

19. Cultural Diversity, Dual-Roles and Well-Being: 353
    A Research Note
    Manfusa Shams

20. Challenges of Research with Seniors 359
    M. Peggy MacLeod

21. Arranged Marriages and Mental Health 363
    Among Immigrant Women
    Lou Heber

22. Ethics and Research 371
    Michael Owen

Contributors

Alan B. Anderson, University of Saskatchewan
B. Singh Bolaria, University of Saskatchewan
Rosemary Bolaria, Saskatchewan Institute on Prevention of Handicaps
Vanaja Dhruvarajan, University of Winnipeg
Alexander M. Ervin, University of Saskatchewan
James S. Frideres, University of Calgary
David I. Hay, Social Planning and Research Council of
    British Columbia, Vancouver
Lou Heber, University of Saskatchewan
Peter S. Li, University of Saskatchewan
M. Peggy MacLeod, University of Saskatchewan
Michael Owen, University of Saskatchewan
Carol Reid, University of Western Sydney, Australia
Manfusa Shams, University of Glasgow, Scotland
Valerie Tarasuk, Ontario Workers' Compensation Institute, Toronto
Frank Trovato, University of Alberta
K. Victor Ujimoto, University of Guelph
James B. Waldram, University of Saskatchewan
Terry Wotherspoon, University of Saskatchewan
Li Zong, University of Saskatchewan

Acknowledgements

We wish to acknowledge the assistance of a number of individuals and organizations who contributed to this project. Most of the papers in this volume were first presented at a conference on Women, Racial Minorities, Medicine and Health and were subsequently revised for publication. Others were specifically written for this volume. We are grateful to all of the authors. The Social Sciences and Humanities Research Council of Canada, Multiculturism and Citizenship Canada, Saskatchewan Health, Health Services Utilization and Research Commission (formerly Saskatchewan Health Research Board) all provided financial assistance. We further acknowledge the financial and institutional support provided by the University of Saskatchewan and by the College of Arts and Science. We wish to thank Vice-President Patrick Browne and Dean David Atkinson. Kathleen Storrie and Bernard Schissel, former Head, Department of Sociology and former Director, Social Research Unit, respectively, were particularly helpful.

Many other individuals were helpful in making the conference a success. G.S. Basran, Kathleen Storrie, Vic Satzewich, Judith Martin, Jock Collins, Wendy Schissel, Katherine Kirk, Ahlam Mansour, James Frideres and Mildred Kerr all kindly agreed to chair sessions at the conference. Office staff, L.A.S. Sather and Helen Meyers, helped in the production of the conference programs and promotion. Romola Trebilcock, Steven Lewis and Michael Owen and many other individuals and community organizations helped to make this project a success.

Eric Cline, M.L.A., by his help in securing funding from Saskatchewan Health, and Pat Lorje, M.L.A., by her address at the opening session, both provided valuable support for the conference. The participation of Priscilla Joseph, Wilma Isbister, Pat Matheson, Victoria Caron, Nayyar Javed, and Cindy Sparvier made it possible to have a session entitled, "In Their Own Behalf: Voices from the Community." Others who contributed to the conference and deserve recognition are: Les Samuelson, Heather MacLean, Rebecca Hagey, Linda Mahood and Bonnie Jeffrey.

Special thanks to Lorna Close for her work in the early stages of the development of the manuscript. We wish to acknowledge the assistance of Kiran Bolaria in conference organization and initial document setup. Thanks also to Noreen Agrey and Kevin Adam for proofreading. Sharon Chapman provided expertise in cover design and final setup of the manuscript for publication. Terry Wotherspoon, Head, Department of Sociology, and Harley Dickinson, Director, Social Research Unit, also helped to see this book through to completion.

Introduction

In recent years, the medical profession, medicine, the structure and delivery of health services, and other aspects of the health-care system have received considerable criticism by medical sociologists and others interested in the health sector. Because of the current fiscal crisis in Canada, the problem of overall health-care costs and the financing of health-care services tend to dominate the discussion. Issues relevant to financing include: federal-provincial cost sharing arrangements, extra-billing, income and wages of health personnel, user fees, pharmaceutical and other institutional costs. This focus on the health sector costs and persistent inequality in health status have brought other aspects of the system under extensive scrutiny. One area which has received considerable attention is the clinical, mechanistic, individualistic, biomedical and reductionist tendencies in medicine. In the realm of medical practice, disease is attributed to malfunctioning of the human body, although, increasingly, social-psychological factors are being recognized as influential in disease processes. The treatment model associated with this conception of disease emphasizes that normal, or healthy, functioning can be restored through mechanical procedures, and technological and pharmacological "fixes." While the clinical model attributes disease to physiological malfunctioning, another reductionist perspective attributes illness to individual lifestyles, behaviours and consumption patterns. In this case, restoration of health lies primarily in changing individual behaviour, lifestyles and patterns of consumption. Although both the biomedical and lifestyle models are effective with regard to some disease processes, critics argue that they obfuscate and obscure the social nature of disease and fail to recognize the important relationships between social, economic, political and environmental conditions in society, and health and illness.

Furthermore, emphasis on disease-centred and curative medicine has tended to undermine, at least until very recently, the public health and social aspects of medicine, such as healthy social environment, health education, promotion and prevention. Also, under debate are the composition of the health sector labour force and the hierarchical organizational structure of health care institutions. Racial, gender and class inequalities continue to permeate the health sector. Women and racial minorities generally occupy the lowest rungs of the medical hierarchy and are often the lowest paid and most highly exploited segments of the health sector workforce. The positions of various social groups in the medical hierarchy and in society have consequences for their health (health status) as well as their experience as consumers of health services (patients). These are manifested in allocation of research efforts and resources toward diseases primarily affecting minority groups and the attitudes of the practitioners toward their illness episodes and symptoms. Critics have argued that research funding for health-related problems of minorities have received low priority. Also, health complaints of women and minorities tend to be trivialized and are often dismissed as psychosomatic. There has also been the tendency to medicalize their problems which not only obscures the social origin of these problems, but also extends further medical control and domination over these groups. Thus, whether as providers or consumers of services, socially subordinated individuals and groups continue to face exploitation, discrimination and even abuse.

Social medicine is primarily concerned with the conditions in the society that produce illness and mortality. Social epidemiology and the environmental approach to health care are in conflict with the biological and individual orientation of the predominant medical paradigm. Several social conditions that generate illness are the focus of this approach. These include material conditions of life, material deprivation and differential opportunity structures and life chances. Despite some variation, the common theme that appears in many of the essays in this volume is that health status and accessibility to and availability of health services is related to racial, social, economic, political and gender inequality.

The broadly defined topic of *Racial Minorities, Medicine and Health* covers a great diversity of issues. This volume, while extensive, does not, of course, cover all the dimensions of this topic. In Part 1, racial and socio-economic dimensions of health and illness are examined. Hay, in Chapter 1, discusses international and Canadian research that examines the relationship between social status and

Introduction

health status. He argues that economic inequalities are among the more important social determinants of health status. Based upon his own research, Hay examines the relationship between *change* in income status and change in health status. The chapter concludes with a critical synopsis of general, methodological, and conceptual issues arising from the literature review, and draws out research and policy implications. Tarasuk, in Chapter 2, examines health issues confronting the homeless population. Three critical features of drop-in members' everyday lives — poverty, homelessness and social isolation — are considered fundamental to the physical, mental and social well-being of this group. Tarasuk argues that these features set the context for other health problems and health care professionals' response to them. In Chapter 3, Bolaria examines the relative effect of individual lifestyle and environmental factors on health and illness and concludes with a discussion of the ideological and policy implications of individualistic and social perspectives.

There is increasing awareness of environmental pollution and hazardous work environments and the linkages between environmental degradation and illness. In Chapter 4, Bolaria and Bolaria examine the links between environmental degradation and health and discuss the differential impact of environmental conditions on individuals and social groups in society. Environmental pollution and degradation and industrial production of health hazards are not confined to a single country or region. Globalization of production has led to globalization of health hazards. This is the subject matter of Chapter 5 by Bolaria and Bolaria.

In the last chapter in this section, Li Zong and Peter Li, using health data from 118 countries around the world, conclude that the racial effects on health disappear when the material conditions of life are taken into account. Their study confirms the importance of economic conditions in accounting for differences in health status.

In Part 2 the health related issues are examined for immigrant populations. Frank Trovato, in Chapter 7, examines the mortality differences between the Canadian-born and foreign-born in Canada, 1985-1987. The findings show that immigrants enjoy a relatively lower level of mortality than the Canadian-born. These observations are consistent with previous studies in other receiving countries such as France, England-Wales, Australia and the United States. The pattern of mortality differences indicates that the advantage for immigrants is largely concentrated in the adult working years, which could be partly a function of health selectivity and other factors such as occupational and lifestyle differences between immigrants and their host populations. The study also shows that relative advantage in survivorship is somewhat greater for immigrant men than for immigrant women.

In Chapter 8, Bolaria and Bolaria examine the health consequences of immigrant status for women and racial minority workers in agriculture, textiles and domestic work and for workers in other service sector jobs. It is argued that the immigrant and migrant workers because of their legal and political vulnerability are subjected to hazardous work environments. Their living and working conditions are dangerous to their health. Gender and race compound workers' disadvantages — minority workers and women are exposed to even more hazardous working environments. In the next chapter, Shams examines the health status and illness patterns among Asian adolescents in Scotland. This pilot study highlights the anthropometric features and health status of 14 and 15 year old Asian-Scottish and Scottish boys and girls. The findings suggest the ways in which Asian assimilation to Scottish health norms may be occurring only selectively and indicates the way to further analysis of the total sample. In Chapter 10, Dhruvarajan uses one aspect of reproductive technologies to illustrate the lived experience of racism and sexism by first generation Hindu Asian Indian women. She contends that targeting of this group for the reproductive technology of fetal sex determination has the potential of making these women an endangered species and the Asian Indian ethnic culture an endangered culture. Ujimoto, in Chapter 11 further explores the issue of culture and health with particular reference to aged populations. The increasing heterogeneity of the Canadian population has important implications for provision of health care services. Ujimoto argues that health care providers must recognize and understand the variations in health beliefs, attitudes, and behaviours in multicultural society, most importantly, the aging ethnic minorities. A culturally sensitive health-care system, Ujimoto argues, will provide some relief to the mental stress experienced in daily life. The last chapter in this section, by Ervin, also explores the factors associated with immigrant well-being and their implications for health promotion and health policy. He argues that the well-being, or physical, psychological, spiritual and social health of immigrants, along with their capacity to integrate and adapt, will depend upon effective, holistic, comprehensive, and multi-sectoral strategies of partnership involving both the immigrant and host communities.

While disparities in health status continue to persist among different socio-economic groups, these disparities are even more pronounced between the Native and non-Native populations. The health status and health care of Aboriginal peoples is the subject of Part 3. Wotherspoon, in Chapter 13, provides an overview of health indicators, which show a serious need for improved health for much of the Native population in Canada. He also examines issues related to jurisdictional reorganization and trends towards the devolution of health care for Canadian Native peoples. Wotherspoon argues that unless self-determination addresses significant socio-economic inequalities and political problems, it is likely that disparities will persist. Frideres, in Chapter 14, also discusses the health status of residents of Indian communities. The data show that their health problems are different from and more severe than in non-Indian communities. This chapter identifies the institutional structure which provides health care services to Indian people, provides a profile of Indian health, and discusses possible explanations of high levels of illness, mortality, and general low quality of life experienced by Natives. Frideres concludes with possible alternative strategies to deal with health issues and conditions on reserve communities. Reid, in Chapter 15, compares the health status of Aboriginal people in Australia and Canada and finds remarkable similarities, not only in health status, but also in their socio-economic status. Reid argues that the health of Aboriginal people in Australia and Canada must always be seen in the context of the political, economic and social conditions of their existence. Anderson, in Chapter 16, focuses on recent trends in health status of Aboriginal people in Saskatchewan, followed by a discussion of policy alternatives to eliminate health status inequalities. Anderson argues that to achieve equality in health it is necessary to address questions of social, economic and political inequality experienced by Aboriginal people and to develop a "culturally sensitive" approach to health care. The final chapter in the section, by Waldram, discussed cultural and socio-economic factors concerning Aboriginal health. Waldram challenges the common assumption that cultural values and norms explain to a large extent their apparent reluctance or inability to use biomedical health care services. He argues that Aboriginal people have suffered from a lumping effect, which assumes that they are not only culturally similar, but also uniformly culturally dissimilar from non-Aboriginal Canadians. Waldram presents evidence that culture *per se* is not an impediment to health care utilization and suggests that their utilization of biomedical services might be better understood by considering both the cultural and socio-economic factors.

In Part 4, various essays examine a number of research issues. Trovato, in Chapter 18, examines substantive and data quality problems and limitations inherent in the study of immigrant mortality using official vital statistics. Shams, in Chapter 19, points out that despite extensive interest in Asian culture and the Asian marriage and family system in Britain, little attention has been given to the gendered division of labour and the influence of the Western work ethic in this group. She also contends that limited attention is given to the feminist movement among diverse socio-cultural groups. Shams identifies some of the salient socio-cultural factors which may enable us to better understand the differences or similarities in dual-role experiences of men and women and the relationship of these experiences to well-being. MacLeod, in Chapter 20, identifies problems in the study of seniors, including sampling bias and ethical considerations and makes recommendations for doing research with people 65 years of age and older.

The increasing cultural heterogeneity of the Canadian population poses challenges and offers opportunities for researchers interested in the health field. In Chapter 21 Heber examines the issue of arranged marriages and mental health among immigrant women from the Philippines, especially those involved in inter-cultural and inter-racial marriages.

Researchers encounter ethical dilemmas in the conduct of their research, according to Owen, especially when projects involve cross-cultural and disciplinary boundaries and impact upon gender and gender relations. While professional associations provide general ethical guidelines for research, these guidelines and protocols may not provide all the necessary information, advice and direction for the conduct of research related to specific areas. Michael Owen addresses some of these issues in Chapter 22. He outlines the role of the Institutional Review Boards (Ethics Committees), discusses general guidelines on research ethics, and concludes with a discussion of issues specifically related to the theme of the conference — Women, Racial Minorities, Medicine and Health.

PART 1:

Racial and Socioeconomic Dimensions of Health and Illness

1

Social Status and Health Status: Does Money Buy Health?

David I. Hay

Introduction

Health policy in Canada affirms the right of equal access to health care services. The introduction of national health insurance in Canada has resulted in a fairer distribution of health care resources among Canadians than at any other time in history. However, the available evidence, although not entirely consistent, suggests that access to health care is still not entirely equitable for Canadians (Badgley, 1991; Badgley et al., 1967; Badgley and Smith, 1979; Barer et al., 1982; Beck, 1973; Beck and Horne, 1976; Boulet and Henderson, 1979; Charles and Badgley, 1987; Enterline et al., 1973; Freedman and Baylis, 1987; Manga, 1978, 1981, 1987; Manga and Weller, 1980; Siemiatycki et al., 1980; Statistics Canada, 1977; Wolfe, 1991).

What if access to health care was more equitable? Would this contribute to greater equity in individual health status? Recent papers (Badgley and Wolfe, 1992; Charles and Badgley, 1987; Manga, 1981, 1987; Manga and Weller, 1980), federal government policy statements (Epp, 1986), and provincial government reports (Government of Ontario, 1987; Ontario Ministry of Health, 1987a, 1987b) suggest that equality of access to health care does not ensure equality of individual health. Differences in individual human biology are not sufficient to produce the vast and patterned health inequalities that exist in our society.

In fact, a relationship between social inequality and health status is difficult to dispute. So durable is the finding of an inverse association between social status and health that one author has proposed using standardized mortality ratios (SMRs), a health status indicator, as an indicator of living conditions (Anson, 1988). If an area has a particularly poor SMR, it would be assumed to also have poor living conditions.

Evidence of inequalities in health have been found in medical and social science literature, at least since the 1800s (D'Arcy, 1988; Illsley, 1987; Townsend, Phillimore and Beattie, 1986). For example, in the 19th century in Britain, the horrendous work and living conditions accompanying rapid industrialization became a major focus of social reformers. Public health studies measured disease death rates in different localities and found a wide variation between upper and lower classes - in some cases members of the upper classes lived three times as long as those in the lower classes (Chadwick, 1842; Engels, 1958). In later years work on area inequalities in health burgeoned (Townsend, Phillimore and Beattie, 1986). Because of this mounting evidence of social and geographic variation in health, and the understanding that a healthy population was not only a benefit to each individual, but also to the community and its economic prosperity, comprehensive population health insurance plans were later advocated to promote equitable health status (Townsend et al., 1986 for Britain; Badgley, 1991 for Canada).

It is evident that health status is not equally distributed among individuals and groups because individual opportunity to achieve health is not equally distributed. An individual's health status and health opportunity depends on a lengthy list of social conditions, and not only on individual biology or access to medical care.

As long ago as 1848 German physician Rudolf Virchow emphasized that economic, social, and cultural reforms were necessary to deal adequately with the causes of a typhus outbreak among a disadvantaged population in Upper Silesia (Taylor and Rieger, 1985). Virchow felt strongly that medicine was a social science, and that improvements in health would only come about through improvements in the social environments of individuals, and not solely through medical intervention.

Since Virchow's time many researchers and policy makers around the world have emphasized social change, rather than improvements to health care services, as a means to reducing health risks (Badgley, 1991; Blaxter, 1983; Block et al., 1987; Bodenheimer, 1989; Buck, 1985; Burke, 1986; Charles and Badgley, 1987; City of Toronto, 1983; 1985; 1991; Dahlgren and Diderichsen, 1986; D'Arcy, 1988; D'Arcy and Siddique, 1985; Doyal and Gough, 1986; Echenberg, 1988; Epp, 1986; Evans and Stoddart, 1990; Gold and Franks, 1990; Gortmaker, 1979; Government of Ontario, 1987; Gray, 1982; Harding, 1987; Hart, 1987; Hartmann, 1982; Hexel and Wintersberger, 1986; Ho, 1982; Hollingsworth, 1981; House, Landis, and Umberson, 1988; Kickbush,

1986; McKeown, 1976; Ontario Ministry of Health, 1987a; 1987b; Patrick et al., 1988; Scott-Samuel, 1986; Syme, 1986; 1988; Townsend, 1981; 1990b; Townsend and Davidson, 1982; Townsend, Davidson, and Whitehead, 1988; Warner and Murt, 1984; Whitehead, 1988; Wilkinson, 1986; 1990; Wolfe, 1991; Zaidi, 1988). The sheer amount of this evidence lends credence to the conclusions. An individual uses health care services because of a suspected health problem. While medical intervention may prevent further individual exposure to health risks, the fact that an individual seeks medical advice generally indicates that illness or disease symptoms are already present. Medical intervention can only attempt to cure individual disease symptoms presented to the health, or more appropriately, 'sick' care system, and hence tends to neglect the prevention of illness.[1]

What are the factors that predispose individuals to illness or disease? Genetic, biological, and behavioural factors can be significant causes of disease. But, as the abundant literature indicates, these factors operate within a social context. The social circumstances of individuals set the stage upon which these other factors act. Thus social factors - income, education, occupation, age, gender, marital status, living conditions, stress, and so on, to some extent determine, through genetic, biological, and behavioural factors, whether or not an individual will be at risk for illness or disease. Health status differences are patterned by these social factors, and are not randomly distributed.

A large body of Canadian and international literature maintains that 'social factors,' related either directly or indirectly to general socioeconomic standing, have a profound effect on health status (D'Arcy, 1988; Macintyre, 1986). Past research on social status and health has used various indicators to measure these concepts. Social status has been measured by indices of social class, socioeconomic status (SES), education, occupation, and/or income. In an attempt to specify or interpret social status and health relationships, other social factors, such as gender, age, region, stress, marital status, social support, and so forth, have been introduced as explanatory variables. Health has been measured primarily by examining aggregate mortality statistics, although there is a body of research which has used morbidity incidence and/or prevalence, either from official records or respondent self-reports. Health status has also been measured in sample surveys with self-reported items such as 'number of illnesses,' 'number of days of disability,' and items tapping the respondent's satisfaction with, or rating of, their health status.

This chapter explores international and Canadian research that examines the relationship between social status and health status. The review concentrates primarily on the literature that examines social status differences (as defined by education, occupation, and/or income differences) in health status.

It has been argued that economic inequalities are among the more important social determinants of health status. Certainly income is a measure of the most significant aspect of economic inequality. As well, many of the specific social factors listed above control or explain income and health status relationships. Therefore, studies that specifically examine relationships between *income* and health are reviewed in a separate section. As well, a study I have recently completed examining the relationship between *change* in income status and *change* in health status is outlined in some detail.

The amount of research on social status and health status, beginning with the nineteenth century British and German studies mentioned above, is so extensive as not to permit detailed review. Furthermore, the general results of these studies are widely known. Almost all of them have found a strong or moderate relationship between social circumstances and health status.

Thus, the literature review begins with a discussion of the *Black Report* (Townsend and Davidson, 1982), one of the most important studies in the inequality and health area. The *Black Report* is important as the publication of the report caused much comment and controversy, and because the report sets out clearly some alternative explanations for the social position - health status linkage. Findings, interpretations of findings, and critiques of the *Black Report* by other authors, are reviewed.

A closing section provides a critical synopsis of general, methodological, and conceptual issues arising from the literature review, and poses a research agenda for further work in this area.

Social Status and Health Status: International Evidence

The *Black Report*

The *Report of the Working Group on Inequalities and Health*, more commonly known as the *Black Report* (published in 1980), has proved to be a watershed regarding inequality and health research. The *Working Group* was a British government sponsored research team charged with investigating the relationship between 'social class' (occupational groupings) and health statistics.

Many commentaries and reinterpretations of the findings presented in the *Black Report* have been published in the last decade. The *Black*

Report renewed research interest in the inequality and health area, as evidenced by the large amount of published material on the subject available in the 1980s. It is important to review the findings of the *Black Report* in order to gain perspective on other research in this area. Townsend (one of the *Working Group's* original members) and Davidson (1982) co-authored a paperback edition of the *Black Report* to make the findings of the report available to a wider audience. This edition is the basis for our review.

The *Black Report* relied on a classification of occupations as its measure of social status. There are criticisms of this reliance, some of which will become clear below. The use of this classification of occupations stems from a tradition of continuously recorded official British government statistics using these measures. Comparable data with measures of education and/or income, from government statistics or periodic health surveys, are unavailable in Britain (Townsend, 1990a).

The *Black Report* presented findings which showed significant differences between occupational groupings on mortality and morbidity measures. In directly relating occupational status and mortality, it was found that the men and women lowest in occupational status had "a two-and-a-half times greater chance of dying before reaching retirement age" relative to those of the highest occupational group (Townsend and Davidson, 1982:51). Controlling for age, the differences were reduced only slightly - to a ratio of two-to-one. In addition to status differences, gender differences in mortality were pronounced. Death rates for men were nearly double that of women for all occupational groups. The most significant social status differences in mortality rates, for men and women, were found for deaths due to accidents and respiratory diseases, both of which are closely related to the socioeconomic environment (Townsend and Davidson, 1982).

In surveying the smaller number of studies investigating the relationship between occupational status and morbidity, similar trends were found to those shown by the mortality data, "though inequalities between occupational classes are more pronounced, and the gradients more uniform, in the case of chronic sickness than in the case of acute or short-term ill-health" (Townsend and Davidson, 1982:64).

In attempting to interpret variability in morbidity and mortality by occupational group, four categories of explanation were proposed (Townsend and Davidson, 1982:12-121):

1. *Artefact explanations* propose that social status and health relationships are artificial products of the research process, and are invalid measures of the actual life conditions of groups of people. Thus, the relationships observed are of little or no causal significance.

2. *Theories of natural or social selection* rest on the assumption that there are certain characteristics of individuals which predispose them to low social status. The implication is that a greater predisposition to ill health is one of these characteristics. Poor health means that an individual cannot adequately compete in societies such as ours - educationally, occupationally, or monetarily. Thus, poor health leads to low status, rather than the reverse.

3. *Materialist - structuralist explanations* emphasize "the role of economic and associated socio-structural factors in the distribution of health and well being" (p. 114). The implication is that a disadvantaged social situation causes ill health.

4. *Cultural - behavioural explanations* lend explanatory power to the attitudes and behaviour of individuals. Behaviour shaped by cultural values, such as those that impact on food and living conditions ('choices'), as well as more specific behaviours such as smoking and excessive drinking, are examples of behavioural factors which might depend on cultural values, and which may place individuals at greater risk of ill health.

Both the materialist - structuralist and the cultural - behavioural explanations assert that low social status, poor social behaviour, and/or our cultural values, can lead to poorer health. Thus both explanations are subsumed under the category of 'social causation' explanations and are in direct opposition to social selection explanations. The *Black Report* lent little credence to the artefact explanation, and also noted that not much evidence existed to support the theories of natural or social selection. The authors of the report favoured social causation explanations. The social context of cultural - behavioural explanations was emphasized and the report supported materialist - structuralist explanations as the most important. It should be emphasized that little research exists (or the *Black Report* failed to review it) which pays attention to 'natural' factors such as inherited or congenital disabilities and their impact on social status or health over time (Joffe, 1989). Investigations of the social transformation and behavioural implications of cultural values on inequalities in health are generally excluded from analyses of administrative data (Baxter and Baxter, 1988).

Critiques of the *Black Report*

A number of analysts have critically reviewed the *Black Report*'s findings and explanations of the relationship between inequalities and health. Gray (1982) acknowledges the importance of the report's findings and summarizes some of the responses to the report. Gray has reservations about the measures of 'health' employed and the extent to which causal direction can be inferred. He questions the use of mortality rates as an indicator of health: "inequalities in death may not be similar to inequalities in health" (1982:373). Gray also feels that the interpretation of causal direction offered by the materialist explanation could have been more fully developed. Gray hypothesizes that defining class in Marxist rather than occupational terms would "have afforded more detailed structural insights into the causation of inequality" (1982:374).

Blane uses the *Black Report*'s framework of explanations of health inequalities and provides an assessment of them with additional evidence from the "literatures of sociology and medicine" (1985:424). Generally, Blane supports the weight accorded to the various explanations by the *Black Report*. The artefact explanation "fails to 'explain away' the association between social class and health" (Blane, 1985:439). The contribution of this explanation is, if anything, in understating social status differences in ill health. While the natural or social selection explanation is assessed as tapping 'real' social processes, "its contribution to social class differences [in health] is small, and limited to particular age groups and movement between particular bands of the social hierarchy" (Blane, 1985:439-440). Blane views social causation explanations as the most plausible in light of the evidence.

Blane (1985) also states that cultural - behavioural explanations of health inequalities are predominantly offered by other authors over materialist - structural explanations of health inequalities. However, Blane feels that material factors have to be further investigated, and that the concept of 'social class' (occupational status) "refers to the combination of many different types of advantage or deprivation, and the summation and interaction of these factors needs to be studied" (Blane, 1985:440).

Bloor and colleagues (1987) offer an assessment of artefact explanations of inequalities in health and conclude "that the role of artefact explanations in mortality differentials is larger, more pervasive, and more complex than Black and his colleagues believed" (Bloor et al., 1987:231). However, the specifics of this more general statement are difficult to interpret. That is, while coding and diagnostic bias may render conclusions based on such data tenuous, there is evidence that suggests the bias may be randomly distributed among the populations under study. Bloor and colleagues (1987) conclude that the possibility of research findings being an artefact of "the measurement process may be construed as both producing and concealing health inequalities" (Bloor et al., 1987:261).

Illsley (1987) and Stern (1983) suggest that the *Black Report* did not give sufficient weight to theories of social selection. Both of these authors maintain that changes in the composition of occupational groupings over time, through inter- and intra- generational mobility of individuals, need to be assessed to adequately estimate the health differences between occupational groups. The suggestion is that the *Black Report*'s finding of historically widening social inequalities in mortality and morbidity may be due to the lack of consideration of the importance of social mobility effects in changing the composition of the various occupational groupings.

Hart (1987) directly challenges Illsley's (1987) arguments by arguing that the data are not available to support such a thesis. To provide evidence of the social selection hypothesis "requires longitudinal data with careful observations on changing health status together with the material and social circumstances of childhood and adult life" (Hart, 1987:19). Hart also cautions that it is difficult to separate personal attributes from their environs. Mobility may be aided by factors other than individual health or fitness. For example, it may be associated with material well-being, such as diet and/or living standards, which promote individual mobility. Focusing on large occupational groupings may obscure these possibly more fundamental material advantages (Hart, 1987).

Fox, Goldblatt, and Jones (1985) found deficiencies in the data examined in the *Black Report*. Specifically, Fox et al. noted potential biases in the mortality statistics examined, as well as arguing that conclusions on trends had been made with what were really different sets of cross sectional data (1985:1). In order to examine the potential contribution of artefact, social selection, or social causation effects on health, they used data from a British longitudinal study which followed a specific population cohort. In general, the findings of Fox and colleagues supported the findings of the *Black Report* "and suggest that major explanations for such [social class] differentials should not be sought from among artefactual or selection theories" (1985:7). However, Fox and colleagues face similar limitations to Black and associates in that the potentially unreliable occupational status measure is employed as the indicator of social position. As well, occupational status is measured at only one point in time and then used to predict mortality five and ten years hence. The status of respondents could easily have changed in this time affecting the interpretation of results (Fox and Goldblatt, 1982).

In a later paper Goldblatt (1990) reiterates the finding of little determinance afforded to social selection explanations of social status differentials in mortality. Goldblatt observes that social status differences in mortality persist over time even though causes of mortality have changed from a predominance of infectious diseases to a predominance of those diseases "most usually associated with lifelong health behaviour" (1990:54). Goldblatt also examines different measures of social status (such as car access and home ownership) and finds similar mortality gradients to those found by Black and associates (Townsend, Phillimore, and Beattie, 1986). These findings would argue against a determining role for social selection theories as a predominant interpretation of mortality differences (Goldblatt, 1990).

Le Grand and Rabin (1986) also have concerns with the way in which data were analyzed by the *Black Report*. First, it is noted that the occupational groupings used to denote 'social classes' may not be as distinct as was thought. For instance, it is shown that weekly earnings of the various occupational groups overlap. Second, the *Black Report* based its main findings on the absolute difference between the standardized mortality ratios (SMRs) of the highest and lowest occupational groups. However, some of the differences in SMRs within occupational 'classes' are greater than the difference observed between the highest and lowest occupational 'classes.' Third, it is noted that not all individuals in the population are included for analysis. The *Black Report* limited its main sample under study to working men and women age 15-64, thereby excluding children, married women at home, retired people, students, the unemployed, and so on. Fourth, it is noted that a large amount of misclassification occurs in placing individuals in occupational groups. What effect this may have on any relationships observed is unknown. Last, it is noted that changes in the actual sizes of the occupational groups could seriously affect the interpretation of results. The actual number of deaths is increasing amongst higher occupational groups while the number of deaths is decreasing for lower occupational groups, because the former are increasing and the latter are shrinking in absolute size. Thus, as mortality *rates* are declining in the higher occupational groups and increasing in the lower occupational groups, simply looking at the number of deaths in each group would reveal a different picture.

However, all these commentators (Blane, 1985; Bloor et al., 1987; Fox, Goldblatt, and Jones, 1985; Goldblatt, 1990; Hart, 1987; Illsley, 1987; Le Grand and Rabin, 1986; Stern, 1983) support, to a greater or lesser extent, social causation explanations. They feel that it is not easy to separate causal mechanisms, especially given the data under examination, and that possibly it may be best to combine the selection and causation explanations as they both could be acting at the same time, or be part of a cyclical relationship (Wolinsky and Wolinsky, 1981). Comprehensive reviews of all these issues can be found in Carr-Hill (1987; 1990) and Marmot, Kogevinas, and Elston (1987). Pereira (1990) provides a bibliography of English language literature which examines the 'economics' of inequalities in health, and methods that may inform the causal debate.

In 1986 Margaret Whitehead was commissioned by the (now defunct) Health Education Council in the United Kingdom to review the burgeoning body of research in the area of inequality and health which had appeared since the publication of the *Black Report*. *The Health Divide* (Whitehead, 1988) was an extensive review of current British literature and data and reached similar conclusions to the *Black Report*. In summary, lower occupational groups were shown to be generally disadvantaged in terms of mortality and morbidity (self-reported and/or 'objectively' measured; chronic and/or acute conditions) relative to higher occupational groups (Whitehead, 1988:227-255). The relationships tended to be linear, although some relationships were characterized by the fact that the very lowest occupational group had much poorer health status than other groups. Two other findings highlight the importance of material well-being in determining health outcomes. First, individuals who were house or flat (apartment) owners, as opposed to tenants, had better health. Both these groups had better health than individuals living in council (government assisted) housing. Second, individuals who were unemployed had poorer mental and physical health than employed individuals. It was also found that women have greater life expectancy than men and "lower mortality rates at every stage of life" (Whitehead, 1988:254), but women also have a higher incidence of reported morbidity than men.

Townsend has responded to criticisms of the *Black Report* findings which has promoted an ongoing debate (Klein, 1988; 1990; 1991; Townsend, 1990a; 1990b; 1991). Part of this debate surrounds the major policy recommendation of the *Black Report* (broad income redistribution), which is seen to be misguided. Critics argue that the policy decisions are based on poor quality data and the ideological inclinations of the authors (Klein, 1990:518-519). Townsend (1990a) responds that the body of research that has appeared in the U.K. since 1980 further supports the findings of the *Black Report*. Townsend also argues that use of the occupational classification as a measure of social position is still valid (1990a:369-371). However, as greater numbers of women enter paid employment, the attribution of social status to family members based on the occupational classification of the 'head of the household' (i.e., the man's) is questionable. Also, occupational status differences in mortality are interpreted to be the result of material deprivation. Social status indicators which better reflect the material circumstances of individuals and families, such as income measures, would more directly test for this interpretation.[2]

Other International Evidence

Investigators in the United States have used various measures of social status. Indices of SES and single variable measures of educational level and/or income are most common. Most studies using measures of income do not control for family size or 'adequacy' of income (i.e., by region or 'cost-of-living') (Liberatos, Link, and Kelsey, 1988). Mortality data are most frequently used as indicators of health, although survey data provide self-reported measures of health status.

The research in the U.S. generally supports the findings of British studies. Mortality rates are higher for individuals living in poor neighbourhoods (Jenkins, 1983; Kitagawa and Hauser, 1973; Rogot et al., 1988). Higher percentages of low income individuals report major activity limitations and more days of disability than high income individuals (Patrick et al., 1988). Dutton reports that "more than three times as many low- as high-income people rate their health status as 'fair or poor'" (1986:37). Residents of a designated poverty area in California experienced higher levels of age/sex/race adjusted mortality in a nine year follow-up, even after a wide range of physical, behavioural, material, and social structural variables were controlled (Berkman and Syme, 1979; Haan, Kaplan, and Camacho, 1986; Marmot et al., 1987). Warner and Smith (1982) found that families of high social status were, over time, able to offset early developmental problems of their children, while families of low social position were not. Mare (1982) found that social status differences (based on indicators of mothers' education and family income) in mortality were as large for persons under the age of 20 as for older adults. The differences were due mainly to a higher risk of accidental death among lower status persons. This would indicate that a poor socioeconomic environment may be causal of mortality (since young people have not had the time to become downwardly mobile). A large number of U.S. government studies (reviewed in Dutton, 1986; Liberatos, Link, and Kelsey, 1988) confirm that social status differences in mortality and morbidity are a persistent feature of U.S. society.

Explanations of health inequalities have generated similar debates in the U.S. as those in Britain. It is recognised that the relation between income and health has a two-way effect: low income can be causal of ill health, while ill health can reduce individual capacity to earn income. Part of this debate rests on the interpretation of the effect of other measures of social status (such as education and occupation) on health. Since patterns of social status inequalities in health tend to be similar, no matter what the measure of social status, social causation explanations are considered primary (Dutton, 1986:32). Comprehensive reviews of these issues in relation to the U.S. literature are in Dutton (1986) and Liberatos, Link, and Kelsey (1988).

Macintyre (1986) has provided an extensive review of British research that shows associations between various social factors and health status. Macintyre proposes that in order to broaden our perspective on the relationships between inequality and health, we have to rethink the nature of the independent variables. That is, variables such as age, gender, marital status, ethnicity, and so forth, have to be investigated simultaneously with variables such as 'social class' or socioeconomic status (SES). This is because SES is an indicator that does not completely summarize the relationship between inequality and health. The interpretation of any SES and health relationships found is also difficult because of the generality, and ambiguity, of the concept of SES. Macintyre argues that uncovering the 'meaning' of SES through the investigation of specific social variables is probably a more fruitful method of investigation than continuing to study SES as a composite indicator of social standing (Macintyre, 1986).

Age is seen as the most important control variable in SES and health relationships as variability in health status is strongly age-related. Generally, older age groups are in poorer states of health than those of younger age. Much of this is due to the cumulative effect of chronic illness for older persons (Conover, 1973; Dutton, 1986). In general, SES inequalities in health remain after controlling for age (Hay, 1988; Townsend and Davidson, 1982). However, there is some inconsistency in the literature as to whether the social status and health relationship is fairly constant across age groups, or is different for different age groups. While some research argues that social status inequalities in health status are not evident for older ages, the most recent review of this literature supports the finding that social status inequalities in health status are evident regardless of age (House, Kessler, and Herzog, 1990).

The literature reviewed indicated large gender differences in mortality and morbidity. Gender is important to include in any model of inequality and health because of the differential distribution of social status and health status between men and women. Waldron (1983) provides a comprehensive review of issues in the area. Generally, women have greater life expectancy and lower mortality than men at all ages. However, women tend to have higher levels of reported morbidity. The possible reasons for these gender differences have been investigated (Verbrugge, 1989). Differential acquisition of health risks, health attitudes, and health reporting behaviour explain some of the gender differences in health.

Marital status is another factor that influences health. While the literature reveals no clear pattern of health status by marital status, whether an individual is married, widowed/divorced/separated, or never married can have an effect on health (Clark et al., 1987; Fletcher, 1988; Macintyre, 1986). One study reported that a married woman's life expectancy and cause of death is associated with her husband's occupational mortality risk, which suggests "that specific occupational risks are transmitted between marital partners, perhaps through psychological mechanisms" (Fletcher, 1988:615). Another study reported that women who were married, with or without children present, had a higher number of bed days than men (Clark et al., 1987). Possible explanations for this relationship include a differential psychological burden of undesirable life events (for example, divorce), or a greater amount of stress experienced by women.

Rimpela and Pukkala (1987) found that some cancers were more common in higher SES groups in Finland. However, the authors note that generally lower SES groups are more susceptible to all forms of illness. In an interesting twist, Mackenbach, Stronks, and Kunst found "that medical care contributed to the widening of the mortality differences between socio-economic groups" in England and Wales, and the Netherlands (1989:369). This is because of the finding that mortality from conditions amenable to medical intervention declined in higher occupational groupings relative to lower occupational groupings, while at the same time it was found that access, utilization, and quality of health care for lower occupational groups was poorer.

Social Status and Health Status: Canadian Evidence

Inequalities in health in Canada include those by SES, gender, region, and age (for reviews see: Adams and Wilkins, 1988; Badgley, 1991; Badgley and Wolfe, 1992; D'Arcy, 1988; 1990). Generally individuals of lower SES have poorer health relative to those individuals of higher SES. Women have lower levels of mortality and greater life expectancy than men at all ages, and the gender difference in life expectancy is greatest for those individuals in the lowest income quintile. Regional differences in life expectancy are declining, although they still exist. Age tends to specify these other relationships in various ways, although generally as an individual ages, health status is poorer.

Marsh and colleagues (1938) conducted the first major analysis of social status and health in Canada. A number of surveys were conducted focusing on the health experiences of employed and unemployed workers and their families. It was reported that various health problems were more prevalent among the unemployed, such as "underweight and malnutrition, decayed teeth and infected gums, rates of deafness and other auditory defects, and abnormal conditions of the nose and throat" (Marsh et al., 1938:62, 71, 76). It was concluded that the availability of medical services would improve this situation, but unless the prior social conditions giving rise to these inequalities were improved, social status differences in health would remain (Marsh et al., 1938:215-216).

Leighton and colleagues (1963) carried out a large scale survey of a rural and small town area of Nova Scotia, the Stirling County study. They constructed an index of psychiatric symptoms in order to measure prevalence of mental disorder in the community. The Health Opinion Survey, as the index is called, was developed for use in the Stirling County studies. Prevalence of mental disorder was identified through hospital records, and a sample of previously hospitalized mental patients were interviewed. In addition, a random sample of community residents were interviewed and scored on the Health Opinion Survey. All respondents were classified by occupation as a measure of social status. Leighton and colleagues found that the risk of psychiatric disorder increases with occupational disadvantage (1963:294). This finding held for both treated patients and individuals surveyed in the community.

The *Canadian Sickness Survey* (1960) was the first nationwide survey of the distribution of health and illness of the Canadian people. The survey was conducted during a twelve-month period from 1950 to 1951. Relationships were reported that showed high income groups had consistently less 'days of disability' than medium and low income groups. The *Canadian Royal Commission on Health Services* (1967) cites the findings of the *Canadian Sickness Survey* (1960) and poses two explanations for them: (1) low status leads to poor housing, nutrition, and sanitation which, in turn, causes poor health; (2) poor health may also restrict individuals' upward mobility.

Bell and Burnside (1972) studied the relationship between 'poverty' and illness using the data of the *Canadian Sickness Survey* (1960). They found that the relationship between SES and illness varied depending on the measure of illness employed. This was true for all measures of SES used: education, occupation, income, and living environment quality. Bell and Burnside conclude that the findings "clearly suggest that, despite statistically significant associations, the amount of variance accounted for by social factors is very modest indeed" (1972, np.). They cite methodological problems with their operationalization of indicators, but still conclude that "standard, simple sociological variables are not adequate" in measuring the complex relationship between poverty and illness (1972, np.).

Roberts and colleagues (1966) studied a disadvantaged area of Montreal and found an inverse linear relationship between occupation and income, and self-reported health status. Roos and Shapiro (1981) studied the elderly in Manitoba and found that low income groups were nearly half again as likely to report health problems, relative to upper income groups. Adams and colleagues (1971), in an investigation of poverty in Canada, and Forcese (1980), in a description of the nature of stratification in Canada, present findings which imply that low social status leads to poor health. Explanations for a greater preponderance of ill health among lower SES groups (based on income measures) include: poor nutrition, a lesser ability in obtaining medical care, interpretation of symptoms as not serious, and generally poorer working and residential conditions (Adams et al., 1971; Forcese, 1980).

Billette and Hill (1977) investigated a random sample of deaths among males aged 25 to 64 in Canada in 1974. Occupation was recoded (using the Blishen-McRoberts (1976) index) from death certificates and coded into quintiles. Taking average mortality as a score of 100, working age males in the lowest occupational quintile had a relative mortality of 145, compared to 75 for those males in the highest occupational quintile. Thus, males in the lowest quintile were at almost twice the risk of dying as those in the highest quintile.

Atkinson, Blishen, and Murray (1980) analyzed a representative sample of the Canadian population with the *Social Change in Canada Survey* data collected in 1977. The focus of the study was on the relationship between physical health status (as measured by self-reported illness symptoms) and perceived health quality (as measured by self-rating of health). However, it was also found that "both education and income are significantly related to perceived [health] status for the entire sample and, more importantly, for the specific age groups" (Atkinson et al., 1980:20).

Gafni and colleagues (1983) studied a random sample of employees of a large steelmaker in Hamilton, Ontario, in order to assess the relationship between income and hypertension. Comparisons of income levels between hypertensives and normotensives (control group) for a five-year period showed a significantly greater rate of increase in mean income level for the normotensive group. Also, comparing treatment and no-treatment hypertensives, it was revealed that hypertensives foregoing treatment lost a significantly greater proportion of income.

Lapierre profiled the health of Canadian women for a Statistics Canada publication in 1984. Work outside the home had a positive effect on women's health. Family income had a positive effect on women's health, but the effect was greater for those women who primarily stay at home. Also, the higher a woman's education level, the better her health (Lapierre, 1984).

The City of Toronto has conducted a number of studies of the health status of its residents in the last decade (1984; 1991). The *Health Inequalities in the City of Toronto* report (1991) summarizes work from two recent studies looking at social status differences in health status. One study examined age-standardized, sex-specific mortality rates for city census tracts which had been rank-ordered based on the percentage of the population of the census tract below the poverty line. The poorest census tracts (the bottom twenty percent) had higher mortality "rates for both men and women for all causes of death combined" and for a number of specific disease causes (City of Toronto, 1991:25). When the average level of occupational status and educational status of each census tract was taken into account, the relative importance of each was identified. For women, level of education (and ethnicity), not degree of poverty, accounted for much of the mortality differences between census tracts. The other study used data from two community health surveys conducted in 1983 and 1988. Evidence was found of inequalities in activity limitation in both survey years, and in levels of reported chronic conditions for the 1983 survey (City of Toronto, 1991:3). When all risk factors (such as age, sex, smoking, and income) were controlled however, few of the bivariate income and health relationships persisted. The report concluded that "it is very difficult and not very efficient to collect the data necessary to address health inequalities with general population surveys at the local level" (City of Toronto, 1991:3).

Echenberg (1988) reviewed community-based literature on health inequalities. Echenberg notes that not one of the documents reviewed "challenged the fundamental and inexorable link between low income on the one hand and higher mortality and morbidity rates on the other" (1988:2). It was felt that poverty and its effects was causal of poor health. The specific effects of poverty identified most often were hunger, poor housing, and stress. It should be emphasized that the literature reviewed by Echenberg was obtained in a call for literature from social advocacy groups. The literature was thus a summary and interpretation of existing evidence by these groups. The nature of this literature thus precluded "detailed comment . . . on methodological considerations, suggested indicators, and data needs" (Echenberg, 1988:1).

The *Canada Health Survey* (Health and Welfare Canada and Statistics Canada, 1981) reports that those individuals of lower income and education status report more health problems than those of higher social status, and that these problems tend to be of the activity-limiting variety. The report stated that lower education and income groups "do not enjoy the same level of health as Canadians of higher social economic status" (1981:114). Women exhibit higher prevalence of almost all reported troubles compared to men. Very young children and older adults and the elderly are the ones reporting most prevalence of health troubles.

Recently in Canada there have been several national health surveys - the *Canadian Health and Disability Survey* of 1983-84 (Statistics Canada and Department of the Secretary of State of Canada, 1987); the *General Social Survey* of 1985 (Statistics Canada, 1987); and the *Health Promotion Survey* of 1985 (Health and Welfare Canada, 1988) - which have confirmed the general trends observed in the *Canadian Sickness Survey* (1960) and the *Canada Health Survey* (Health and Welfare Canada and Statistics Canada, 1981). Reports of these surveys are reviewed in Badgley and Wolfe (1992).

Hay (1988) analyzed *Canada Health Survey* data (Health and Welfare Canada and Statistics Canada, 1981) to examine the relationship between SES and physical and mental health status. A direct positive relationship between SES and health status was found. SES and health findings remained when age was controlled. Income was found to be the most consistent correlate of health status, relative to education and occupation. The low income group invariably had the poorest health status.

Wilkins (1988; see also Rootman, 1986) analyzed the relationship between social status (educational level and income level) and health status with data from the 1985 Canada *Health Promotion Survey*. Wilkins improved on past measures of income by operationalizing an income measure based on the Statistics Canada low income cut-offs (or 'poverty lines') in order to control for the adequacy of income. However, since regional information was unavailable from the survey, low income cut-offs for various family sizes according to city populations of 500,000 and over were used. As community size greatly affects the low income cut-off level, many respondents may have been misclassified on the income measure. The analysis showed that people with less income and/or education, the unemployed, and/or individuals who reported they were primarily housekeepers, had the poorest health. Those groups highest in education, occupation, and/or income status had the highest health status. Wilkins notes the similarity of these findings with those found in previous work (Hirdes et al., 1986; Wilkins and Adams, 1983).

Income and Health Status: International Evidence

Previous studies of SES and health have identified income as the crucial component of SES related to health (Blaxter, 1990; Townsend and

Davidson, 1982; Wilkinson, 1986). As well, a number of writers have identified the importance of disaggregating SES to examine the separate relationships that the components of SES have with health (Kessler, 1982; Liberatos, Link, and Kelsey, 1988; Macintyre, 1986; Rodgers, 1979). Of all the components of SES, income is the most easily interpretable. Income directly represents opportunity in materialist consumer 'market' societies like ours. The amount of income individuals can command directly affects their everyday lives.

A number of international studies examine the relationship between income and health using aggregate level data. The findings indicate large differences in mortality risk/life expectancy between income groups at all ages, and between men and women. However, earlier aggregate international comparisons indicated no relationship between level of economic development/Gross National Product per capita (GNP p.c.) and mortality rates. More recent research indicates that when individual level income data are used (rather than GNP p.c.) and related to mortality/life expectancy data, income inequality is related to inequality in mortality/life expectancy. Specific review of some of these studies follows.

Wilkinson (1986; 1990) maintains that it is important to study the specific relationship between income and health in order to assess the material explanation of health inequalities. He presents evidence (1986) that lower levels of occupational income, pension income, and household income, are all related to lower levels of health. From this evidence Wilkinson concludes that income redistribution would lead to a five times greater improvement in mortality risk for the poorest group relative to worsening risk for the richest group. Also, economic development per se, in terms of increasing wealth for top level income earners, may produce greater mortality risk for the lowest income group as *relative* economic well-being deteriorates (Townsend and Davidson, 1982). In fact, life expectancy is highest in those developed countries where income is distributed most equally, rather than in countries that are simply the richest (Wilkinson, 1990:391). This is an important finding as it would suggest that *the level of inequality* existing and not necessarily absolute levels of income are significant (Rodgers, 1979; Wilkinson, 1990).

Blaxter (1990) presents findings from an analysis of British cross-sectional data on individual income and health from the *Health and Lifestyles Survey*. Income was measured by self-reported gross weekly household income. Three measures of self-reported health were used: an index of disease and/or disability, an index of illness symptoms, and an index of psycho-social health. An inverse relationship between income and all three measures of health was observed. However, the relationship was not directly linear. Individuals with the lowest income were in the poorest health, but individuals at the higher levels of income also reported poorer health. Ill health decreased up to a maximum level of income (£250 per week) and then started to increase for higher income levels. These findings suggest, like Wilkinson's (1986; 1990) work, that relative income distribution, rather than absolute levels of income, may be an important factor in determining health. Blaxter concluded "that the apparently strong association of social class [occupational status] and health is primarily an association of income and health" (1990:72).

Duleep (1986) investigated the effect of income on mortality using longitudinal administrative health record data in the United States. In her literature review, Duleep notes that previous work found a small negative effect of income on mortality (Hadley and Osei, 1982 - see below) or an insignificant and even positive effect (Auster et al., 1969; Fuchs, 1965; Grossman, 1972; Silver, 1972). Duleep surmises that these findings were limited in interpretation precisely because of the aggregate nature of the data under study. Duleep overcomes this limitation of previous work by linking data sets that combine information on individual health status, income, education, and mortality. Controlling for health status, and regressing income, education, and age in an equation to predict the probability of death, it was found that "a strong inverse relationship between income and mortality risk persists, up to an average level of income, even when disability is controlled for" (Duleep, 1986:242). Duleep concluded that changes in income affect changes in probability of death. This is most likely through the effect of income on other variables. A further point raised is that, in this study, higher education was not associated with a reduction in mortality risk. In fact those with less schooling had lower mortality risk.

Hadley and Osei (1982) studied U.S. census 'county groups,' census areas of approximately 250,000 people (county groups may cross state boundaries). Populations among the county groups were divided into three age groups, by gender and by race (white/black), thus producing twelve cohorts. Seven types of income measures (as well as other socio-demographic information) were constructed by aggregating individual data, of each cohort, from a two percent sample from the 1970 census. The dependent variable was the all-causes mortality rate, disaggregated by age, gender, and race. The results supported the hypothesis that high income is related to lower mortality rates, although the observed effect was small, and the strength of the effect depended mainly on which age cohort was being observed.

Newacheck and colleagues (1980) investigated the relationship between income and illness using data from the 1977 *Health Interview*

Survey of the National Center for Health Statistics in the United States. The sample was divided into age-specific poor and non-poor groups (based on the poverty level of a family of four). Restricted activity days, bed disability days, and limitation of activity due to chronic conditions were the measures of health employed. It was found that the 'gap' in illness rates among the poor and non-poor can be attributed almost entirely to activity limiting chronic conditions. There are some weaknesses with the analysis however. Although large poor/non-poor differences were shown, age is the only control used. Also income is not standardized for family size, and data were only collected at one point in time.

Rodgers (1979) investigated the importance of income and inequality as determinants of mortality. The rationale for this study was that while other factors such as sanitation, education, occupation, and so forth, may be factors to consider, they are difficult to study. This is because the variables tend to be collinear, as well as being associated with many other factors, making their causal isolation difficult. Thus, while it may be desirable to study all these factors, it may not be critical in understanding mortality changes. "For behind these specific variables, the overall economic status of individuals is likely to dominate health changes - through nutrition and other aspects of consumption, and also because economic status is a close correlate and determinant of many of the more specific variables noted above" (Rodgers, 1979:343). While this statement is relevant for all countries, it should be pointed out that Rodgers is referring to fairly large income changes in developing countries. Income change is not as likely to produce such a great mortality change in more developed countries. Several different models are proposed of the relationship between community/national life expectancy and individual income level (for an elaboration of these models see Rodgers, 1979). Using income quintile distributions and Gini coefficients to indicate income inequality, and life expectancy at birth and infant mortality as health variables, it was found that greater inequality, rather than any absolute national average level of income, is associated with higher mortality (Wilkinson, 1986; 1990).

Cochrane and colleagues (1980) review and reanalyse aggregate data to assess the socioeconomic determinants of mortality. Per capita income is negatively associated with mortality and positively associated with life expectancy for all studies reviewed, independent of health service factors. When compared with other socioeconomic determinants of mortality, literacy and other measures of education are more closely related to mortality than is income. Subsequent multivariate analysis shows that the importance of literacy is reduced as the level of development of the country under study rises. The more developed the country, the more important the role of income becomes, relative to literacy and education, as a predictor of mortality.

Ho (1982:1) has cogently summarized the income and health relationship:

> There is a close interactive relationship between health and the level of income. The attainment of a higher income level affords an individual access to better health. He [sic] may not necessarily choose to maximize his health status (given his taste for commodities such as cigarettes or 'junk food,' for example) but he at least has the means to attain improved health. In general, health levels do improve with increases in income levels . . . .

Income and Health Status: Canadian Evidence

Hirdes and colleagues (1986) analyzed data from the *Ontario Longitudinal Study of Aging* to examine the relationship between income and health status. Two thousand 45 year old males, who were active in the labour force, were interviewed annually from 1959 through 1978. Self-reported income was divided into three categories based on a frequency distribution of respondents' income levels. Twenty percent of respondents were placed in the 'low' income category, sixty percent in the 'middle' income category, and the remaining twenty percent in the 'high' income category. The percentage of respondents reporting 'good' health was the dependent variable. Two specific questionnaire items asked respondents if their income and/or health had changed from the year prior to survey.

Income was found to be related to health status independent of education and/or smoking effects (Hirdes et al., 1986). It was also found that *changes* in income were related to *changes* in health status. From their analysis, Hirdes et al. conclude that income changes precede health changes. The explanations offered for this finding include increased "stress, reduced purchasing patterns, and/or changes in social and physical activities," although these explanations were not directly investigated (Hirdes et al., 1986:201).

Two limitations of the Hirdes and colleagues (1986) findings should be noted. First, the dropout rate of respondents in the study was nearly 50 percent. It is not clear how this high dropout rate might have affected the findings. Second, smoking consumption and years of education were the only other 'non-income' independent variables employed in the study. Thus the opportunities for explanation of the relationship between income and health status were restricted.

Using national Canadian mortality statistics, Wigle and Mao (1980) reported differential life expectancy according to census tract average income status. Wilkins and Adams (1983) combined *Canada Health Survey* data (Health and Welfare Canada and Statistics Canada, 1981) and national mortality statistics to report differences in 'health expectancy' between census tract average income groups. Health expectancy is an index comprised of mortality measures and institutionalized and non-institutionalized morbidity measures. The findings from these two studies were similar: persons from high income families could expect to live six (Wigle and Mao, 1980) to seven (Wilkins and Adams, 1983) years longer than persons from low income families.

Wilkins, Adams, and Brancker (1989) recently updated the work of Wigle and Mao (1980). Individual death certificates were matched to census tracts of individuals' usual place of residence, and then related to the income of census tracts for the 1971 and 1986 census. Income was measured by taking the percentage of census tract residents below the poverty line (based on family and community size) and ranking census tracts, based on this percentage. An inverse relationship between income and all causes of mortality was found in both time periods, but the gap between income groups seemed to be declining. Mortality rates for specific disease groups were also differentially distributed by average income. The gap between income groups was increasing, decreasing, or had not changed, depending on the specific causes of mortality.

Ugnat and Mark (1987) used 1984 mortality data from the *Canadian Mortality Database* to investigate the relationship between mortality, income, gender, and age. Income was measured by taking the median household income of the census tracts of Canada's census metropolitan areas (CMAs) and then ranking the tracts into quintiles. Life expectancy at each age level for men and women by income quintile was tabulated using various epidemiological techniques. It was stated, "the difference in life expectancy by income level was greater for men than women at all ages. The difference for each gender was greatest at birth, relatively constant up to age 35 and declines rapidly after age 45. For women over 55 and men over 75, this difference is less than one year" (Ugnat and Mark, 1987:12). However, Ugnat and Mark are commenting on the actual differences in years (i.e., a five year difference at birth, or a one year difference at age 70). If percentage differences are calculated, a different picture emerges. For men, the difference is greatest in the 55-59 age group (life expectancy for the highest income quintile is nearly 13 percent higher than the lowest income quintile) and least at birth (nearly 8 percent). For women the difference is a constant three percent which begins to decline to less than two percent after age 75.

The importance is the continuity of the income difference in mortality for both men and women at all ages.

The previous four studies reviewed (Ugnat and Mark, 1987; Wigle and Mao, 1980; Wilkins and Adams, 1983; Wilkins, Adams, and Brancker, 1989) are widely quoted in Canada as evidence of a relationship between income and health. Thus, it is important to mention their limitations. Mortality statistics are indisputable (although not necessarily re: *cause* of death) and therefore little in doubt as to their validity. However, inequalities in death may not be similar to inequalities in health (Gray, 1982). As well, while these studies claim to be reporting inequalities in mortality in Canada *as a whole*, large percentages of the population were excluded from analysis. Specifically, only deaths in urban Canada were reported, as only deaths of residents of census metropolitan areas (CMAs) were examined. CMAs are communities of 100,000 or more population, and thus represented only 60 percent of the Canadian population in 1986 and only 54 percent of the Canadian population in 1971 (Wilkins, Adams, and Brancker, 1989). Additionally, not all deaths matched to CMAs were included for analysis. For various reasons, approximately nine percent of deaths were excluded in 1971, and over 12 percent in 1986 (Wilkins, Adams, and Brancker, 1989). The other limitation of these studies is in their matching of census tract income characteristics to the individual mortality data. In order to obtain income levels of census tracts, residents of census tracts were sampled (1 in 3 residents in 1971 and 1 in 5 residents in 1986). As mentioned above, Ugnat and Mark (1987) simply take the *median* census tract income level and relate this to individual mortality. Wilkins, Adam, and Brancker (1989) introduce controls for family and community size to rank census tracts based on the percentage of sample residents below Statistics Canada's low income cut-offs (the 'poverty lines'). The underlying problem with all these approaches, however, is the possibility of the ecologic fallacy (Robinson, 1950). It is unknown how accurately grouped income data represent the conditions of individuals. It is known that it can only be an approximation of individuals' 'true' income level.

Wolfson, Rowe, Gentleman, and Tomiak (1990) recently examined the relationship between income and mortality using longitudinal administrative data from the *Canada Pension Plan* (CPP). The CPP get their employment income information from Revenue Canada Taxation. Thus, income is measured at the individual level and represents earnings histories of 100 percent of the paid labour force. Year and month of death are recorded and included in the same data base. Although individual, not family, income is used, and controls for family and community size are absent, the measures are generally of high quality and this is the most methodologically rigorous study done on the topic of income and mortality in Canada. It was found that higher incomes in the decades prior to age 65 were significantly associated with lower mortality in the following nine years. The findings are limited to males of a certain age group and even though longitudinal data were examined, "the causal pathways by which these socio-economic status variables influence mortality are generally unknown" (Wolfson et al., 1990:14).

An Explication of the Relationship Between Income and Health

I recently completed a study looking into the relationship between income and health (Hay, 1992). What was unique about this study was its focus on the relationship between *change in income* and *change in health* using *longitudinal* data. The findings from the study were somewhat unexpected, and contrary to widely held beliefs about social status and health. The following reviews and discusses the findings from the study in some detail.

The data for the analysis were from the 1977, 1979, and 1981 *Social Change in Canada Surveys*, conducted by the Institute for Behavioural Research at York University, Toronto. The surveys provided national cross-sectional data for each year, and a panel (longitudinal) study, of quality of life in Canada (N=3300, Panel N=1700).

A poverty line index (PLI) was the primary measure of income explored in the study. The PLI was a measure of family income expressed as a percentage of the Statistics Canada Low Income Cut-offs. Consequently the PLI measure controlled for family and community size.

The measure of health status employed was an index composed of a number of self-reported questionnaire items. The items covered specific health states, disability or impairment, and general self-reported states of health and physical fitness. The index included measures of both chronic ailments and acute events.

The findings are summarized as they relate to the following specific hypotheses that were tested:

1. Low income groups have poorer health status than other income groups.
2. Older respondents have poorer health status than younger respondents, but low income groups have poorer health at all ages.
3. Women have poorer health status than men, but lower income is related to poorer health for both men and women.

4. Change in income status is causal of change in health status.
5. The relationships between income and health are partially explained or interpreted through the influence of income on a variety of 'intermediate' social variables.

Hypotheses 1, 2, and 3

The 1977 data were first examined in depth to test the first three hypotheses. Bivariate and multivariate analyses confirmed that: 1) low income groups have poorer health status than do other income groups; 2) older respondents have poorer health status than do younger respondents, but income differences remain across age groups, with the result that older, low income respondents have the poorest health; and 3) women have poorer health status than do men, but lower income is related to health status for both men and women.

Regression analysis with the 1977 data revealed that for men and women together, age, gender, educational level, and income, in that order, were the strongest predictors of health status. However, when regressions were performed separately for men and women, quite a different picture emerged. Age and income were the strongest predictors of health for men, while age and education were the strongest predictors of health for women.

Hypothesis 4

Data from 1977, 1979, and 1981 were used to explore the income change - health change relationship. Health status in 1981 was the dependent variable, and it was regressed on 1977 health status (to control for prior health status), 1981 income, 1977-81 income change, and 1981 age, gender, educational level, and marital status. As expected, prior health status was a very strong predictor of health status, two and four years hence. The addition of the income variables did not further aid our explanation of health changes over two or four years. Considering all independent variables together (other than prior health status), only age was a significant predictor of change in health over four years.

It was possible that a more direct examination of respondents who experienced an income change and/or a health change would improve our understanding of the relationship between income and health. Three separate analyses were undertaken to explore this possibility.

First, specific sub-groups of respondents, those who reported a change in income and/or a change in health status between 1977 and 1981, were investigated to determine if they differed from respondents not experiencing an income and/or health change. We explored the possibility that important relationships between respondents with income change and health change were being obscured by the large number of respondents with little or no income or health change. Frequency distributions and means of several socio-demographic variables were explored for nine specific sub-groups (based on increase, decrease, or no change in income, and better, worse, or no change in health). While there were some small differences between groups on some of the socio-demographic variables, no discernible pattern emerged.

Of note was that respondents with the best health in 1977 were not affected by increases or decreases in their income status between 1977 and 1981. For those respondents with poor health in 1977, their 1981 health status tended to decline further, while respondents reporting moderate health in 1977 showed an improvement in their 1981 health status - *regardless* of whether income increased or decreased from 1977 to 1981 for these respondents.

Second, the possibility that different aspects of health (i.e., chronic or acute conditions) would be more or less sensitive to income change was investigated. Each component variable of the health index in 1981 was regressed on the corresponding 1977 component variable, 1981 income, 1977-81 income change, and 1981 age, education, and marital status, for men and women separately. Current income, and income change, did not explain change in any of the component variables of the health index.

A third possibility existed that there were certain points in individuals' lives at which their health was more or less susceptible to changes in income. We wondered if the health status of older or younger respondents was affected differently by changes in income. We investigated this possibility by using the regression methods for analyzing change, for men and women separately, and for four age groups. The analyses did not support the idea of 'crucial age points.' Changes in income were not predictive of changes in health status for any of the age groups.

Hypothesis 5

The study investigated the effects of the explanatory variables (housing conditions, neighbourhood conditions, satisfaction with surroundings, and life satisfaction) on health status. It was hypothesized that the explanatory variables would further specify income and health relationships (for cross-sectional 1977 data). The findings confirmed that housing conditions, neighbourhood conditions, and life satisfaction, while having unique effects on health, do partially act as intervening factors linking income (for men), and education (for women), with health status.

Since there was no relationship between income change and health change, the explanatory variables could not further our understanding of this relationship. However, it was possible that the explanatory variables themselves were predictive of health change. The findings confirmed that housing conditions and life satisfaction are related to change in health status between 1977 and 1981, for both men and women.

Discussion: Income Change and Health Change

It was expected that changes in respondents' income levels over two or four years would be related to changes in their health status over the same time periods. As was reported, the results of our analyses clearly show that change in income does not contribute to our understanding of change in health status, over the periods 1977-1979, 1979-1981, or 1977-1981.

How may these findings be interpreted? It is possible that the time lag is too short, i.e., two or four years is not enough time for changes in income to effect health status. This raises two questions:

1. How much time would have to elapse for changes in income to effect changes in health status?

2. Does this finding mean that advocates of programs to redistribute income to equalize social conditions are misguided?

To answer the first question, data from individuals over a longer time period would be required. Statistical techniques and/or longitudinal studies that could better isolate the effects of income change on health change would also be needed. Longitudinal, or a combination of retrospective and longitudinal studies, would be required to fully assess the effects of social conditions on *children*, and to examine if income or education, or some other social variable, alone or in combination, did 'fix' a health trajectory early in life.

Our results did demonstrate that social status (income for men; education for women) was related to health status with cross-sectional data. Individuals of lower social status had poorer health status than their higher social status counterparts. When examining respondent health status between 1977 and 1981, health status tended to further decline for those already in poorer health; tended to improve for those in moderate health; and tended to stay the same for those individuals already with above average health status - regardless of whether social status improved, declined, or stayed the same.

A synthesis of findings from a number of other studies, in combination with the findings presented here, suggest that various life events, and material and social circumstances, *over time* select individuals into various social strata (Hertzman, 1991). Thus, from birth, because of opportunities either realized or denied, or because of capabilities either developed or constrained, a number of social status attributes become constitutive of the person. With these assets and liabilities a person then enters an already stratified labour market. Subsequently, individual movement within the labour market is, to some extent, constrained by the individual's point of entry. Therefore the social status attributes that are consequential for health may be difficult to modify as they develop over a number of years and are reinforced by the organization of our western industrialized societies.

Income, Education, and Health for Men and Women

Previous research has identified the importance of education as a predictor of health status for women (City of Toronto, 1991; Kandrack et al., 1991; Kessler, 1982; Lapierre, 1984; Verbrugge, 1989; Waldron, 1983). Our study demonstrated that education, rather than income, was related to health status for women. The reverse was true for men - income, rather than education, was important.

It is possible to suggest an explanation for the income/education difference between men and women based on previous findings relating income inequality to health. Wilkinson (1990) reported findings that life expectancy is highest in those developed countries where income is distributed most equally, rather than in countries that are simply the richest. This finding would suggest that the degree of income inequality, and not necessarily the absolute level of income, is significant in explaining income and health relationships (Rodgers, 1979). Cheal (1991) reported on a study that demonstrated that income distribution *within* families was highly unequal (on average 50 percent of families studied) across a number of different family types (one earner, dual earner, and dual career). The assumption in previous studies that all members of a family benefit equally from family income may not be tenable (Lazear and Michael, 1988). Also, one would assume that men, rather than women, have the most control over family income.

Income may not be a factor in explaining variability in health for women as family income may not be indicative of the amount of income that is available to women. In our sample we were unable to account for the income distribution within families. It is likely that the degree of income inequality in families would be dispersed throughout our sample distribution of family income. If income inequality within a family is more important than absolute income level in producing health deficits for women, our understanding of these income and health relationships would be obscured by our lack of knowledge of the distribution of income within families.

We could further suggest that the higher a woman's educational level, the more likely it is that the woman would be in a family with a lower level of income inequality. This is because a higher educational level would provide the woman with the skills necessary to formulate a distribution of income within the family that would be more favourable to her. If not, it is possible that a woman's higher educational level at least provides a buffer to the effects of family income inequality.

Although these speculations are plausible, the income/education difference between men and women is still somewhat perplexing. It is difficult to understand how the material well-being of a family is not shared among all individual members. That is, all individuals within a family would share the food, shelter, housing conditions, neighbourhood amenities, and so forth. But it may be that control over the discretionary portion of income (i.e., the resources available to family members after essentials have been covered) is the issue that is consequential for health. Inequalities in the *control* of these resources may contribute to inequalities in health outcomes. Individuals that have little or no control over the discretionary portion of their family income may have relatively poorer health than family members with greater control, all other things being equal (Lerner, 1986).

It must be acknowledged that the above discussion on the differences between men and women as to income/education and health relationships is speculative. But, the notion of the possible importance of degree of control over income, rather than the amount of family income, does deserve further exploration.

Summary and Policy and Research Implications

The findings from this chapter's review of the international and Canadian literature can be summarized as follows:

1. Lower social status groups have poorer health. The consistency of this finding despite a variety of conceptions and measures of social status and health status is substantial.

2. As age increases, the number of illnesses (chronic and acute) increases. However, social status differences in health status are evident at all age levels.

3. The international literature highlights age, gender, living and work environment, inadequate nutrition, inadequate housing, social support networks, stress, and marital status, as possible explanatory variables for social status and health relationships.

Some of the policy and research implications of this review are discussed below.

Policy Implications

Most studies examined the influence of 'current' income on health status. However, it seems likely that current health status depends more on the *cumulative effect of income over time* than the effect of present income on present health status (Hay, 1992). In this view health status at any one point in time, always, to some extent, reflects the effect of prior income status, as well as current income status, on health. Thus, lifetime access to (income related) resources, beginning in childhood, may be particularly crucial in its influence on health.

One consequence, if this implication is correct, is that the improvement of the social conditions of children in lower income families is a public policy challenge. If conditions can be improved it is more likely that consequences such as poor health will not become 'fixed' early in life, as the earlier a child experiences poor health, the greater the possibility that the child will be susceptible to poorer health throughout its life (Marmot et al., 1987).

From a practical perspective such a preventive approach brings the possibility of a long-term saving in health care and other associated social service costs (Ross and Shillington, 1990). The money that is saved on health care and other social services is then available for other more 'productive' uses (Evans and Stoddart, 1990). That is, we are talking about preventing ill-health and enhancing human potential, rather than curing ill-health and repairing human weaknesses.

This discussion leads one to conclude that the equalization of social and economic conditions *is* important, although a superficial reading of the income change - health change results of my study (Hay, 1992) might indicate otherwise. If lifetime income trajectories, and particularly family conditions during childhood, are important determinants of health status, then we may need long-term programs to raise lower income levels, rather than short-term attempts to improve health status.

Research Implications

The literature has pointed to the difficulties in measuring and interpreting occupational status as a measure of inequality. Apart from problems with potential misclassification of individuals who are able to be classified, there is the far greater problem that many individuals are completely unable to be classified at all. Women, children, retired people, students, unemployed persons, and so on, are regularly excluded from studies of occupational inequality and health.

A further difficulty with operationalizing a measure of occupational status is the problem of ordering occupations hierarchically. Particular characteristics of occupations, such as average educational requirements and income levels, have to be at least implicitly incorporated in order to rank them. Thus, a rank ordering of occupations will be confounded with education and income levels.

The literature review highlighted many forms of material deprivation as the most probable explanations of health inequalities. The effects of material deprivation on health would be more directly examined using measures of income. There would seem to be less of a problem with using income, rather than occupation, as a measure of social status. However, our review highlighted the problems of using such measures of income as census tract averages and Gross National Product per capita, and the difficulty in relating this information to individual health data. If individual level income data are collected there are many forms of income that may be important. Income from employment, pension income, government transfer payments such as unemployment and welfare benefits, income from property such as rental income, income from savings and investments, and income from other family or household members, should all be included to provide a measure of the total amount of income available to an individual. This is particularly important for older persons who may get the major proportion of their income from pensions, savings, and investments. What sources are used in obtaining income information are also important. Income tax data would be the most reliable (although far from being perfect), while self-reported income data may be subject to a higher degree of reporting error.

There are also important factors which affect the adequacy of income and these need to be considered when constructing measures of income in future research. It is important to control for factors that have a bearing on the amount of income actually available to individuals when investigating the relationship between income and health. Family size, community size, region, and the degree of income inequality within the family are factors known to greatly affect the adequacy of income. A further issue with the adequacy of income is the importance of using a poverty line criterion, even though the decision as to what that poverty line is, and hence the adequacy of income, is inherently arbitrary. Use of a poverty line criterion does oblige a researcher to address the issue of income adequacy.

It would seem to be important to explore the extent of income inequality within families, and hence the possible importance of the degree of control over family income, and its possible relationship with health. This type of investigation would begin to explore issues of control and powerlessness, and the link between material conditions, social psychological processes, and health. For example, the *meaning* of income, rather than income itself may be consequential for health. This type of model would link income level - (dis)satisfaction with income level - feelings of lack of control or powerlessness - stress - and health. This model would most likely be in addition to the straight material conditions - health model, as explanations of social status and health relationships.

To further improve our understanding of the relationship between income change and health change it is important to study the relationship with longitudinal data over longer time periods. This will enable a closer look at lifetime patterns of income - health relationships. Much of what we generally study has been *current* income, but this neglects the importance of prior income (more than four years previous) on current health status.

Patterns of income change over time may be differentially consequential for health. Therefore there is a need to study income over the lifetime - this would include parental income, and past and current income - and their interactions with health. Further study of income change and health change is important as it has ramifications for advocates of policies to change social conditions in order to change health status.

It is also important to investigate the relationship between social conditions and health with children. This is necessary to test the effect of social conditions on children, and at what stage in the lives of individuals social conditions may permanently 'fix' their subsequent health status.

As our societies become more economically unstable, there may be many points in the lives of individuals where income will be fluctuating widely. Thus, future studies of income and health should also consider the interaction of individual income status with the performance of the economy. Individual income status is obviously dependent on a well functioning economy. A poor economy could mean an overall reduction in the income status of the population, and hence an overall reduction in population health status. The relationships between economic cycles, unemployment, and health have been examined previously, but not conclusively (Adams, 1981; Bartley, 1988; Brenner, 1977; Brenner and Mooney, 1983; Dooley and Catalano, 1984; Forbes and McGregor, 1987; Grayson, 1989; Soderstrom; 1986). Studying income and health relationships among, and between, population groups (such as the employed and unemployed) rather than among individuals, may also improve our understanding of the mechanisms linking income and health.

Measures of education are less subject to reporting error than are income measures. The major difficulty with using education measures is the ability to interpret differences between educational levels. For example, what would be the difference between an individual with 10 years of schooling and an individual with 13 years? And what is it about this difference that may be consequential for health? The other problem with measures of education is their relatively weaker relationship to material well-being. We all know of the examples of Ph.D. graduates who are underemployed driving taxis, and the owners of businesses who never completed high school. This is the problem of social 'status inconsistency' (Smith, 1980).

Liberatos, Link, and Kelsey (1988) provide a comprehensive, critical review of the measurement of 'social class' in health related research. In their review, Liberatos et al. are unable to recommend any one indicator over another. The use of either, or all, of education, occupation, or income measures depends on the goals of the particular research project.

There are particular methodological concerns when using longitudinal data sources which should be noted. Whether or not the same respondents are present at each point of data collection is obviously important. The degree of respondent 'drop-out' over time could greatly affect the interpretation of results. It is very likely that respondents that drop-out would differ from those still included on measures such as social status and health status. Whether or not all variables are measured in the same way, and at each time, is important for conceptual and methodological rigor. As well, measures such as income should be standardized to reflect inflation and cost of living changes during the period of data collection.

It would also seem to be important to examine the relationship between social status and health status separately for men and women (Hay, 1992). The puzzling differences between men and women regarding income and education and their relationships with health require detailed further study.

Le Grand (1986:115-124) proposed a research agenda for inequalities in health based on the following five questions:

1. *How much ought there to be?* These are equity/justice issues and are more properly addressed by delving into moral and political philosophy through concepts such as needs, basic welfare, and so forth.

2. *How great are they?* Le Grand states that the *Black Report* is not the definitive word on the subject. Measures of health need attention - i.e., should measures of mortality be employed?; should specific disease states be studied, although general levels of health seem to vary across diseases by social group?; the measure of health has to be made appropriate to what relationships are under study. Measures of social group should focus on factors other than occupation (i.e., income; gender; race; region; and so on).

3. *What causes them?* The structural primacy of explanations is argued by Le Grand. That is, behaviour is guided through material circumstances - again, the importance of studying income is stressed, and its social effects which may influence health status. Much of the necessary explanations can only be wrought from large (Le Grand's words) samples with longitudinal data. If a relationship is established - "it is desirable to explore in depth - using a much smaller sample - the exact way in which the factors indicated operate" (Le Grand, 1986:119). For example, does income affect health through lack of material goods, or indirectly by influencing tastes for healthy or unhealthy things?

4. *What consequences do they have?* What effect do health inequalities have on employment; income; 'quality of life'; also on attitudinal differences between groups?

5. *What can be done (policy implications)?* This follows from the conclusions to the previous questions, however, it is an avenue of study in its own right.

Le Grand (1986) outlines the importance of: using income as a primary indicator of social status; utilizing a 'social factors' approach whereby all independents are allowed to co-vary; using longitudinal data; and, using morbidity, rather than mortality, indicators as measures of health status.

A detailed understanding of the relationship between income and health is a formidable assignment. It is clear that relationships between social status and health status are complex. While it is evident that lower social status is related to lower health status, a better understanding of the mechanisms operating in this relationship is still needed. However, this review has raised a number of important issues relative to our understanding of income and health relationships, for both social policy and research.

Notes

1. The medical profession would maintain that physical checkups, patient screening, case finding, and so on, are methods that physicians regularly use to provide preventive health services to patients (Hay, 1990a; 1990b). Two points can be raised. First, when physicians identify 'at risk' patients, the resulting intervention usually involves the prescription of drugs or the promotion of lifestyle change. This hardly ever gets at the root of the problem that produces the risk. Second, despite the rhetoric, preventive activity by physicians on behalf of their patients is a very small fraction of physicians' daily practice. Physicians are not equipped, nor necessarily should they be, to practice prevention to the fullest extent.

2. Part of this debate rests on the political inclinations of the researchers, as Klein has identified in his labelling of Townsend. Those researchers inclined to left of centre, progressive politics - such as Townsend, Hart, Gray, Wilkinson - tend to favour social causation explanations. Those researchers inclined to liberal or conservative politics - such as Klein, Illsley, Le Grand - tend to favour selection or 'not enough evidence' explanations for health inequalities.

References

Adams, I. et al. 1971. *The Real Poverty Report.* Edmonton: M.G. Hurtig.

Adams, O.B. 1981. *Health and Economic Activity: A Time-series Analysis of Canadian Mortality and Unemployment Rates.* Statistics Canada, Catalogue 82-539E, Ottawa: Minister of Supply and Services.

Adams, O. and Wilkins, R. 1988. *Social Inequalities in Health in Canada: A Review of Current Research, Data and Methodological Issues.* Ottawa: Health Division, Statistics Canada.

Anson, J. 1988. "Mortality and Living Conditions: Relative Mortality Levels and their Relation to the Physical Quality of Life in Urban Populations." *Social Science and Medicine* 27(9): 901-910.

Atkinson, T., B. Blishen and M. Murray. 1980. *Physical Status and Perceived Health Quality.* Report from the Social Change in Canada Project, Institute for Behavioural Research, York University.

Auster, R. et al. 1969. "The Production of Health, An Exploratory Study." *Journal of Human Resources* 4: 411-436.

Badgley, R.F. 1991. "Social and Economic Disparities Under Canadian Health Care." *International Journal of Health Services* 21(4): 659-671.

Badgley, R.F. et al. 1967. "The Impact of Medicare in Wheatville, Saskatchewan." *Canadian Journal of Public Health* 58: 109-116

Badgley, R.F. and R.D. Smith. 1979. *User Charges for Health Services*. Toronto: Ontario Council of Health.

Badgley, R.F. and S. Wolfe. 1992. "Equity and Health Care." In C.D. Naylor (ed.), *Medicine and the State*. Montreal: McGill-Queens University Press.

Barer, M.L. et al. 1982. *Income Class and Hospital Use in Ontario*. Toronto: Ontario Economic Council.

Bartley, M. 1988. "Unemployment and Health: Selection or Causation - A False Antithesis?" *Sociology of Health and Illness* 10(1): 41-67.

Baxter, C. and D. Baxter. 1988. "Racial Inequalities in Health: A Challenge to the British National Health Service." *International Journal of Health Services* 18(4): 563-571.

Beck, R.G. 1973. "Economic Class and Access to Physicians' Services Under Public Medical Care Insurance." *International Journal of Health Services* 3: 341-355.

Beck, R.G. and J.M. Horne. 1976. "Economic Class and Risk Avoidance: Experience Under Public Medical Care Insurance." *Journal of Risk and Insurance* 43: 73-86.

Bell, N.W. and R.W. Burnside. 1972. "Poverty and Illness." Paper presented to the Annual Meeting of the Canadian Sociology and Anthropology Association.

Berkman, L.F. and S.L. Syme. 1979. "Social Networks, Host Resistance, and Mortality: A Nine-Year Follow-Up Study of Alameda County Residents." *American Journal of Epidemiology* 109(2): 186-204.

Billette, A. and G.B. Hill. 1977. *Inegalities sociales de mortalite au Canada*. Ottawa: Health and Welfare Canada.

Blane, D. 1985. "An Assessment of the Black Report's 'Explanations of Health Inequalities.'" *Sociology of Health and Illness* 7(3): 423-445.

Blaxter, M. 1983. "Health Services as Defense Against the Consequences of Poverty in Industrialized Societies." *Social Science and Medicine* 17(16): 1139-1148.

Blaxter, M. 1986. "Longitudinal Studies in Britain Relevant to Inequalities in Health." in R.G. Wilkinson (ed.), *Class and Health*. London: Tavistock, Pp. 125-215.

Blaxter, M. 1990. *Health and Lifestyles*. London: Routledge.

Blishen, B.R. 1958. "The Construction and Use of an Occupational Class Scale." *Canadian Journal of Economics and Political Science* 24: 519-531.

Blishen, B.R., and H.A. McRoberts. 1976. "A Revised Socio-Economic Index for Occupations in Canada." *Canadian Review of Sociology and Anthropology* 13(1): 71-79.

Blishen, B.R. et al. 1987. "The 1981 Socioeconomic Index for Occupations in Canada." *Canadian Review of Sociology and Anthropology* 24(4): 465-488.

Block, F. et al. 1987. *The Mean Season*. New York: Pantheon Books.

Bloor, M. et al. 1987. "Artefact Explanations of Inequalities in Health: An Assessment of the Evidence." *Sociology of Health and Illness* 9(3): 231-264.

Bodenheimer, T.S. 1989. "The Fruits of the Empire Rot on the Vine: United States Health Policy in the Austerity Era." *Social Science and Medicine* 28(6): 531-538.

Boulet, J.A. and D.W. Henderson. 1979. *Distributional and Re-distributional Aspects of Government Health Insurance Programs*. Ottawa: Economic Council of Canada.

Brenner, M.H. 1977. "Health Costs and Benefits of Economic Policy." *International Journal of Health Services* 7: 581-623.

Brenner, M.H. and A. Mooney. 1983. "Unemployment and Health in the Context of Economic Change." *Social Science and Medicine* 17: 1125-1138.

Buck, C. 1985. "Beyond Lalonde - Creating Health." *Canadian Journal of Public Health* 76(supplement 1 May/June): 19-24.

Burke, M.A. 1986. "Changing Health Risks." *Canadian Social Trends*. Summer: 22-26.

Canadian Sickness Survey. 1960. *Illness and Health Care in Canada*. Ottawa: The Queen's Printer.

Canadian Council on Social Development 1984. *Not Enough: The Meaning and Measurement of Poverty in Canada*. Report of the CCSD National Task Force on the Definition and Measurement of Poverty in Canada, Ottawa: Canadian Council on Social Development.

Carr-Hill, R. 1987. "The Inequalities in Health Debate: A Critical Review of the Issues." *Journal of Social Policy* 16(4): 509-542.

Carr-Hill, R. 1990. "The Measurement of Inequities in Health: Lessons From the British Experience." *Social Science and Medicine* 31(3): 393-404.

Chadwick, E. 1842. *Report to Her Majesty's Principal Secretary of State for the Home Department from the Poor Law Commissioners on an Enquiry into the Sanitary Condition of the Labouring Population of Great Britain*. M.W. Flinn (ed.) (1965), Edinburgh: Edinburgh Press.

Charles, C. and R.F. Badgley. 1987. "Health and Inequality: Unresolved Policy Issues." In S.A. Yelaja (ed), *Canadian Social Policy*. 2nd edition, Waterloo: Wilfrid Laurier University Press, Pp. 47-64.

Cheal, D. 1991. "Family Finances: Money Management in Breadwinner/Homemaker Families, Dual Earner Families, and Dual Career Families." Winnipeg Area Study Research Reports No. 38, Department of Sociology, Winnipeg: University of Manitoba.

City of Toronto 1983. *The Unequal Society: A Challenge to Public Health*. Report submitted to the Board of Health and adopted by Toronto City Council, mimeograph.

City of Toronto 1984. *The City of Toronto Community Health Survey: A Description of the Health Status of Toronto Residents 1983*. Department of Public Health, Toronto: Board of Health.

City of Toronto 1985. *The Unequal Society*. Toronto: Department of Public Health.

City of Toronto 1991. *Health Inequalities in the City of Toronto*. Summary Report, Toronto: City of Toronto, Department of Public Health.

Clark, W.A.V. et al. 1987. "The Influence of Domestic Position on Health Status." *Social Science and Medicine* 24(6): 501-506.

Cochrane, S.H. et al. 1980. *The Effects of Education on Health*. World Bank Staff Working Papers Number 405, Washington, D.C.: The World Bank.

Conover, P. 1973. "Social Class and Chronic Illness." *International Journal of Health Services* 3(3): 357-368.

Dahlgren, G. and F. Diderichsen. 1986. "Strategies for Equity in Health: Report from Sweden." *International Journal of Health Services* 16(4): 517-537.

D'Arcy, C. 1988. *Reducing Inequalities in Health*. Health Services and Promotion Branch Working Paper, Catalogue HSPB 88-16, Ottawa: Health and Welfare Canada.

D'Arcy, C. 1990. "Reducing Inequalities in Health in Canada? Trends and Implications." Paper presented at the Annual Meeting of the Canadian Sociology and Anthropology Association, Victoria, Canada.

D'Arcy, C., and C.M. Siddique. 1985. "Unemployment and Health: An Analysis of Canada Health Survey Data." *International Journal of Health Services* 15(4): 609-635.

Dooley, D. and R.A. Catalano. 1984. "The Epidemiology of Economic Stress." *American Journal of Community Psychology* 12: 387-409.

Doyal, L. and I. Gough. 1986. "Human Needs and Socialist Welfare." *Praxis International* 6(1): 43-69.

Duncan, G.J. 1984. *Years of Poverty, Years of Plenty*. Ann Arbor: Institute for Social Research, University of Michigan.

Duleep, H.O. 1986. "Measuring the Effect of Income on Adult Mortality Using Longitudinal Administrative Record Data." *Journal of Human Resources* 21: 238-251.

Dutton, D.B. 1986. "Social Class, Health, and Illness." In L.H. Aitken and D. Mechanic (eds.), *Applications of Social Science to Clinical Medicine and Health Politics*. New Brunswick, N.J.: Rutgers University Press, Pp. 31-62.

Echenberg, H. 1988. *Reducing Inequalities*. Health Services and Promotions Branch Working Paper, Catalogue HSPB 88-7, Ottawa: Health and Welfare Canada.

Engels, F. 1958. *The Condition of the Working-Class in England in 1844*. London: Methuen.

Enterline, P.E. et al. 1973. "The Distribution of Medical Services Before and After 'free' Medical Care: The Quebec Experience." *New England Journal of Medicine* 289: 1174-1178.

Epp, J. 1986. *Achieving Health For All: A Framework for Health Promotion*. Ottawa: Health and Welfare Canada.

Evans, R.G. and G.L. Stoddart. 1990. "Producing Health, Consuming Health Care." *Social Science and Medicine* 31(12): 1347-1363.

Fletcher, B.C. 1988. "Occupation, Marriage and Disease-Specific Mortality Concordance." *Social Science and Medicine* 27(6): 615-622.

Forbes, J.F. and A. McGregor. 1987. "Male Unemployment and Cause-Specific mortality in Postwar Scotland." *International Journal of Health Services* 17(2): 233-240.

Forcese, D. 1980. *The Canadian Class Structure*. (2nd Ed.) Toronto: McGraw-Hill Ryerson.

Fox, A.J. and P.O. Goldblatt. 1982. *Socio-demographic Mortality Differentials: Longitudinal Study 1971-75*. OPCS Series LS No.1, London: HMSO.

Fox, A.J., P.O. Goldblatt and D.R. Jones. 1985. "Social Class Mortality Differentials: Artefact, Selection or Life Circumstances?" *Journal of Epidemiology and Community Health* 39: 1-8.

Freedman, B. and F. Bayliss. 1987. "Purpose and Function in Government-Funded Health Coverage." *Journal of Health Politics, Policy and Law* 12(1): 97-112.

Fuchs, V. 1965. *Some Economic Aspects of Mortality in the United States*. New York: National Bureau of Economic Research.

Gafni, A. et al. 1983. "Is There a Trade-Off Between Income and Health? The Case of Hypertensive Steelworkers in Canada." *Inquiry* 20: 343-349.

Gersten, J.C. et al. 1976. "Life Dissatisfactions, Job Dissatisfactions and Illness of Married Men Over Time." *American Journal of Epidemiology* 103(3): 333-341.

Gold, M.R. and P. Franks. 1990. "The Social Origin of Cardiovascular Risk: An Investigation in a Rural Community." *International Journal of Health Services* 20(3): 405-416.

Goldblatt, P. 1990. "Social Class Mortality Differentials." In C.G.N. Mascie-Taylor (ed.), *Biosocial Aspects of Social Class*. Oxford: Oxford University Press, pp. 24-58.

Gortmaker, S.L. 1979. "Poverty and Infant Mortality in the United States." *American Sociological Review* 44: 280-297.

Government of Ontario 1987. *Toward a Shared Direction for Health in Ontario: Report of the Ontario Health Review Panel*. J.R.Evans (chair), Toronto: Government of Ontario.

Gray, A.M. 1982. "Inequalities in Health. The Black Report: A Summary and Comment." *International Journal of Health Services* 12(3): 349-377.

Grayson, J.P. 1989. "Reported Illness After a CGE Closure." *Canadian Journal of Public Health* 80(1): 16-19.

Grossman, M. 1972. *The Demand for Health: A Theoretical and Empirical Investigation*. New York: Columbia University Press.

Haan, M., G.A. Kaplan and T. Camacho. 1987. "Poverty and Health: Prospective Evidence From the Alameda County Study." *American Journal of Epidemiology* 125: 989-998.

Hadley, J. and A. Osei. 1982. "Does Income Affect Mortality? An Analysis of the Effects Of Different Types of Income on Age/Sex/Race-Specific Mortality Rates in the United States." *Medical Care* 20(9): 901-914.

Harding, M. 1987. "The Relationship Between Economic Status and Health Status and Opportunities: A Synthesis." Report Prepared for The Ontario Social Assistance Review Committee, Toronto: M. Harding Consulting.

Hart, N. 1987. "The Health Divide: Social Class Still Reigns." *Poverty* 67: 17-19.

Hartmann, J. 1982. "Health and Social Welfare." *Eurosocial Newsletter* 25: 9-13.

Hay, D.I. 1985. *Socioeconomic Status and Health Status: A Study of Males in the Canada Health Survey.* M.Sc. Thesis, Department of Community Health, University of Toronto.

Hay, D.I. 1988. "Socioeconomic Status and Health Status: A study of Males in the Canada Health Survey." *Social Science and Medicine* 27(12): 1317-1325.

Hay, D.I. 1992. *An Explication of the Relationship Between Income and Health.* Ph.D. thesis, Department of Community Health, University of Toronto.

Hay, W.I. 1990a. "Prospective Care of Elderly Patients in Family Practice Part 1: Health Maintenance for the Elderly." *Canadian Family Physician* 36: 910-914.

Hay, W.I. 1990b. "Prospective Care of Elderly Patients in Family Practice Part 2: Is Screening Worthwhile?" *Canadian Family Physician* 36: 1121-1126.

Health and Welfare Canada 1988. *Canada's Health Promotion Survey: Technical Report.* Ottawa: Minister of Supply and Services Canada.

Health and Welfare Canada & Statistics Canada 1981. *The Health of Canadians: Report of the Canada Health Survey.* Ottawa: Minister of Supply and Services & Minister of National Health and Welfare.

Hertzman, C. 1990. "Where Are the Differences Which Make a Difference? Thinking About the Determinants of Health." CIAR Population Health Working Paper No. 8, Canadian Institute for Advanced Research, Toronto.

Hertzman, C. 1991. Personal communication, Vancouver, August.

Hexel, P.C. and H. Wintersberger. 1986. "Inequalities in Health: Strategies." *Social Science and Medicine* 22(2): 151-160.

Hirdes, J.P. et al. 1986. "The Association Between Self-Reported Income and Perceived Health Based on the Ontario Longitudinal Study of Aging." *Canadian Journal on Aging* 5(3): 189-204.

Ho, T.J. 1982. *Measuring Health as a Component of Living Standards.* Living Standards Measurement Study Working Paper No.15, Washington, D.C.: The World Bank.

Hollingsworth, J.R. 1981. "Inequality in Levels of Health in England and Wales, 1891-1971." *Journal of Health and Social Behavior* 22: 268-283.

House, J.S., R.C. Kessler and A.R. Herzog. 1990. "Age, Socioeconomic Status, and Health." *Milbank Quarterly* 68(3): 383-411.

House, J.S., K.R. Landis, and D. Umberson. 1988. "Social Relationships and Health." *Science* 241: 540-545.

Illsley, R. 1987. "The Health Divide: Bad Welfare or Bad Statistics?" *Poverty* 67: 16-17.

Illsley, R. 1990. "Comparative Review of Sources, Methodology and Knowledge." *Social Science and Medicine* 31(3): 229-236.

Jenkins, C.D. 1983. "Social Environment and Cancer Mortality in Men." *New England Journal of Medicine* 308(7): 395-398.

Joffe, M. 1989. "Social Inequalities in Low Birth Weight: Timing of Effects and Selective Mobility." *Social Science and Medicine* 28(6): 613-619.

Kandrack, M.A., K.R. Grant and A. Segall. 1991. "Gender Differences in Health Related Behaviour: Some Unanswered Questions." *Social Science and Medicine* 32(5): 579-590.

Kessler, R.C. 1982. "A Disaggregation of The Relationship Between Socio-Economic Status and Psychological Distress." *American Sociological Review* 47: 752-764.

Kickbush, I. 1986. "Lifestyles and Health." *Social Science and Medicine* 22(2): 117-124.

Kitagawa, E.M. and P.M. Hauser. 1973. *Differential Mortality in the United States: A Study in Socioeconomic Epidemiology.* Cambridge, Mass.: Harvard University Press.

Klein, R. 1988. "Acceptable Inequalities." In D. Green (ed.), *Acceptable Inequalities? Essays on the Pursuit of Equality in Health Care.* London: Institute of Economic Affairs Health Unit.

Klein, R. 1990. "Research, Policy, and the National Health Service." *Journal of Health Politics, Policy and Law* 15(3): 500-523.

Klein, R. 1991. "Making Sense of Inequalities: A Response to Peter Townsend." *International Journal of Health Services* 21(1): 175-181.

Lapierre, L. 1984. *Canadian Women: Profile of Their Health.* Statistics Canada, Catalogue 82-542E, Ottawa: Minister of Supply and Services.

Lazear, E.P. and R.T. Michael. 1988. *Allocation of Income Within the Household.* Chicago: University of Chicago Press.

Le Grand, J. 1986. "Inequalities in Health and Health Care: A Research Agenda." In R.G. Wilkinson (ed), *Class and Health.* London: Tavistock, pp. 115-124.

Le Grand, J. and M. Rabin. 1986. "Trends in British Health Inequality, 1931-83." In A.J. Culyer and B. Jonsson (eds.), *Public and Private Health Services.* Oxford: Basil Blackwell, pp. 112-127.

Le Riche, W.H. 1974. *The Downtown Toronto Health Attitude Survey.* Toronto: School of Hygiene, University of Toronto.

Leighton, D.C. et al. 1963. *The Character of Danger.* New York: Basic Books.

Lerner, M. 1986. *Surplus Powerlessness.* Oakland, California: The Institute for Labour and Mental Health.

Liberatos, P., B.G. Link and J.L. Kelsey. 1988. "The Measurement of Social Class in Epidemiology." *Epidemiologic Reviews* 10: 87-121.

Lipset, S.M. 1977. "Observations on Economic Equality and Social Class." In I.L. Horowitz (ed.), *Equity, Income, and Policy.* New York: Praeger, pp. 278-286.

Lundberg, O. 1986. "Class and Health: Comparing Britain and Sweden." *Social Science and Medicine* 23(5): 511-517.

Mackenbach, J.P., K. Stronks and A.E.Kunst. 1989. "The Contribution of Medical Care to Inequalities in Health: Differences Between Socio-Economic Groups in Decline of Mortality from Conditions Amenable to Medical Intervention." *Social Science And Medicine* 29(3): 369-376.

Macintyre, S. 1986. "The Patterning of Health by Social Position in Contemporary Britain: Directions for Sociological Research." *Social Science and Medicine* 23(4): 393-415.

Macintyre, S. and C. Pritchard. 1989. "Comparisons Between the Self-Assessed and Observer-Assessed Presence and Severity of Colds." *Social Science and Medicine* 29(11): 1243-1248.

Manga, P. 1978. *The Income Distribution Effect of Medical Insurance in Ontario.* Toronto: Ontario Economic Council.

Manga, P. 1981. "Income and Access to Medical Care in Canada." In D. Coburn, et al. (eds.), *Health and Canadian Society: Sociological Perspectives.* Markham, Ontario: Fitzhenry and Whiteside, pp. 325-342.

Manga, P. 1987. "Equality of Access and Inequality in Health Status: Policy Implications of a Paradox." In Coburn, D. et al. (eds.), *Health and Canadian Society: Sociological Perspectives.* (2nd edition), Markham, Ontario: Fitzhenry and Whiteside.

Manga, P. and G.R. Weller. 1980. "The Failure of the Equity Objective in Health: A Comparative Analysis of Canada, Britain, and the United States." *Comparative Social Research* 3: 229-267.

Mare, R.D. 1982. "Socioeconomic Effects on Child Mortality in the United States." *American Journal of Public Health* 72(6): 539-547.

Marmot, M.G., M. Kogevinas and M.A. Elston. 1987. "Social/Economic Status and Disease." *Annual Review of Public Health* 8: 111-135.

Marmot, M. and T. Theorell. 1988. "Social Class and Cardiovascular Disease: The Contribution of Work." *International Journal of Health Services* 18(4): 659-674.

McKeown, T. 1976. *The Modern Rise of Populations*. London: Arnold.

McQueen, D.V. and J. Siegrist. 1982. "Social Factors in the Etiology of Chronic Disease: An Overview." *Social Science and Medicine* 16: 353-367.

Michael, R.T. 1972. "The Effect of Education on Efficiency in Consumption." Occasional Paper No. 116, New York: National Bureau of Economic Research.

Newacheck, P.W. et al. 1980. "Income and Illness." *Medical Care* 18(12): 1165-1176.

Ontario Ministry of Health 1987a. *Health For All Ontario: Report of the Panel on Health Goals for Ontario*. R.A. Spassoff (chair), Toronto: Ontario Ministry of Health.

Ontario Ministry of Health. 1987b. *Health Promotion Matters in Ontario: A Report of the Minister's Advisory Group on Health Promotion*. S. Podborski (chair), Toronto: Ontario Ministry of Health.

Patrick, D.L. et al. 1988. "Poverty, Health Services, and Health Status in Rural America." *Milbank Quarterly* 66(1): 105-136.

Pearce, N.E. et al. 1985. "Social Class, Ethnic Group and Male Mortality in New Zealand, 1974-1978." *Journal of Epidemiology and Community Health* 39: 9-14.

Pereira, J. 1990. "The Economics of Inequality in Health: A Bibliography." *Social Science and Medicine* 31(3): 413-420.

Rimpela, A.H. and E.I. Pukkala. 1987. "Cancers of Affluence: Positive Social Class Gradient and Rising Incidence Trend in Some Cancer Forms." *Social Science and Medicine* 24(7): 601-606.

Roberts, J. et al. 1966. *Social and Mental Health Survey: Summary Report*. Montreal: Urban and Social Redevelopment Project.

Robinson, W. S. 1950. "Ecological Correlations and the Behaviour of Individuals." *American Sociological Review* 15(3): 351-357.

Rodgers, G.B. 1979. "Income and Inequality as Determinants of Mortality: An International Cross-Section Analysis." *Population Studies* 33(2): 343-351.

Rogot, E. et al. 1988. *A Mortality Study of One Million Persons by Demographic, Social, and Economic Factors: 1979-1981 Follow-up*. U.S. Department of Health and Human Services, NIH Publication No. 88-2896.

Roos, N.P. and E. Shapiro. 1981. "The Manitoba Longitudinal Study on Aging." *Medical Care* 19: 644-657.

Rootman, I. 1986. *Inequality and Health: Some Preliminary Findings from the 1985 Canada Health Promotion Survey*. Ottawa: Health Promotion Directorate, Health and Welfare Canada.

Rootman, I. 1988. "Inequities in Health: Sources and Solutions." *Health Promotion* 26(3): 2-8.

Ropers, R.H. and R. Boyer. 1987. "Perceived Health Status Among the New Urban Homeless." *Social Science and Medicine* 24(8): 669-678.

Ross, D.P. and R. Shillington. 1989. *The Canadian Fact Book on Poverty-1989*. Ottawa: Canadian Council on Social Development.

Ross, D.P. and R. Shillington. 1990. "Child Poverty and Poor Educational Attainment: The Economic Costs and Implications for Society." Appendix I of *Children in Poverty: Toward a Better Future*, Ottawa: Standing Senate Committee on Social Affairs, Science and Technology, Pp. 57-86.

Royal Commission on Health Services. 1967. *The Health of the Canadian People*. Ottawa: The Queen's Printer.

Scott-Samuel, A. 1986. "Social Inequalities in Health: Back on the Agenda." *The Lancet* May 10: 1084-1085.

Segall, A. and J. Goldstein. 1989. "Exploring the Correlates of Self-Provided Health Care Behaviour." *Social Science and Medicine* 29(2): 153-161.

Segovia, J. et al. 1989. "An Empirical Analysis of the Dimensions of Health Status Measures." *Social Science and Medicine* 29(6): 761-768.

Siemiatycki, J.L. et al. 1980. "Equality in Medical Care Under National Health Insurance in Montreal." *New England Journal of Medicine* 303: 10-15.

Silver, M. 1972. "An Econometric Analysis of Spatial Variations in Mortality Rates by Race and Sex." In V.R. Fuchs (ed.), *Essays in the Economics of Health and Medical Care*. New York: Columbia University Press.

Smith, R.D. 1980. *Social Class and Health Behaviour*. Vol. I & II, Ph.D. dissertation, Department of Sociology, University of Toronto.

Soderstrom, L. 1986. "The Effect of Unemployment on the Health of Unemployed Married Women." Paper presented to the Conference of the Canadian Health Economics Research Association, Winnipeg, Manitoba.

Starrin, B., G. Larrson and S. O. Brenner. 1988. "Regional Variations in Cardiovascular Mortality in Sweden - Structural Vulnerability in the Local Community." *Social Science and Medicine* 27(9): 911-917.

Statistics Canada 1977. *Distributional Effects of Health and Educational Benefits in Canada* (1974). Ottawa: Queen's Printer.

Statistics Canada 1982. *Income Distributions by Size in Canada, 1980*. Ottawa: Minister of Supply and Services.

Statistics Canada 1987. *Health and Social Support, 1985*. Ottawa: Minister of Supply and Services.

Statistics Canada and Department of the Secretary of State of Canada. 1986. *Report of the Canadian Health and Disability Survey*. Ottawa: Minister of Supply and Services Canada.

Stern, J. 1983. "Social Mobility and the Interpretation of Social Class Mortality Differentials." *Journal of Social Policy* 12(1): 27-49.

Syme, S.L. 1986. "Strategies for Health Promotion." *Preventive Medicine* 15(5): 492-507.

Syme, S.L. 1988. "Social Epidemiology and the Work Environment." *International Journal of Health Services* 18(4): 635-645.

Syme, S.L. and L.F. Berkman. 1976. "Social Class, Susceptibility and Sickness." *American Journal of Epidemiology* 104(1): 1-8.

Taylor, R. and A. Rieger. 1985. "Medicine as Social Science: Rudolf Virchow on the Typhus Epidemic in Upper Silesia." *International Journal of Health Services* 15(4): 547-559.

Townsend, P. 1981. "Towards Equality in Health Through Social Policy." *International Journal of Health Services* 11(1): 63-75.

Townsend, P. 1990a. "Widening Inequalities of Health in Britain: A Rejoinder to Rudolph Klein." *International Journal of Health Services* 20(3): 363-372.

Townsend, P. 1990b. "Individual or Social Responsibility for Premature Death? Current Controversies in the British Debate about Health." *International Journal of Health Services* 20(3): 373-392.

Townsend, P. 1991. "Evading the Issue of Widening Inequalities of Health in Britain: A Reply to Rudolf Klein." *International Journal of Health Services* 21(1): 183-189.

Townsend, P. and N. Davidson (eds.). 1982. *Inequalities in Health: The Black Report*. Harmondsworth, England: Penguin (Pelican edition) Books.

Townsend, P., N. Davidson and M. Whitehead. 1988. "Introduction to *Inequalities in Health*." In P. Townsend, N. Davidson (eds.) and M. Whitehead, *Inequalities in Health: The Black Report and The Health Divide*. Harmondsworth, England: Penguin Books, pp. 1-27.

Townsend, P., P. Phillimore and A. Beattie. 1986. *Inequalities in Health in the Northern Region*. Bristol / Newcastle, U.K.: University of Bristol / Northern Regional Health Authority.

Ugnat, A. M. and E. Mark. 1987. "Life Expectancy by Sex, Age, and Income Level." *Chronic Diseases in Canada* 8(1): 12-13.

Verbrugge, L.M. 1989. "The Twain Meet: Empirical Explanations of Sex Differences in Health and Mortality." *Journal of Health and Social Behavior* 30: 282-304.

Waldron, I. 1983. "Sex Differences in Illness Incidence, Prognosis and Mortality: Issues and Evidence." *Social Science and Medicine* 17(16): 1107-1123.

Warner, E.E. and R.S. Smith. 1982. *Vulnerable But Invincible: A Longitudinal Study of Resilient Children and Youth.* New York: McGraw-Hill.

Warner, K. and H.A. Murt. 1984. "Economic Incentives for Health." *Annual Review of Public Health* 5: 107-133.

West, P. 1988. "Inequalities? Social Class Differentials in Health in British Youth." *Social Science and Medicine* 27(4): 291-296.

Wheaton, B. 1978. "The Sociogenesis of Psychological Disorder: Re-Examining the Causal Issues With Longitudinal Data." *American Sociological Review* 43: 383-403.

Wheaton, B. 1990. "Life Transitions, Role Histories, and Mental Health." *American Sociological Review* 55: 209-223.

Whitehead, M. 1988. "The Health Divide." In P. Townsend and N. Davidson (eds.) and M. Whitehead, *Inequalities in Health: The Black Report and The Health Divide.* Harmondsworth, England: Penguin Books, pp. 215-356.

Wigle, D.T. and Y. Mao. 1980. *Mortality by Income Level in Urban Canada.* Ottawa: Health and Welfare Canada.

Wilkins, R. 1987. "Health Inequalities in Canada: Some Policy Implications." Heart Health Inequalities Workshop Report, December 3, 1987, Pp. 5-10.

Wilkins, R. 1988. *Special Study on the Socially and Economically Disadvantaged.* Canada's Health Promotion Survey, Technical Report Series, Health and Welfare Canada, Ottawa: Minister of Supply and Services.

Wilkins, R. and O. Adams. 1983. *Healthfulness of Life.* Montreal: Institute for Research on Public Policy.

Wilkins, R. and O. Adams. 1988. "Measurement of Health Equity: Examples of Indicators, Sources, Strengths, Weaknesses." Background material prepared for *Equity in Health* session, Ontario Public Health Association Annual Meeting.

Wilkins, R., O. Adams and A. Brancker. 1989. "Changes in Mortality by Income in Urban Canada from 1971 to 1986." *Health Reports* 1(2): 137-174.

Wilkinson, R.G. 1986. "Income and Mortality." In R.G. Wilkinson (ed.), *Class and Health.* London: Tavistock, pp. 88-114.

Wilkinson, R.G. 1990. "Income Distribution and Mortality: A Natural Experiment." *Sociology of Health and Illness* 12(4): 391-412.

Wolfe, S. 1991. "Ethics and Equity in Canadian Health Care: Policy Alternatives." *International Journal of Health Services* 21(4): 673-679.

Wolfson, M. et al. 1990. "Earnings and Death - Effects Over a Quarter Century." Internal Document No. 6B, Program in Population Health, Canadian Institute for Advanced Research, Toronto.

Wolinsky, F.D. and S.R. Wolinsky. 1981. "Background, Attitudinal and Behavioural Patterns of Individuals Occupying Eight Discrete Health States." *Sociology of Health and Illness* 3(1): 31-48.

Zaidi, S.A. 1988. "Poverty and Disease: Need for Structural Change." *Social Science and Medicine* 27(2): 119-127.

2

Poverty, Homelessness and Health

Valerie Tarasuk

Introduction

The homeless are perhaps the most impoverished and disenfranchised sub-group of the estimated four million people who currently live in poverty in Canada (National Council of Welfare, 1992). Homelessness is defined as the lack of secure, adequate and affordable housing (McLaughlin, 1987). In urban Canadian settings, it might be argued that the homeless constitute the fastest growing visible minority at risk of ill health. Although the difficulty in monitoring such a transient and often "invisible" group means that there are no good census data, some indication of the prevalence of homelessness in Canada comes from the widespread and ever-growing demand for emergency relief services such as shelters, soup kitchens, and drop-in centres. A 1986 survey of shelter usage revealed that as many as 250,000 different people spent at least one night in a shelter that year. The number underestimated the true prevalence of homelessness as it omitted people living "on the street" or in accommodations which were inadequate, insecure and/or unaffordable. More recently, the 1991 Canadian census included enumeration in shelters and soup kitchens across the country. Unfortunately, however, results of this survey are not going to be released to the public[1] so prevalence estimates of homelessness in Canada remain elusive.

Severe and chronic poverty, the shortage of affordable housing, and the deinstitutionalization of psychiatric patients without the provision of adequate community support have been identified as the underlying causes of homelessness both in Canada (McLaughlin, 1987; Syrotuik, 1990) and in the United States (Youssef, Omokehinde and Garland, 1988; Hodnicki, 1990; Chaftez, 1988). Homelessness has been a topic of little study in Canada, but some insight into the nature of this problem can be gleaned from a review of U.S. studies. Although it could be argued that social policies in Canada lessen the prevalence of homelessness in this country, the disenfranchisement associated with homelessness implies that the experience of being homeless is probably fairly similar in Canada and the United States. Cross-sectional, descriptive studies of U.S. homeless populations in urban centres illustrate the links between the underlying structural issues of poverty, affordable housing crises, and desinstitutionalization, and individuals' situations (Bassuk, Rubin and Lauriat, 1984; Benda and Dattalo, 1988; Breakey et al., 1989; Malloy, Christ and Hohloch, 1990; Rossi et al., 1987; Roth and Bean, 1986; Sosin, 1989). In addition, there is some evidence that social factors such as previous physical and sexual abuse (Ritchey, La Gory and Mullis, 1991; Winkleby et al., 1992), substance abuse (Breakey et al., 1989; Linn, Gelberg and Leake, 1990), increased family breakdowns (Susser, Struening and Conover, 1987; Syrotuik, 1990), and social isolation (Benda and Dattalo, 1988; Breakey et al., 1989; Rossi et al., 1987) may contribute to homelessness. However, it is difficult to determine whether factors such as addictive and psychiatric disorders precede homelessness or are consequences of it (Benda and Dattalo, 1988; Winkleby et al., 1992), particularly given the lack of longitudinal data.

This chapter presents an examination of critical health issues confronting one group of homeless adults and explores possible directions for responses. It is based on insights gained during the course of a two-year health promotion project which was conducted at a drop-in centre in downtown Toronto. At the time of this project, the drop-in centre was used by 80-120 people ("members")[2] per day. Over 90 percent of the members were male, and 37 percent were native. Members spanned a wide range of ages, from youth to senior citizens; the average age was 34 years. The health promotion project was initiated to develop innovative methods to promote health among what was recognized as a highly vulnerable but traditionally "hard to reach" population. Through the experience of program development, delivery, and evaluation, a heightened understanding of the principal health issues confronting this population group emerged.

The process evaluation of the health promotion project was based on a combination of qualitative and quantitative research methods. Insights gained from two specific components of the evaluation form the basis of this paper. The first is basic descriptive data on program participants which was obtained from a 15-item interviewer-administered survey. No identification was included on the surveys, and no attempt was made to link individual responses with other data collected during the project. Forty-nine individuals completed the survey.

The second and principal source of insights presented here is the analysis of longitudinal case studies developed on 25 drop-in members. Sampling for the case studies was purposive to ensure that the full range of ages, housing situations, ethnicity (native and non-native), psychiatric health, and gender present in the drop-in membership were represented. Of necessity, members known to be extremely transient or inarticulate were excluded. Potential participants were identified in consultation with the drop-in staff. Participation was by informed consent and was entirely voluntary. Data collection spanned two to twelve months, depending on the duration and regularity of individuals' attendance at the drop-in. Up to three semi-structured interviews were conducted with each participant. (Twenty-one completed the first two interviews, and seventeen completed the third. The others were lost to follow-up.) Interview guides were designed to assist interviewers in eliciting information about individuals' personal histories, present living situations, responses to specific program methods, perceptions of the relevance of health promotion program initiatives to their own lives, and actions or attitudes stimulated by specific initiatives. Drop-in staff also maintained ongoing "significant event logs" on case study participants to permit documentation of any major changes in individuals' situations which occurred between interviews. A content analysis of interview notes and "significant event log" entries was conducted. Through the systematic examination of data on specific content-related themes, patterns were identified both within individuals and across groups of individuals.

A summary of one case study is presented below to illustrate the nature of health issues experienced by individuals in this setting as such issues arise in the context of everyday life. The case study is not intended to represent the experience of all homeless people, but to highlight the emergence and intertwining of critical health issues within the life of one individual.

"Dave" - A Case Study

Dave is now 30 years old. At the age of three, he was removed from his family home and placed under the care of the Children's Aid Society. The rest of Dave's childhood was spent moving in and out of group homes - a pattern he explained by the fact that he kept "running away." As an adolescent, Dave sought out and made contact with both natural parents, but the encounters were difficult and disappointing. Dave has had no contact with his parents since this time.

Dave was first incarcerated at the age of 16, when he was caught stealing a car. He continued to move in and out of the prison system for the next ten years, being convicted repeatedly on charges of theft and assault. It was in prison that Dave gained his only work experience, doing janitorial work and factory work using a metal press. At the time of writing this paper, Dave had been out of prison for three and a half years. This was the longest time period in which he had ever lived outside of an institution. Dave often contrasted his current circumstances to living conditions in prison and sometimes toyed with the thought of returning to prison (e.g., to live during the winter months). It was as if this one option would always be available to him, and he derived some comfort from that thought.

When Dave first came to the drop-in centre, he was illiterate. When linked to a local adult literacy program, he began to learn to read and write. Although his attendance eventually became sporadic, Dave's progress in the program indicated almost certainly that his illiteracy was not the result of learning disabilities but a reflection of severely disrupted schooling as a child.

Another problem which appears to have its roots in Dave's childhood is his drug addiction. During this project, Dave's drug of choice was cocaine but he also used glue, crack, and marijuana. Dave first tried drugs when he was nine years old, and he has struggled with a drug addiction for his entire adult life. He recognized that his drug use was harmful to his health and expressed particular concern about the increased risk of AIDS which he understood to be associated with his intravenous drug use. However, Dave's drug use was also a central focus of his life, shaping his social interactions and his sense of identity. He differentiated himself from higher income addicts, pointing out how they frequently define their addictions as problems which lead to disruptions in their careers, family and/or married life, and accumulation of material wealth. For Dave, who has never known any of these things, both the nature of the problem and the process of recovery were framed differently.

Dave had several experiences of addiction treatment during the course of this project. His brief stays in detoxification units and longer term residential treatment programs provided an important respite when street living and chronic substance use became too exhausting. He sometimes described his attendance in these programs as opportunities to recuperate from the ravages of extensive drug abuse, explaining that "the body can only take so much." At other times, he spoke at length of his desire to "straighten out" his life. The programs did not appear to have any lasting impact on his drug addiction, however.

When he first began coming to the drop-in centre, Dave was squatting in a shed. With the help of drop-in staff he eventually secured accommodation in a rooming house. Three months later the rooming house was destroyed by a fire which left one tenant dead. When the fire broke out, tenants who were on the premises apparently tried to use the fire alarm and fire extinguishers, only to discover that none of these were functional. The experience left Dave badly shaken and homeless once again. It also marked the beginning of a three-year period of instability in which Dave would cycle between brief stints in rooming houses or other shared accommodations, street living, and time in addiction treatment programs. He never again managed to retain housing for as long as three months. Given his dependence on welfare for financial support, Dave could afford little more than rooms "the size of jail cells." His difficulty retaining housing appeared to be linked to his drug habits and his inability to keep up with rent payments.

At the time of Dave's last interview, he was living in a park. He slept in a sleeping bag with a plastic cover over it, moving into a bus shelter when it rained. During the day he carried his belongings around in a bag, or left them in the drop-in centre's storage area for safekeeping. He took showers and did laundry using facilities at the drop-in centre. He also consumed most of his meals there, using the centre's kitchen facilities to prepare food that he generally obtained from local charitable food assistance agencies. This food was sometimes supplemented by foods purchased with cash obtained from pan-handling and by food stolen from local merchants. His social network was comprised of service providers (e.g., drop-in staff) and other members.

Critical Features of Everyday Life

Poverty, homelessness and social isolation characterized the everyday lives of drop-in members and were central to their health and well-being. What follows is a discussion of each issue as it has been understood from the analysis of case studies, but with reference to demographic data on drop-in members and pertinent literature on homelessness and poverty. Just as in the case study of "Dave," these three features of everyday life appear to be complex and intertwined, yet fundamental to health.

1. Poverty

The majority of drop-in members were either financially dependent on social assistance programs (55 percent) or had no source of income at all (29 percent). Only 12 percent of members reported receiving income from employment earnings. While no attempt was made in this project to obtain data on members' actual incomes, it can be assumed that all were below the Statistics Canada low-income cut-offs (the "poverty line"). Low-income cut-offs define relative poverty in Canada, representing gross levels of income where people must spend a disproportionate amount for food, shelter and clothing (National Council of Welfare, 1992). Depth of poverty is indicated by the extent to which the income of a family or individual falls below these levels. Social assistance rates for unattached individuals deemed employable (vs. disabled) averaged 47 percent of the low-income cut-off levels in 1989 in Ontario (National Council of Welfare, 1990). No member interviewed or surveyed reported being employed on a full-time basis; even those reporting some employment income were very unlikely to be receiving sufficient income to be living above the poverty line.

The relatively low proportion of members receiving employment earnings must be interpreted in terms of the exhausting, all-encompassing and crisis-ridden nature of lives characterized by extreme poverty and homelessness. Many members were locked in a daily struggle simply to meet basic survival needs for food and shelter. There were additional barriers to employment even for members not currently facing such severe poverty. Only 6 of the 25 case study participants had remained in school long enough to graduate from high school; a seventh participant graduated later, completing courses in adult upgrading programs. Furthermore, few had had the opportunity to receive job skills training. Other barriers to employment included psychiatric and physical disabilities, substance abuse problems, and the social stigma associated with personal histories which included periods in psychiatric or correctional institutions. The cumulative effect of such barriers to employment was particularly limiting in the current climate of fierce competition for unskilled and semi-skilled jobs which had been created by high local unemployment levels. The unemployment rate in Toronto increased by 156 percent between, 1987 and 1992, rising to 11.7 percent in 1992 (Committee of Planning and Coordinating Organizations, 1992).

The picture of extreme poverty among drop-in users is echoed by national statistics on poverty among unattached individuals. In 1990, unattached men under the age of 65 who were living in poverty in Canada had incomes which were on average 56 percent of the poverty line; the incomes of women in the same category were slightly higher, but still only 57.3 percent of the poverty line (National Council of Welfare, 1992). Only 19 percent of poor unattached individuals were working full time, but 54 percent reported working part time (National Council of Welfare, 1992). The higher prevalence of employment among poor unattached individuals nationally than among those in our study implies that the homeless population, which is the focus of this study, likely lived even further below the poverty line than is the norm for unattached individuals in general.

2. Homelessness

Fifty-one percent of members surveyed were homeless in an absolute sense - living on the street or staying in hostels or with friends. Those who were housed lived in boarding homes, rented rooms and apartments - in accommodations which for the most part were insecure and inadequate. At the time of this study, only 10 percent of members lived in rent-geared-to-income housing. Members' homelessness reflected both the inavailability of safe, affordable, personally acceptable housing (Committee of Planning and Coordinating Organizations, 1992; McLaughlin, 1987) and the lack of supportive housing opportunities which are targetted to single adults.

Individuals with psychiatric or physical disabilities, severe addiction problems, or lengthy histories of extreme poverty and social isolation require a variety of personal supports if they are to obtain and sustain housing. Although the development of effective models of support in housing is a focus of considerable interest and continued research (e.g., Boydell and Everett, 1992; Pomeroy, Cook, Benjafield, 1992), in reality such housing opportunities are scarce (McLaughlin, 1987). For the homeless adults encountered in this project, the critical lack of supportive and supported housing options in the nonprofit sector meant that many often found themselves in inappropriate housing situations and unsupported in their endeavors to live independently. Like "Dave," many members consequently had lengthy histories of failure in their attempts to get "off the street" and out of hostels.

The lack of affordable, appropriate housing caused members to sometimes translate treatment programs that included a residential component into temporary housing opportunites. For example, several members had substance abuse problems, and many of them had extensive experience in detox units and residential addiction treatment programs. The programs appeared to play a vital function in providing food and shelter during winter months or at times when street living and extensive substance abuse became too exhausting. In fact, as part of one health promotion program on housing, members rated local detox units in terms of the quality of lodgings they offered. These units and other addiction treatment programs available to members appeared to have little long-lasting impact on severe addiction problems, however.

Members' income and housing situations were key determinants of the nature of their daily lives. Many wandered daily between soup kitchens, social service agencies, temporary employment agencies, and hostels or other forms of shelter. Their impoverished circumstances invariably necessitated a dependence on charitable food assistance programs for the bulk of their food. This pattern of food acquisition may have compromised the nutritional quality of individuals' intakes, placing them at increased risk of ill health. Poverty also meant additional health risks for members with drug and alcohol addictions as they sought out less and less expensive intoxicants. The consumption of potentially lethal substances such as non-beverage sources of alcohol was common among some members. Others were known to inhale gasoline or glue - substances which can cause serious neurological damage.

Although no objective measures of health were collected in the course of this project, it is likely that members' health was compromised by their poverty and homelessness. A recent survey of 458 homeless people in the City of Toronto detailed a wide range of chronic and acute health problems reported by this group (Ambrosio et al., 1992). These included respiratory problems, gastrointestinal problems, accidents and injuries, physical and sexual assault, stress-related symptoms, and poor mental health. Absolute homelessness ("living on the street") appears to impart health risks which are in addition to those associated with poverty (Gelberg and Linn, 1989). The threat of physical and sexual abuse is particularly high for homeless women; one U.S. study estimated homeless women to be 20 times as likely to be assaulted sexually as U.S. women in general (Wright and Weber, 1987 in Ritchey et al., 1991).

In their survey of Toronto's homeless, Ambrosio and colleagues (1992) also documented the practical difficulties homeless people encounter in practicing preventive health care, carrying out treatments and following health advice. For example, two-thirds of individuals requiring special diets had been unable to follow dietary advice because they could not afford the recommended foods or had no place to store food. This same survey also identified substantial structural and attitudinal barriers to homeless persons' access to health care services (Ambrosio et al., 1992). Vladeck (1990) has suggested that the excess morbidity and premature mortality among homeless people may largely be due to the barriers to treatment of illness which accompany homelessness.

3. Social Isolation

Social isolation is fundamental to homelessness and extreme poverty (Malloy et al., 1990; Rossi et al., 1987), and it was a key theme in the case studies. Members' social isolation appeared to have been associated with a number of interrelated issues. One factor common to almost all case study participants was the lack of family support. In times of personal crisis, most had been unable to obtain financial or emotional support from family members, and instead had been forced to turn to social asistance programs and charitable services for help. As in the case of "Dave," the absence of family support in adulthood was for many members simply an extension of childhood experiences. One-quarter of case study participants had spent their childhoods being shunted between foster homes or group homes. Of those raised by one or both natural parents, most described turbulent childhood homes, often characterized by violence, alcoholism, and chronic poverty. Their stories suggest that some members had been victims of physical and/or sexual abuse as children. Other studies which have included an examination of homeless adults' personal histories have also documented disadvantaged backgrounds and histories of abuse (Breton and Bunston, 1992; Susser et al., 1987; Winkleby et al., 1992). A survey of 1437 homeless adults in northern California found that 10 percent of men and 17 percent of women had been placed in foster care before the age of 18, 6 percent of men and 33 percent of women reported sexual abuse as children, and 13 percent of men and 28 percent of women reported physical abuse (Winkleby et al., 1992).

A further implication of the poverty and homelessness which characterized members' lives and contributed to their social isolation was their marginalization in the larger community. To be poor and homeless is to be denied access to mainstream society and to be made acutely aware of one's inadmissibility. Marginalization occurs in a physical sense as homeless persons (who by definition lack secure private space) are denied access to all but the most unattractive and inhospitable of public spaces. It is telling, for example, that "Dave" slept in a park but could not spend his days there; his access to this public space was restricted to the hours when others would not be likely to make use of it. Their extreme poverty prohibited members from enjoying equal access to goods and services taken for granted by the majority and from participating in everyday social processes. Marginalization, coupled sometimes with blatant discrimination, shaped individual members' interactions with health care professionals, landlords, police officers, social service workers, and merchants.

For some members, the profound sense of isolation which

accompanies marginalization in the larger community was exacerbated by social barriers associated with particular psychiatric and/or physical disabilities, drug and alcohol addictions, and lengthy histories of psychiatric or correctional institutionalization. For those who were native, social isolation was often compounded by racial prejudice. Low literacy levels and communication barriers arising from disrupted educational histories, learning disabilities, mental health problems, and the lack of opportunity to develop social and life skills also contributed to some members' social isolation.

Conclusions

As illustrated in the case history of "Dave," the health issues confronting homeless adults are complex and intertwined. Three critical features of drop-in members' everyday lives - poverty, homelessness, and social isolation - have been described here. Regardless of whether health is defined in purely physical terms or more broadly, as the state of complete physical, mental and social well-being, these three features are fundamental to it. They set the context for other health problems (e.g., substance abuse), and shape both the subjective experience of such problems and health care professionals' responses to them. Furthermore, poverty, homelessness, and social isolation are themselves inherently "unhealthy." Social policies and programs which respond to (rather than exacerbate) the structural issues underlying poverty and homelessness are urgently needed. These need to be recognized both as preventive health measures and as health promoting programs for those currently experiencing poverty and homelessness.

Health care services and health promotion programs targetted towards homeless adults must recognize and respond to the interrelated nature of the health issues which confront them. To address individual problems or risk factors in isolation of the broader context in which they arise and are dealt with is to offer nothing more than superficial, "band-aid" solutions to the problems. The need for an integration of services to respond to the multiple and interrelated needs of the homeless has been noted elsewhere (Chaftez, 1988; Gelberg and Linn, 1988; Roth and Bean, 1986), and it is perhaps best illustrated in the example of substance abuse. While often regarded as a behavioural problem whose solutions lie in individual counselling and support groups, programs to address the addiction problems of homeless adults must deal with the contextual issues of severe and chronic poverty, homelessness, and social isolation as well. Otherwise, there is little incentive for homeless adults to commit themselves to treatment programs and little support to maintain substance-free living upon program completion. For individuals like "Dave," with a history of substance abuse dating back to childhood, extremely limited literacy skills, no work experience outside the prison system, and limited social supports, the prospect of an addiction-free lifestyle must have been terrifying. While on the surface his drug addiction may appear to be the greatest barrier to his good health and full participation in society, it is simply "the tip of the iceberg."

A final issue apparent from "Dave's" story and from the analysis of other case histories collected in the course of this project is the tremendous disadvantage inflicted upon some individuals by their childhood experiences. The lack of education and job skills among many homeless adults is perhaps the most obvious result of their disadvantaged childhoods. Other possible associations not investigated in this study include the links between childhood histories of neglect and abuse and current problems of substance abuse. While there is a need for further research into these links, there is a more pressing need for Canadians to re-examine the social supports and services available to children in troubled homes. "Dave's" story clearly reflects our society's failure to respond effectively to the needs of some children - a failure whose consequences remain with them long into adulthood.

The foregoing discussion is based on research conducted during a two-year health promotion project at The Meeting Place, St. Christopher House, Toronto, Ontario. The project was funded by a grant from the Health Innovations Fund, Ontario Premier's Council on Health, Well-being, and Social Justice. The author assumes full responsibility for the analysis and interpretations expressed in this paper.

Notes

1. Giles, Philip. Statistics Canada, Ottawa. Personal communication. February, 1993.

2. People coming to this particular drop-in centre are routinely referred to as "members," a term chosen to foster a sense of belonging and acceptance among all those who enter the centre. The term is retained throughout this paper.

References

Ambrosio, Eileen, Dilin Baker, Cathy Crowe and Kathy Hardill. 1992. The Street Health Report. A Study of the Health Status and Barriers to Health Care of Homeless Women and Men in the City of Toronto. Toronto.

Bassuk, Ellen L., Lenore Rubin and Alison Lauriat. 1984. "Is Homelessness a Mental Health Problem?" *American Journal of Psychiatry* 141:1546-1550.

Benda, Brent B. and Patrick Dattalo. 1988. "Homelessness: Consequence of Crisis or a Long-Term Process?" *Hospital and Community Psychiatry* 39:884-886.

Boydell, Katherine M. and Barbara Everett. 1992. "What Makes a House a Home? An Evaluation of a Supported Housing Project for Individuals with Long-term Psychiatric Backgrounds." *Canadian Journal of Community Mental Health* 10:109-123.

Breakey, William R., Pamela J. Fischer, Morton Kramer, Gerald Nestadt, Alan J. Romanoski, Alan Ross, Richard M.Royall and Oscar C. Stine. 1989. "Health and Mental Health Problems of Homeless Men and Women in Baltimore." *Journal of the American Medical Association* 262:1352-1257.

Breton, Margot and Terry Bunston. 1992. "Physical and Sexual Violence in the Lives of Homeless Women." *Canadian Journal of Community Mental Health* 11:29-43.

Chaftez, Linda. 1988. "Perspectives for Psychiatric Nurses on Homelessness." *Issues in Mental Health Nursing* 9:325-335.

Committee of Planning and Coordinating Organizations. July, 1992. *A Social Report for Metro.* Toronto, Ontario: Social Planning Council of Metro Toronto.

Gelberg, Lillian and Lawrence S. Linn. 1988. "Social and Physical Health of Homeless Adults Previously Treated for Mental Health Problems." *Hospital and Community Psychiatry* 39:510-516.

Gelberg, Lillian and Lawrence S. Linn. 1989. "Assessing the Physical Health of Homeless Adults." *Journal of the American Medical Association* 262:1973-1979.

Hodnicki, Donna R. 1990. "Homelessness: Health-Care Implications." *Journal of Community Health Nursing* 7(2):59-67.

Linn, Lawrence S., Lillian Gelberg and Barbara Leake. 1990. "Substance Abuse and Mental Health Status of Homeless and Domiciled Low-Income Users of a Medical Clinic." *Hospital and Community Psychiatry* 41:306-310.

McLaughlin, MaryAnn . 1987. *Homelessness in Canada. The Report of the National Inquiry.* Ottawa: Canadian Council on Social Development.

Malloy, Catherine, Mary Ann Christ and Faith J. Hohloch. 1990. "The Homeless: Social Isolates." *Journal of Community Health Nursing* 7(1):25-36.

National Council of Welfare. 1990. *Welfare Incomes 1989.* Ottawa, Ont.: Minister of Supply and Services Canada.

National Council of Welfare. 1992. *Poverty Profile, 1980-1990.* Ottawa, Ont.: Minister of Supply and Services Canada.

Pomeroy, Edward, Bruce Cook and John Benjafield. 1992. "Perceived Social Support in Three Residential Contexts." *Canadian Journal of Community Mental Health* 11:101-107.

Ritchey, Ferris J., Mark La Gory and Jeffrey Mullis. 1991. "Gender Differences in Health Risks and Physical Symptoms Among the Homeless." *Journal of Health and Social Behavior* 32:33-48.

Rossi, Peter H., James D. Wright, Gene A. Fisher and Georgianna Willis. 1987. "The Urban Homeless: Estimating Composition and Size." *Science* 235:1336-1341.

Roth, Dee and Gerald J. Bean. 1986. "New Perspectives on Homelessness: Findings from a Statewide Epidemiologic Study." *Hospital and Community Psychiatry* 37:712-719.

Sosin, Michael R. 1989. "Homelessness in Chicago." *Public Welfare* Winter:22-28.

Susser, Ezra, Elmer L. Struening and Sarah Conover. 1987. "Childhood Experiences of Homeless Men." *American Journal of Psychiatry* 144:1599-1601.

Syrotuik, Jim. 1990. "Modelling the Production Process of Homelessness in London, Ontario." *Ontario Geography* 35:1-13.

Vladeck, Bruce C. 1990. "Health Care and the Homeless: A Political Parable for Our Time." *Journal of Health Politics, Policy and Law* 15:305-317

Winkleby, Marilyn A., Beverly Rockhill, Darius Jatulis and Stephen P. Fortmann. 1992. "The Medical Origins of Homelessness." *American Journal of Public Health* 82:1395-1298.

Youssef, Fatma A., Maize Omokehinde and Iven M. Garland. 1988. "The Homeless and Unhealthy: A Review and Analysis." *Issues in Mental Health Nursing* 9:317-324.

3

Lifestyles, Material Deprivation and Health

B. Singh Bolaria

Introduction

There are currently a number of issues being debated about the Canadian health-care system. One area which continues to receive considerable attention is the relative effect of individual lifestyle and environmental factors on health and illness. In this debate a distinction is often made between environmental and social factors beyond one's control which influence health and factors over which the individual presumably has control and can make "healthy" choices. Proponents of the former approach focus on structural conditions in society, such as material deprivation, which produce illness, while proponents of the latter approach emphasize individual behaviour and consumption patterns, such as exercise and diet. It is argued that since the major risk factors causing much of mortality are under the personal discretion of the individuals, there would be considerable reduction in mortality if individuals would focus their attention on changing those aspects of their lifestyles which are injurious to their health. On the other hand, as the studies from the historical materialistic epidemiological perspective focus on illness-generating conditions in society, it is argued that the solution lies in changing the social and environmental conditions that produce illness and mortality.

As these contending paradigms have important implications in health decisions, health policy and provision of health care, they merit serious consideration. This chapter addresses the issues involved in this debate and concludes with a discussion of the ideological and policy implications of the individualistic and social perspectives.

Background to Reductionism in Medicine

Many aspects of medical practice including the structure and delivery of health services are receiving extensive scrutiny. One area which has received considerable attention is the individualistic, biomedical and reductionist tendencies in medicine.

This section evaluates the implications of the clinical paradigm, widely accepted in medical practice, that defines health and illness in individual terms, independent of the social context in which they occur. Turshen (1977:46) states: "This paradigm takes individual physiology as the norm for pathology (as contrasted with broader social conditions) and locates sickness in the individual's body." Contemporary medicine operates on a mechanistic and individualistic model in which individuals are "atomized" and decontextualized for treatment (McKeon, 1965:38). This approach basically ignores the fact that much ill health is rooted in the structure of society itself. Many diseases are considered to have a "specific etiology"; that is, the specific causes are sought in the body's cellular and biochemical systems. This individual-centred concept of disease has led to an essentially curative orientation, whereby people can be made healthy by means of "technological fixes" (Renaud, 1975). Technical solutions are offered to many problems which stem from social conditions (Fee, 1977).

Furthermore, the major response to many of the psychological disorders has been pharmacological — antidepressants, anti-anxiety agents, stimulants, and tranquilizers (Waldron, 1977; Katz, 1972; Stroufe and Stewart, 1973; Fee, 1977). These are generally prescribed to women, who consume large quantities of these drugs (Fee, 1977; Harding et al., 1977; Miller and Findlay, 1994).

Many diseases are viewed as malfunctions, mere technical defects in the body's machinery, and many treatments are oriented toward restoring the "normal" functioning of the human body. Rather than removing the external causes of illness, medical technology is used to destroy the capacity of the body to register reaction to these causes (Eyer and Sterling, 1977:34).

There has been increasing criticism of the clinical paradigm, especially as applied to psychiatric treatment (Illich, 1976; Dubos, 1968; Powels, 1973; Szasz, 1961; Laing, 1970; Doyal and Pennell, 1979; Waitzkin, 1983; Navarro, 1986). Nonetheless, this orientation has a pervasive and continuing influence in medical practice (Turshen, 1977).

Much of the research into non-psychological, or physical, illnesses reflects this orientation as well. There has been heavy emphasis on individual treatment and etiology of disease rather than on social and environmental factors, such as occupational and environmental exposure to pollutants, chemicals, and other harmful agents.

In some areas of medicine this individual etiology is taking extreme forms. For instance, in the area of occupational health, genetic screening is being done in some petrochemical industries in order to detect those workers whose genetic makeup may make them more susceptible to various toxins. The assumption made in genetic screening programmes is that certain workers get ill because of their genetic background and structure rather than because of exposure to toxins at the workplace. This shifts the responsibility for disease back onto the individual, promoting a victim-blaming epidemiology (Navarro, 1984:113).

Similarly, in the case of some cancer research, the major emphasis, both in research and educational campaigns, is often placed on individual responsibility and behaviour, such as smoking and personal habits (Greenberg and Randal, 1977). Little attention is given to environmental factors, such as pollutants and carcinogens, which are more and more being recognized as the agents most responsible for cancer: it is estimated that environmental factors are involved in the etiology of about 80 percent of all cancers (Waitzkin, 1983). Yet in many educational campaigns the emphasis is on the individual preserving his or her own health. Information on environmental and occupational carcinogens is rarely included in these campaigns.

This mechanistic-individualistic conception of disease, which engenders a disease-centred, high technology, medical orientation, is pervasive in medical practice and research. This reductionist orientation absolves the economic and political systems from the responsibility for disease, and denies its social foundations. A similar reductionist approach has emerged, which emphasizes individual lifestyle. In Canada in 1974, the publication of Lalonde's paper gave prominent attention to health risks associated with individual lifestyles and consumption patterns (Lalonde, 1974). Lifestyle was also one of the foci of another official policy paper (Epp, 1986). While the clinical model attributes disease to the malfunctioning of the human body, this reductionism introduces the idea that the causes of disease lie in individual lifestyles and behaviours. In the former case, the normal functions of the human body can be restored through "technological fixes," while in the latter the solution lies primarily in changing individual behaviours and patterns of consumption. This approach, too, obscures the social nature of disease and fails to recognize the important relationships between social and work environments and health and sickness.

Individual Lifestyles and Material Deprivation

The reductionist perspectives are criticized on ideological and empirical grounds. This emphasis on lifestyles over social environment is symptomatic of what William Ryan has called "blaming the victim" syndrome. More importantly, as Berliner (1977:119) maintains, "focusing on lifestyles serves only to reify the lifestyles as an entity apart from the social conditions from which it arises." Berliner (1977:119) further argues: "Discussing changes in lifestyle without first discussing the changes in the social conditions which give rise to them without recognizing that the lifestyle is derivative, is misleading and, in effect, is victim blaming."

It may also be noted that this approach to analyzing "social problems" is not confined to the health sector alone. It has been used in the sociological study of racism, education, inequality, welfare, and poverty. For instance, sociologists, for the most part, focused on the poor, analyzing their attributes and their way of life (culture) and lifestyles. Rather than looking into the socio-political and economic conditions which create inequality, poverty is explained in terms of personal attributes and deficiencies of the poor and their inappropriate ways of life. This view is best represented in Oscar Lewis' "culture of poverty" thesis (Lewis, 1966). Numerous variations of this perspective appear in other areas in the form of functionalist theory, the I.Q. argument, achievement syndrome, and personal pathologies, to mention just a few (Davis and Moore, 1945; Rosen, 1956; Davis, 1975; see also Bolaria, 1991a).

Despite the prevalence of this approach which conceals the social context of disease, there is considerable evidence which suggests that many diseases are environmentally generated, by the workplace in particular.

Workers constantly face hazardous working conditions, conditions which can hardly be attributed to their lifestyles. Workplace-related illnesses and accidents cost millions of dollars and account for millions of days of lost work in Canada and often far exceed the number of days lost due to strikes and lockouts (Rinehart, 1987; Jangula, 1986; Statistics Canada, 1991, 1992; Shields and Dickinson, 1994; Labour Canada, 1991). Thousands of workers work in unhealthy environments, where they are exposed to poor ventilation, inadequate safety, excessive dirt, radioactive dusts, and other pollutants. Some of these pollutants are directly linked to various debilitating and fatal diseases such as asbestosis, silicosis, and black lung. In addition to these pulmonary diseases, many types of cancer are associated with environmental conditions (Cairns, 1975; Hammond, 1974; Goff and Reasons, 1986; Harding, 1994; Bolaria, 1991b).

Occupational diseases are, for the most part, environmentally determined. The priority of profits over occupational safety and workers' satisfaction is clearly responsible for disease-causing work environments (Miller, 1975; Waitzkin, 1983).

The nature and organization of work, job factors, and job attributes appear to have important relationships to the individual's general well-being (Coburn, 1975). Bosquet (1977:102) writes:

> So deep is the frustration engendered by work that the incidence of heart attacks among manual workers is higher than that in any other stratum of society. People "die from work" not because of it is noxious or dangerous . . . but because it is intrinsically "killing."

Other investigators have shown a correlation between general economic conditions, such as the unemployment rate, and cardiovascular and other mortality (Eyer, 1975, 1977; Brenner, 1971). Research evidence shows substantial health differences between the employed and the unemployed. The unemployed, for instance, report higher levels of psychological distress, more symptoms of depression, higher anxiety levels, and generally more health problems than the employed (Grayson, 1985). This observation is particularly significant in view of the continued high unemployment situation in Canada. The high unemployment rates in Canada are accompanied by increases in long-term unemployment — that is, for six months or longer (Parliament, 1987). The number of Canadians experiencing long-term unemployment more than tripled between 1980 and 1983. In 1985, 28 percent of unemployed Canadians were in the long-term unemployment category (Parliament, 1987). There was a dramatic drop in employment levels for men aged 55-64 between 1975 and 1985 (Lindsay, 1987). Because of the ever-present threat of unemployment, many workers may be reluctant to complain about conditions at the workplace. Under these circumstances, workers are faced with a choice between working in an unsafe and unhealthy workplace or not working at all.

Many factors in the work environment serve to produce conditions which are widely known as "stress-related diseases." Many of these stress-related diseases, such as heart disease, can be seen as originating from the needs of the production process itself.

The competitive nature of the production process, the continuous demand for an increase in efficiency, the need for a flexible and free labour force, unemployment, and job security, all contribute to general stress in the population. This is evident in the disruption of the social environment. Eyer and Sterling (1977) argue that economic and cultural forces in capitalist society, which mould competitive, striving individuals and disrupt communal ties, create stress. Increasingly, stress is being recognized as a variable in the creation of ill health. Stressful effects of disruption of co-operative relationships and traditional cultures are manifested in high blood pressure and increases in blood cholesterol and fat levels (Sterling and Eyer, 1981; Waldron et al., 1982). Elevated blood fats and cholesterol levels increase the risk of cardiovascular diseases, which dominate modern excess mortality.

While competitiveness often leads to success in the capitalist work environment, at the same time much research has shown that it is a prime determinant of heart disease. Individual behaviour patterns have been identified as one of the strongest risk factors in heart disease. In the literature, studies have shown that the chance of a person with "Type A" behaviour (aggressive, competitive) having a heart attack is two to five times higher than that of a person with "Type B" behaviour (co-operative, easy-going, relaxed, passive). The Type A behaviour pattern has become common and is associated with an increase in mortality from coronary heart disease (Rosenman et al., 1970,1975). Independent of the effect of other risk factors, Type A alone increases the risk of coronary heart disease (Jenkins and Zyzsanski, 1980).

This indicates a contradiction between the needs of the economic system and what is healthy for the individual. It is in the interest of the individual, then, to practice Type B behaviour, but the interest of the system demands that individuals maintain Type A behaviour (Eyer, 1975). This suggests that the health effects of individual behaviour must be examined in the context of the social conditions from which the behaviour arises.

Competitiveness and orientation towards achievement become ideals; this is achieved through socialization in schools, religion, education, and cultural values (Bowles and Gintis, 1977). As noted earlier, social disruptions are the price of maintaining a free and flexible labour force. To correct for such disruptions would hinder the capitalist pursuit of profits and productivity. Similarly, as Eyer and Sterling (1977:37) state, "mass relaxation by the majority of men who share coronary-prone behaviour patterns would undermine productivity, the profits of capitalist firms, and thence the growth process itself"

Those in this society who do not exhibit competitive achievement orientation may be considered as "maladjusted," and the individuals blame their failure on their own lack of initiative. Therefore, the primary adaptation is competitive achievement orientation. There are those who cannot adapt or for whom the cost of adaptation is too high. The cost takes many forms other than coronary heart disease. The massive social and personal stresses engendered by the capitalist system may lead to drug and substance abuse. For instance, alcohol consumption is higher among groups with higher rates of unemployment, family breakup, and migration (Eyer, 1977; Egger, 1980). Other work-induced problems are ulcers, mental illness, and even suicide (Eyer and Sterling, 1977).

There is also evidence (including studies reported in this volume) which reinforces the conclusion that the dominant cause of inequalities in health status is social inequality and material deprivation.

Epidemiological data clearly demonstrates the differential health status of the population by socio-economic status. The health gap between the rich and the poor continues to exist in Canada, where the principle of universality was a major impetus to the introduction of medical care in the sixties (National Council of Welfare, 1990; Grant, 1988). Upper income Canadians live longer, healthier, and disability free lives on the average than poor Canadians. This gap in health status is primarily due to the "debilitating conditions of life that poverty forces upon people" (National Council of Welfare, 1990:6). Social and material conditions of existence such as poor housing, poor nutrition, poor neighbourhoods and poor environment all contribute to high mortality in the low income population. High mortality levels in poor neighbourhoods are well documented (Thomson, 1990; National Council of Welfare, 1990). Evidence indicates that the poorer the area, the shorter the life expectancy of both men and women. Data also show that children of parents in the poorest neighbourhoods have twice the infant mortality rates of children in the richest neighbourhoods. High mortality, high disability and the low health status of Natives is associated with environmental, economic, social, and living conditions of the population (Borsellino, 1990; Mao et al., 1992). Other studies lend support to the general conclusion that low-income poor people not only have high mortality and morbidity, but low utilization of health services (Driver, 1991; Shah et al., 1987; Wilkins et al., 1991; Grant, 1988).

A number of studies show the relationship between low incomes and inadequate diets (Nutrition Canada, 1975; Myers and Kroetsch, 1978; Reid and Miles, 1977). Poverty, nutrition, and hunger are also closely linked to health status (Epp, 1986; Wilkins and Adams, 1983; Wigle and Mao, 1980). A report published by the Minister of Health revealed that "men in the upper income groups can expect 14 more disability-free years than men with a low income; in the case of women, the difference is eight years" (Epp, 1986:398). Other evidence associates poverty with malnutrition, psychomotor and growth retardation, emotional disturbances, and visual difficulties. These problems are even more acute among Native people (Shah and Farkas, 1985).

The adverse health effects of poverty for children have their beginning during pregnancy; they have significant impact on complications during pregnancy, low birth weight of children, handicaps, poor growth, and intellectual and emotional disorders (National Council of Welfare, 1975). Child mortality rates are higher for poor children than their wealthy peers (Fine, 1989).

The cumulative effect of poverty, malnutrition, hunger, and ill health is the extensive reproduction of poverty. All of these things influence poor children's learning ability and performance in school (National Council of Welfare, 1975), which subsequently affect job prospects, employment patterns, and earnings. As a report by the National Council of Welfare (1975:1) states: "To be born poor in Canada does not make it a certainty that you will live poor and die poor — but it makes it very likely."

Low income and poverty forces upon people many debilitating conditions which produce poor health, shorter lives, high infant mortality, and other physical and mental health problems for the disadvantaged. Dependency on food banks further these disadvantages (Bolaria, 1994). In this context, one of the questions most frequently raised is whether the food banks meet the diet and nutritional needs of their clients. While Canadian studies which provide systemic evidence on this subject are lacking, the evidence from elsewhere suggests that the provision of food assistance in itself cannot be equated with nutritional and dietary adequacy (Rauschenbach et al., 1990; Emmons, 1987; Laven and Brown, 1985; Carrillo et al., 1990; Reuler, 1989; Wood and Valdez, 1991). Poverty and homelessness is also likely to increase as "disadvantages" accumulate for individuals and groups, and with differential social status and power relations and differential medical and nutritional needs of the individuals. For instance, even in the food bank population, women and children are likely to be at a higher risk than men. The reference here is to women's reproductive health (Martin, 1989; Pollock, 1988; Trypuc, 1988), nutritional health needs during pregnancy, and children's nutritional needs. Abuse and violence against women and children also puts them at a greater health risk.

The effects of malnutrition and vitamin deficiencies have begun to appear in some cases. Mo Ali, physician and hematologist, points out in this regard:

> We're seeing more patients who suffer from blood diseases by lack of vitamins. One of the vitamins is folic acid, and that's present in fresh vegetables and fresh fruit. People who are living on canned food from food banks are the people we are starting to see in age groups I have not seen before, people in their 20s and 30s. They become anemic. They become weak and tired. They have to walk and line up for food, jobs, clothing, shelter. It is really sad what is happening (*Globe and Mail*, Tuesday, December 22, 1992: A4).

Folic acid, for instance, also prevents neural tube defects (Laxdal, Habbick and Bolaria, 1993).

There is also differential impact of environmental degradation by socio-economic status and race (Bolaria, 1991a; Frideres, 1994). Native people are subject to more pollutants than the general population because they frequently live in environmentally unsafe areas. Mercury poisoning of rivers and lakes at some Indian reserves in Ontario has received a great deal of publicity (Castrilli, 1982; Smith and Smith, 1975). The Native people of the White Dog and Grassy Narrows reserves were found to have 40 to 150 times more mercury in their blood than the average Canadian (McDonald, 1975; Moore, 1975). This problem is not confined to northwestern Ontario. The Medical Post reported that there were 15 badly contaminated areas in Canada (Cassels, 1975). The release of toxic chemical wastes is creating a physical environment harmful to public health.

Poor housing, a polluted environment, poor working conditions, unemployment, and poverty — all elements of material conditions of life and deprivations — are important social determinants of health irrespective of individual lifestyles (for a review of evidence, see Townsend, 1990).

In summary, the focus on individual lifestyle and self-imposed risks tends to downgrade the importance of social and environmental factors in the production of illness. As noted above, massive social disruptions, unemployment, conditions in the workplace, requirements of the production process, and stress account for a great deal of illness. In the face of this evidence, this singular emphasis on individual etiology and individual solutions has important ideological and policy implications, which are discussed below.

Ideological and Policy Implications

It must be pointed out that the individual centred approach — individual etiology and individual solutions — has received considerable support in many Western countries. For example, a DHSS (1976:62-63) report in Britain stated:

> The prime responsibility for his own health falls on the individual. The role of the health professions and of government is limited to ensuring that the public have access to such knowledge as is available about the importance of personal habit and at the very least, no obstacles are placed in the way of those who decide to act on that knowledge.

This message that health depends upon what we choose to do and not to do is being promoted in other papers and publications (see Cohen, 1987; Association of American Medical Colleges, 1984; White, 1987; Carlson, 1975; Vickery and Fries, 1976).

In times of economic constraints, when the situation becomes even more critical and the health-care crisis deepens, government programmes promoting this type of individual emphasis gain dominance over others. An attempt is made "to shift the responsibility for disease back onto the worker, in this case through victim-blaming epidemiology and of individual solutions for the workers" (Berliner, 1977:119). As Doyal and Pennell (1979:296) put it: "Thus it is said that individuals are to blame for their own health problems and it is up to them to adopt a healthier life-style. The Victorian notion of 'undeserving poor' is being replaced by the equally inappropriate notion of 'the undeserving sick.'" This has strong implications for health care policy. And as Ryan states: "It is a brilliant ideology for justifying a perverse form of social action designed to change, not society, as one might expect, but rather society's victim (Ryan, 1971:7).

The health promotion strategies and educational campaigns are primarily oriented toward changing individuals and their lifestyles. Relatively little attention is given to the transformation of the physical and social environment and the health-care system. For instance, Epp's policy paper says relatively little about creating a healthy environment (McDowell, 1986), and Epp considers "health promotion as an approach that complements and strengthens the existing systems of health care" (Epp, 1986:396). The need for legislative action to curb the harmful effects of the environment and to have a critical look at the health-care system is increasingly being recognized.

Change of individual behaviour and promotion of "self-care prevention" through health education are an important part of the strategy to reduce health-care costs. The DHSS (1976:22) Priorities Report stated: "Preventive medicine and health education are particularly important when resources are tightly limited, as they can often lead to savings in resources in other areas." Similarly, Epp, in his health policy promotion paper, (1986:406-7) stated that there is the question of allocating resources during times of scarcity. The availability of financing is obviously a critical question for each of us. Canada has performed fairly well in controlling the growth of health care costs; however, cost control is a matter of continuing concern. The pressure created by an aging population and the growth of incidence of disabilities in our society will take a heavy toll on our financial resources. We believe, however, that the health promotion approach has the potential over the long term to slow the growth in health care costs.

This response to crises in health care strengthens "the ideological construct of bourgeois individualism by which one is responsible for one's wealth or lack of it, for one's work or lack of it, and for one's health or lack of it" (Navarro, 1978:206), and thus it masks the social nature of disease. By focusing on workers' lifestyles and habits it diverts attention from unhealthy and unsafe work environments; by concentrating on safe driving and seat belts it ignores the automobile industry and unsafe cars, and by concentrating on individual diet it diverts attention from food monopolies and potentially harmful food additives (Berliner, 1977).

However, a focus on social, economic, and political institutions will bring into question the legitimacy of the whole system and its health sector. By promoting individual responsibility this strategy serves as a legitimizing function and distracts attention from the illness generating economic and social environment.

The policies are primarily geared toward changing lifestyles; this is achieved through educational campaigns. Popularization of this strategy, in the long run, would be instrumental in preparing the populace to accept further reductions in health services — "to tighten their medical care belts" (Berliner, 1977:116). It is likely to have adverse effects. Healthy lifestyles, "wise living," and self-care are fine, but cannot substitute for professional health services when they are required (Waitzkin, 1983). With regard to Epp's health promotion policy paper, McDowell (1986:448) states: "Self-care and the assistance of neighbours are laudable, but are made here to sound like a cheap alternative to professional health care . . . . Epp is trying to reduce the demand for health services, rather than the need for them."

Therefore, the burden of health crises may be borne by individuals to the extent that they are willing to accept the proposition that what are actually to a great extent socially, economically, and politically caused conditions can be solved individually either by medical intervention or by self-care and changes in lifestyle. This approach promotes a policy of "health education in prevention and clinical medicine in cure," rather than drawing attention to the organization of health care delivery systems, or the nature, function, and composition of the health sector in this society and the overall economic and political forces which determine the state of healthiness.

Conclusions

In this chapter we have presented an analysis of one of the strategies — focus on lifestyles and self-imposed risks — being largely popularized by the state and media at the present time in the area of health care. The promotion of this strategy in the context of the current health debate is more than coincidental. Our discussion indicates that this approach is consistent with the basic tenets of "bourgeois individualism and freedom of choice," and its singular emphasis on the individual obscures the extent to which health and illness are perceived as arising from socially determined ways of life. Thus, responsibility for health and illness depends on behaviour modification by individuals rather than on changing the existing social, economic, and political institutions and the health sector.

At a broader political level, this strategy serves to legitimate existing class relations and the dominant political and economic structures. The popularization of this ideology, in the long run, would be instrumental in preparing the population to alter its expectations regarding health care and, perhaps, accept reductions in health services (Crawford, 1977). On the other hand, challenging existing social, economic, and political institutions is likely to bring into question the legitimacy of the whole system and the health sector.

The burden of health crises may therefore be borne by individuals to the extent that they accept the proposition that illnesses that are actually the result of environmentally induced conditions can be solved individually by self-care or "wise living."

A final point must be made. In this chapter we are not presenting a social deterministic behaviour model. It would be absurd to argue that individuals have no control over their lives and that individual lifestyle has no significance whatsoever for individual health. What is important, however, is the recognition that individual lifestyle choices are not made in a vacuum. Instead, individual choices are limited by structural conditions — social, political, and economic forces. Many individuals live and work in unhealthy environments. Changes in personal lifestyle can do nothing to correct the unhealthy surroundings. For the unemployed, their joblessness and associated health problems can hardly be blamed on their lifestyles. Unemployment is causally related to a number of physical and mental illnesses and to numerous social problems. It is also crucial to note that lifestyle modification campaigns have been more effective in modifying the health-related behaviour (smoking cessation, for instance) of better-educated and higher-income groups; these are also likely to have stable employment patterns, healthy workplace environments, better nutrition, and perhaps more leisure and relaxation time. There are grounds to believe that changing "at risk" behaviour of certain individuals may improve their state of health. However, this cannot be used as a substitute for improving the social and economic conditions that are responsible for so many of their health problems. Therefore we have criticized the political and ideological undercurrents inherent in the approach which continues to "atomize both causation and solution to illness" and the policy implications of changing individual behaviour and not the social and economic environment.

A revised version of this chapter also appeared in *Sociology of Health Care in Canada*, B. Singh Bolaria and Harley D. Dickinson (eds.). Toronto: Harcourt Brace Jovanovich, 1988.

References

Association of American Medical Colleges. 1984. "Physicians for the Twenty-First Century. Report of the Project Panel on the General Professional Education of the Physician and College Preparation for Medicine." *Journal of Medical Education* 59(11): 1-208.

Berliner, Howard S. 1977. "Emerging Ideologies in Medicine." *Review of Radical Political Economics* 9(1): 116-24.

Berliner, Howard S. 1975. "A Large Perspective on the Flexner Report." *International Journal of Health Services* 5 : 573-92.

Blackburn, R., ed. 1973. *Ideology in Social Science*. New York: Random House.

Bodenheimer, Thomas S. 1989. "The Fruits of Empire Rot on the Vine: United States Health Policy in the Austerity Era." *Social Science and Medicine* 28(6): 531-538.

Bolaria, B. Singh. 1988. "The Politics and Ideology of Self-Care and Lifestyles." Pp. 537-550 in *Sociology of Health Care in Canada*. Edited by B. Singh Bolaria and Harley D. Dickinson. Toronto: Harcourt Brace Jovanovich.

Bolaria, B. Singh. 1991a. "Introduction: Social Issues and Contradictions." Pp. 1-12 in *Social Issues and Contradictions in Canadian Society*. Edited by B. Singh Bolaria. Toronto: Harcourt Brace Jovanovich.

Bolaria, B. Singh. 1991b. "Environment, Work and Illness." Pp. 222-246 in *Social Issues and Contradictions in Canadian Society*. Edited by B. Singh Bolaria. Toronto: Harcourt Brace Jovanovich.

Bolaria, B. Singh. 1994. "Income Inequality, Food Banks and Health." Pp. 245-255 in *Health, Illness and Health Care in Canada*. Edited by B. Singh Bolaria and Harley D. Dickinson. Toronto: Harcourt Brace.

Borsellino, M. 1990. "Poor Health Care Housing Blamed For Native's High Disability Rate." Medical Post March 27:20.

Bosquet, M. 1977. *Capitalism in Crisis and Everyday Life*. Sussex: Harvest Press.

Bowles, Samuel, and Herbert Gintis. 1977. *Schooling in Capitalist America*. Basic Books.

Brenner, M. Harvey. 1977. "Economic Changes and Heart Disease Mortality." *American Journal of Public Health* 61: 60-71.

Brenner, M. Harvey. 1977. "Health Costs and Benefits of Economic Policy." *International Journal of Health Services* 7:581-623.

Cairns, J. 1975. "The Cancer Problem." *Scientific American* 233 (18):64-72.

Canada. Senate. 1971. Special Senate Committee on Poverty. *Poverty in Canada*. Ottawa.

Carillo, T., A. Gilbride and M. M. Chan. 1990. "Soup Kitchen Meals: An Observation and Nutrient Analysis." *Journal of the American Diet Association* 90: 989-991.

Carlson, Rick. 1975. "The End of Medicine." New York: Wiley/Interscience.

Cassels, Derek. 1975. "Minamata." *Medical Post* 30 September.

Castrilli, J. 1982. "Control of Toxic Chemicals in Canada: An Analysis of Law and Policy." *Osgoode Hall Law Journal* 2(June): 322-401.

Coburn, David. 1975. "Job-Worker Incongruence: Consequences for Health." *Journal of Health and Social Behavior* 16: 198-212.

Coburn, David. 1978. "Work and General Psychological and Physical Well-Being." *International Journal of Health Services* 8(3): 415-35.

Cohen, Lynn. 1987. "Responsibility for Health Shift From Doctors and Hospitals, Conference Told." *Canadian Medical Association Journal* 136(3): 282-85.

Crawford, Robert. 1977. "You are Dangerous to Your Health: The Ideology and Politics of Victim Blaming." *International Journal of Health Services* 7(4): 663-80.

Davis, Kingsley and Wilbert E. Moore. 1945. "Some Principles of Stratification." *American Sociological Review* 10(April): 242-9.

Davis, Nanette J. 1975. *Deviance*. Dubuque, Iowa: Wm. C. Brown Co.

Department of Health and Social Security (DHSS). 1976. *Prevention and Health: Everybody's Business*. London: HMSO.

Department of Health and Social Security. 1976. *Priorities for Health and Personal Social Services in England*. London: HMSO.

Department of Health and Social Security. 1977. *The Way Forward*. London: HMSO.

Doyal, Lesley and Imogen Pennell. 1979. *The Political Economy of Health*. London: Pluto Press.

Drietzel, Hans Peter, ed. 1979. *The Social Organizations of Health*. New York: MacMillan Co.

Driver, D. 1991. "Poverty Linked to Higher Risks of Poor Health, Death." *Medical Post* September 17: 81.

Dubos, R. 1968. *Man, Medicine and Environment*. Harmondsworth: Penguin Books.

Egger, G. 1980. "Psychosocial Aspects of Increasing Drug Abuse: A Postulated Economic Cause." *Social Science and Medicine* 14A: 163-170.

Ehrenreich, Barbara, et al. 1974. "Health Care and Social Control." *Social Policy* (May-June).

Emmons, L. 1987. "Relationship of Participation in Food Assistance Programs to the Nutritional Quality of Diets." *American Journal of Public Health* 77: 856-858.

Epp, Jake. 1986. "Achieving Health For All: A Framework for Health Promotion." *Canadian Journal of Public Health* 77(6): 393-407.

Eyer, Joseph. 1979. "A Diet-Stress Hypothesis of Coronary Heart Disease Causation." *International Journal of Health Services* 9: 161-68.

Eyer, Joseph. 1984. "Capitalism, Health and Illness." In *Issues in the Political Economy of Health Care*. Edited by John B. McKinlay. New York: Tavistock Publications.

Eyer, Joseph. 1975. "Hypertension as a Disease of Modern Society." *International Journal of Health Services* 5: 539-58.

Eyer, Joseph. 1977. "Prosperity as a Cause of Death." *International Journal of Health Services* 7(I): 125-50.

Eyer, Joseph. 1980. "Social Causes of Coronary Heart Disease." *Psychotherapy and Psychomatics* 34: 75-87.

Eyer, Joseph and Peter Sterling. 1977. "Stress-Related Mortality and Social Organzation." *Review of Radical Political Economics* 9(1): 1-44.

Fee, Elizabeth. 1977. "Women and Health Care: A Comparison of Theories." In *Health and Medical Care in the U.S.: A Critical Analysis*. Edited by Vicente Navarro, 115-32. New York: Baywood Publishing Co.

Fine, S. 1989. "Poor Children More Likely to Die Than Wealthy Peers, Study Finds." *Globe and Mail* 25 July:A5.

Friders, J.S. 1994. "Racism and Health: The Case of Native People." Pp.202-220 in *Health Illness and Health Care in Canada*. Edited by B. Singh Bolaria and Harley D. Dickinson. Toronto: Harcourt Brace.

Fuchs, Victor. 1972. "Health Care and the United States Economic System." *Milbank Memorial Fund* Quarterly 50(2, part 1): 21 1-37.

Fuchs, Victor. 1974. *Who Shall Live?* New York: Basic Books.

Globe and Mail. 1975. "Miller Fed Up." 16 October.

Grant, K. R. 1988. "The Inverse Care Law in Canada: Differential Access Under Universal Free Health Insurance." *Sociology of Health Care in Canada*. Edited by B. S. Bolaria and H. D. Dickinson. Toronto: Harcourt Brace Jovanovich. 118-134.

Greenberg, D.S. and J.E. Randal. 1977. "Waging the Wrong War on Cancer." *Washington Post* 1 May.

Goff, Colin H. and Charles E. Reasons. 1986. "Organizational Crimes Against Employees, Consumers, and the Public." In *The Political Economy of Crime*. Edited by Brian D. MacLean. Scarborough, Ontario: Prentice-Hall.

Grayson, Paul. 1985. "The Closure of a Factory and Its Impact Upon Health." *International Journal of Health Services* 15(1): 69-93.

Hammond, E.C. 1974. "Epidemiologic Basis for Cancer Prevention." *Cancer* 33(6).

Harding, Jim. 1994. "Environmental Degradation and Rising Cancer Rates: Exploring the Links in Canada." Pp. 649-667 in *Health, Illness and Health Care in Canada*. Edited by B. Singh Bolaria and Harley D. Dickinson. Toronto: Harcourt Brace.

Harding, J., N. Wolf, and G. Chan. 1977. "A SocioDemographic Profile of People Being Prescribed Mood-Modifying Drugs in Saskatchewan." Regina: Alcoholism Commission of Saskatchewan, November.

Hinch, Ronald and Walter DeKeseredy. 1994. "Corporate violence and Women's Health at Home and in the Workplace." Pp. 326-344 in *Health, Illness and Health Care in Canada*. Edited by B. Singh Bolaria and Harley D. Dickinson. Toronto: Harcourt Brace.

Illich, Ivan. 1976. *Limits to Medicine: Medical Nemesis, The Expropriation of Health*. New York: Pantheon.

Jangula, Gordon. 1986. "Occupational Health and Safety: A Human Rights Perspective." In *The Struggle For Justice: A Multi-Disciplinary Approach*. Edited by Dawn Currie and Brian MacLean, 24-55. Saskatoon Social Research Unit.

Jenkins, C.D. and S.J. Zyzsanski. 1980. "Behavioral Risk Factors and Coronary Heart Disease." *Psychotherapy and Psychosomatics* 34:149.

Katz, R.L. 1972. "Drug Therapy: Sedatives and Tranquilizers." *New England Journal of Medicine* 286.

Kotelchuk, David, ed. 1976. *Prognosis Negative: Crisis in the Health Care System*. New York: Vintage.

Labour Canada. 1991. *Occupational Injuries and Their Costs in Canada, 1987-1989*. Ottawa.

Laing, R.D. 1970. *The Politics of Experience and The Bird of Paradise*. Harmondsworth: Penguin Books.

Lalonde, Marc. 1974. *A New Perspective on the Health of Canadians*. Ottawa: Information Canada.

Laven, G. T. and K. C. Brown. 1985. "Nutritional Status of Men Attending a Soup Kitchen: A Pilot Study." *American Journal of Public Health* 75: 875-878.

Laxdal, O. E., B. Habbick, and R. Bolaria. 1993. "Folic Acid Prevents Neural Tube Defects." *Saskatchewan Medical Journal* 4.1: 11-14 (March).

Lewis, Oscar. 1966. *La Vida*. New York: Random House.

Lindsay, Colin. 1987. "The Decline in Employment Among Men Aged 55-64, 1975-85." *Canadian Social Trends* (Spring): 12-15.

Mahler, H. (Director-General of WHO). 1986. "Address At the Opening Ceremony of the International Conference on Health Promotion in Industrialized Countries, Ottawa, 17-21 November 1986." *Canadian Journal of Public Health* 77(6):387-89.

Mao, Y., B. Moloughney, R. M. Semenciw, and H. Morrison. 1992. "Indian Reserves and Registered Indian Mortality in Canada." *Canadian Journal of Public Health*. 83: 350-353.

Martin, S. L. 1989. *Women's Reproductive Health.* Canadian Advisory Council on the Status of Women.

McClelland, D. 1961. *The Achieving Society.* New York: Free Press.

McDonald, Marie. 1975. "The Massacre at Grassy Narrows." *Maclean's* 20 October.

McDowell, Ian. 1986. "National Strategies for Health Promotion." Letters to *Canadian Journal of Public Health* 77(6):448.

McKeon, T. 1965. *Medicine in Modern Society.* London: Allen and Unwin.

McKinlay, John B., ed. *Issues in the Political Economy of Health.* New York: Tavistock Publications.

Miller, A. 1975. "The Wages of Neglect: Death and Disease in the American Work Place." *American Journal of Public Health* 65(11):1217-20.

Miller, Lawrence G. 1975. "Negative Therapeutics." *Social Science and Medicine* 9: 673-77.

Miller, Leslie and Deborah Findlay. 1994. "Through Medical Eyes: The Medicalization of Women's Bodies and Women's Lives." Pp. 276-306 in *Health, Illness and Health Care in Canada.* Edited by B. Singh Bolaria and Harley D. Dickinson. Toronto: Harcourt Brace.

Moore, Steve. no date. *Mercury Poisoning, Native People and Reed Paper Company.* Toronto Alliance Against Racism and Political Repression, Pamphlet No. 1.

Myres, A. W. and D. Kroetsch. 1978. "The Influence of Family Income on Food Consumption Patterns and Nutrition Intake in Canada." *Canadian Journal of Public Health* 69. 3: 208-21.

National Council of Welfare. 1975. *Poor Kids.* Ottawa: Ministry of Supply and Services.

National Council of Welfare. 1990. *Health, Health Care and Medicare.* Ottawa: Supply and Services Canada (Autumn).

Navarro, Vicente. 1978. "The Crisis of the Western System of Medicine in Contemporary Capitalism." *International Journal of Health and Services* 8(2).

Navarro, Vicente. 1986. *Crisis, Health, and Medicine.* New York: Tavistock Publications.

Navarro, Vicente. 1977. *Health and Medical Care in the U.S.: A Critical Analysis.* New York: Baywood Publishing Co.

Nutrition Canada. 1975. Survey Report on Indians and Eskimos. Ottawa: Information Canada.

Parliament, Jo-Anne. 1987. "Increase in Long-Term Unemployment." *Canadian Social Trends* (Spring): 16-19.

Pollock, S. 1988. "Feminism and Reproduction." In *Sociology of Health Care in Canada.* Edited by B. S. Bolaria and H. D. Dickinson. Toronto: Harcourt Brace Jovanovich. 167-182.

Powels, J. 1973. "On the Limitations of Modern Medicine." *Science, Medicine and Man* 1(1):1-30.

Rauschenbach, B. S., E. A. Frongillo, F. E. Thompson, E. J. Y. Anderson, and D. Spicer. 1990. "Dependency on Soup Kitchens in Urban Areas of New York State." *American Journal of Public Health* 80.1: 57-60.

Reid, D. L. and J. E. Miles. 1977. "Food Habits and Nutrition Intakes of Non-Institutionalized Senior Citizens." *Canadian Journal of Public Health* 68. 2: 154-58.

Renaud, Marc. 1975. "On the Structural Constraints to State Intervention in Health." *International Journal of Health Services* 5(4): 559-71.

Reuler, J. B. 1989. "Health Care for Homeless in a National Health Program." *American Journal of Public Health* 79.8: 1003-1035.

Rinehart, James W. 1987. *The Tyranny of Work*. Toronto: Harcourt Brace Jovanovich.

Rosen, Bernard C. 1956. "The Achievement Syndrome: A Psychocultural Dimension of Social Stratification." *American Sociological Review* 21: 203-11.

Rosen, Bernard C. 1959. "Race, Ethnicity, and the Achievement Syndrome." *American Sociological Review* 24: 47-60.

Rosen, R., M. Friedman, R. Strauss, C. Jenkins, S. Zyzsanski, and M. Wurm. 1970. "Coronary Heart Disease in the Western Collaborative Group Study: A Follow Up Experience of Four and One Half Years." *Journal of Chronic Diseases* 23: 173.

Rosenman, R., R. Brand, C. Jenkins, M. Friedman, R. Strauss, and M. Wurm. 1975. "Coronary Heart Disease in the Western Collaborative Group Study: The Final Follow Up Experience of Eight and One Half Years." *Journal of the American Medical Association* 233: 872.

Ryan, William. 1971. *Blaming the Victim*. New York: Vintage Books.

Saskatchewan Public Health Association (Position Paper). 1994. "The Determinants of Health." Regina, Saskatchewan.

Shah, C.P. and C.S. Farkas. 1985. "The Health of Indians In Canadian Cities: A Challenge to Health-Care System." *Canadian Medical Association Journal* 133: 859-63.

Shah, C. P., M. Kahan, and J. Krauser. 1987. "The Health of Children of Low Income Families." *Canadian Medical Association Journal* 137, September 15: 485-490.

Shields, John and Harley Dickinson. 1994. "Health for Sale: The Political Economy of Occupational Health and Safety." Pp. 668-683 in *Health, Illness and Health Care in Canada*. Edited by B. Singh Bolaria and Harley D. Dickinson. Toronto: Harcourt Brace.

Smith, E.W. and A. Smith. 1975. *Minamata*. New York: Holt, Rinehart and Winston.

Statistics Canada. 1991. *Work Injuries — 1988-1990*. Ottawa.

Statistics Canada. 1992. *Canada Yearbook, 1992*. Ottawa: Supply and Services Canada.

Statistics Canada. 1994. *The Daily*. March 25.

Statistics Canada and Health and Welfare Canada. 1981. *The Health of Canadians: Report of the Canadian Health Survey*. Catalogue 82-538E. Ottawa.

Sterling, P. and J. Eyer. 1981. "Biological Basis of Stress-Related Mortality." *Social Science and Medicine* 15E: 3-42.

Stroufe, L.A. and M.A. Stewart. 1973. "Treating Children with Stimulant Drugs." *New England Journal of Medicine* 289: 409.

Szasz, T. 1961. *The Myth of Mental Illness*. New York: Harper and Row.

Thomson, M. 1990. "Association Between Mortality and Poverty." *B. C. Medical Journal* 32.8 (August).

Townsend, Peter. 1990. "Individual or Social Responsibility for Premature Death? Current Controversies in the British Debate About Health." *International Journal of Health Services* 20(3): 373-392.

Trypuc, J. B. 1989. "Health Care for Homeless in a National Health Program." *American Journal of Public Health* 79.8: 1033-1035.

Turshen, Meredith. 1977. "The Political Ecology of Disease." *The Review of Radical Political Economies* 9(1): 45-60.

United States. Special Task Force to the Secretary of Health, Education and Welfare. 1973. *Work in America*. Cambridge, Mass.: M.I.T. Press.

Vickery, D.M. and J.F. Fries. 1976. *Take Care of Yourself: A Consumer's Guide to Medical Care*. Reading, Mass.: Addison-Wesley.

Waitzkin, Howard. 1983. *The Second Sickness*. New York: Free Press.

Waldron, I. 1977. "Increased Prescribing of Valium, Librium, and Other Drugs — An Example of the Influence of Economic and Social Factors on the Practice of Medicine." *International Journal of Health Services* 7(1): 37-62.

Waldron, I., M. Nawotarski, M. Freimer, J. Henry, N. Post, and C. Wittin. 1982. "Cross-Cultural Variation in Blood Pressure: A Quantitative Analysis of the Relationships of Blood Pressure to Cultural, Salt Consumption and Body Weight." *Social Science and Medicine* 16: 419-30.

White, Franklin. 1987. "The Environment of Medicine in the 21st Century: Implications for Prevention and Community Approaches." *Canadian Medical Association Journal* 136(6): 571-75.

White, Franklin. 1986. "A Voluntary Perspective on Health Promotion — The Role of Non-Government Organizations, Particularly in the Voluntary Sector." *Canadian Journal of Public Health* 77: 431-36.

Wigle, D.T. and Y. Mao. 1980. *Mortality by Income Level in Urban Canada*. Ottawa: Health and Welfare Canada.

Wilkins, R. and O. Adams. 1983. *Healthfulness of Life*. Montreal: Institute on Public Policy.

Winkleby, M. A. 1990. "Comparison of Risk Factors for Ill Health in a Sample of Homeless and Nonhomeless Poor." *Public Health Reports* 105.4: 404-409.

Wood, D. and B. Valdez. 1991. "Barriers to Medical Care for Homeless Families Compared with Housed Poor Families." *American Journal of Diseases in Children* 145: 1109-1115.

4

Inequality and Differential Health Risks of Environmental Degradation

B. Singh Bolaria and Rosemary Bolaria

Introduction

The clinical paradigm that defines health and illness in individualistic terms independent of the social contexts in which they occur has been widely accepted in medical practice. While the clinical model attributes disease to the malfunctioning of the human body, another individualistic perspective attributes illness to individual lifestyles, behaviour and consumption patterns. Critics argue that these approaches obscure the social nature of disease and fail to recognize the important relationship between the physical and social environment and health and sickness. Recent studies from the historical materialistic epidemiological perspective have focused on illness generating conditions. Rather than focusing on individual etiology, this approach is primarily concerned with the social and environmental conditions in society that produce mortality and illness. Recent studies provide persuasive evidence that links social class, economic cycles, social organization, work environment, production process and environmental pollution to illness and disease (Waitzkin, 1983; Navarro, 1986).

This chapter primarily focuses on the links between environmental degradation and health and discusses the differential impact of environmental conditions on individuals and social groups in society.

State of the Environment

Environmental degradation has taken several forms. The following description of the various forms of pollution, causes, and the contributing substances provides a glimpse of the extent and severity of the problem.

In any discussion of environmental damage and workplace hazards, the chemical industry occupies a central place. While scientific advances in chemistry and other basic sciences laid the foundation for many technological innovations, the Second World War accelerated the production and application of these products (Kazis and Grossman, 1982:199-208; Freudenberg, 1989). Currently there are thousands of chemicals on the market. For instance, it is estimated that in Saskatchewan alone there may be as many as 10,000 potentially hazardous chemicals in use. The use of these chemicals may be generating as much as 50,000 tonnes of hazardous waste yearly (*Star-Phoenix*, October 17, 1989:10). In the United States over one million pounds of synthetic organic chemicals are produced per day, and are released into the environment. To these chemical pollutants, new substances are added every year. Many of these chemicals are added to products used in homes (e.g., detergents), in construction and insulation, fertilizers, plastics, cloth fibres and many other products. The public is exposed to many of these toxic substances (Eitzen and Zinn, 1989:96-100; Parenti, 1988:116; Kazis and Grossman, 1982).

There are a number of ways by which many chemicals end up polluting the environment. The use of agricultural chemicals provides a good example. There has been a dramatic increase in the use of pesticides which are predominantly used in agriculture. For instance, there was a four-fold increase in the total annual sales of pesticides from 1971 to 1982. Data also show an extensive use of herbicides in Canada (Bird and Rapport, 1986). These chemicals leach into the surface water and seep into soil and ground water.

Spills, accidents, and disposal of toxic waste are other ways that chemicals are released into the environment. For example, the chlorine gas spill caused by a train derailment in Mississauga (November, 1979), and the release of poisonous gases at the Union Carbide plant in Bhopal, India (December, 1984), serve to show potential risks associated with accidents. In many instances, toxic waste ends up in waterways and in unsafe dump sites. Thus, chemicals and the chemical industry cause environmental pollution in various forms.

Air quality has been another environmental concern. Waste from industrial production, automobile emissions, smelters, and aerosols all contribute to air pollution. More and more of these pollutants are added to the environment every year with increasing environmental degradation.

Recently attention has been focused on acid rain as a serious air pollution problem. Acid rain is produced when sulphur dioxide and nitrogen oxide emissions are converted in the atmosphere to acidic compounds (sulphuric and nitric acids), returning to earth as precipitation in the form of raindrops or snowflakes. The primary sources of sulphur dioxide and nitrogen oxide are smelter smokestacks and automobile emissions. These acids pose a threat to forests and agriculture and are even damaging steel and concrete structures (Environment Canada, 1986:16; Eitzen and Zinn, 1989:101-103).

Two other phenomena associated with air pollution are considered even more dangerous than acid rain — the greenhouse effect and ultraviolet radiation. The greenhouse effect is contributing to the warming of the earth and climate change. This occurs when such gases as carbon dioxide and chlorofluorocarbons accumulate in the atmosphere in sufficient volume to act like the roof of a greenhouse, which traps the earth's heat and prevents it from escaping into the outer environment. Air pollution is also depleting the ozone layer which filters out the sun's deadly ultraviolet radiation. Importantly, acid rain affects areas far away from the sources of origin. The effects of acid rain are observed on forests in sites downwind from smelters and other industrial plants that release large volumes of air pollutants (Bird and Rapport, 1986:54). Studies of air quality indicate that ozone pollution (smog) levels are high in many Canadian cities (Bueckert, 1989:B11). Thus, acid rain and the associated greenhouse effect and ultraviolet radiation pose a serious environmental threat and are damaging to forests, agriculture, animals, birds and human life.

Many industries and chemical products that contribute to air pollution also pollute the waters and threaten aquatic life. Environment Canada (1986:8-9) identifies the following sources of contaminants: eutrophication, acidification, toxic chemicals, municipal sewage and industrial effluents. Because of the depletion of oxygen supply in water due to eutrophication and acidification, many lakes and rivers can no longer support aquatic life. Furthermore, such rivers and lakes would take many years to recover even if acid precipitation ceased immediately (Environment Canada, 1986).

Toxic substances originating from various sources, such as municipal sewage and industrial waste and heavy metals such as lead and mercury all contribute to water pollution. Untreated sewage is a central source of bacterial and viral contamination.

Besides municipal sewage, many industries dump their waste into the rivers, streams, lakes and oceans. Of all the industries, pulp and paper mills and petroleum and chemical refining industries have particularly large volumes of discharge (Environment Canada, 1986). Shipments of hazardous and toxic substances and oil tankers always carry potential risks of accidents and spillage.

Canadians are exposed daily to radiation from natural sources, such as building materials, soil and cosmic radiation. The growth of the nuclear industry has added greatly to these sources which place more people at risk of radiation exposure. Fallout from nuclear weapons, nuclear accidents, radioactive spills, and nuclear waste, have all increased the risk of radiation pollution.

The safety record of the nuclear power plants is not very reassuring. In 1980, for example, 69 licenced reactors in the United States reported about 3,800 mishaps, including equipment failure and malfunction, leaks and spills (*New York Times*, July 28, 1981:B4). Another survey of 50 plants by the Nuclear Regulatory Commission in 1981 found fifteen "below average" in maintenance, fire protection and overall compliance with operation regulations (*New York Times*, Sept. 13, 1981:48). There was a recent spill of radioactive water at the Bruce Nuclear Power Plant in Ontario (*StarPhoenix*, January 25, 1990:B14). In addition, an accident in 1989 in Pickering exposed two workers to excessive radiation at an Ontario Hydro nuclear generating station (*StarPhoenix*, August 11, 1989:A19). These cases from different locations indicate the potential hazards faced by workers and the community from radioactive spills in power plants.

Uranium mining also poses environmental and occupational health risks. A newspaper article on November 10, 1989 indicated that there were 153 uranium mine spills, most of them radioactive, at three mines in Saskatchewan since mid-1981 (Yanko, 1989:A7). The size of these spills varied from 1,000 litres to 350,000 litres, and they contained a variety of hazardous substances including contaminated water, diesel fuel, mill tailings and sulphuric acid.

As hazardous and serious as these spills are, the "accidents" in nuclear power plants pose the most serious danger to the environment. Some of these accidents are well known: Windscale, England (1957), Three Mile Island, Pennsylvania, USA, (1979), and Chernobyl, USSR (1986). The Windscale plant fire released four hundred times more radioactivity into the atmosphere than what was released in the 1979 accident at Three Mile Island (Adkins, 1984:15).

Apart from accidents, a notable environmental problem associated with the nuclear industry is the disposal of radioactive waste. Tonnes of this waste are produced every year by nuclear power plants and other sources. Consequently, safe disposal and storage of this waste remains a serious environmental issue.

The above discussion indicates that chemical, air, water and radiation contamination have contributed to environmental degradation and pollution. Chemical and other pollutants only exacerbate the health status of those whose social and material conditions of existence already have adverse effects on their health.

Environment and Health: Differential Exposure to Risks

There is a growing awareness in this country of environmental pollution and the association between environmental degradation and health (Environment Canada, 1988; Synergistics and Environics, 1990; Health and Welfare Canada, 1992). Public opinion polls during the past few years show that Canadians are deeply concerned about their environment, primarily because of its effect on human health. In a 1988 survey, a very large majority of the Canadians (over 90 percent) believed that there were probably many unknown environmental hazards damaging to human health and just under 90 percent felt that pollution had already affected the health of many Canadians (Environment Canada, 1988). In a 1990 survey, 98 percent of the respondents expressed concern about environmental pollution and human health and safety (Synergistics and Environics, 1990). In other opinion surveys, over the years, Canadians have consistently shown their concern about environmental conditions, in particular, about toxic chemicals, acid rain, and water and air pollution (Health and Welfare Canada, 1992). Surveys also reveal that Canadians continue to be very conscious of the relationship between environment and health. Some of these findings are reported in a Health and Welfare Canada Report (1992:8):

- 82 percent of the respondents recognized that the natural environment is very important in helping people to be healthy;
- 73 percent believed that pollution is a major cause of cancer;
- 85 percent believed that pollution problems threaten the survival of the human race (Health and Welfare Canada, 1992).

This awareness among Canadians of environmental conditions and health corresponds to a growing body of literature that provides evidence of linkages between environmental degradations and illness (Bolaria, 1991). One area which has received considerable attention is the link between chemicals in the environment and health risks.

Increasing production and use of chemicals since World War II means that public exposure to these toxic substances is escalating. Toxic dump sites, seepage of chemicals into water, the entry of chemicals into the food chain, and other forms of exposure to these hazardous substances endanger the health of millions of people. Many of these chemicals are linked to "adverse ecological or human health effects" (Bird and Rapport, 1986:174). These chemicals also pose risks to aquatic species and wildlife. Most notably, these chemicals are linked to the increase of cancers. According to a *Newsweek* article:

> The introduction of new chemical products into the environment since World War II parallels the increased cancer rates since them. Experts now believe that is no coincidence. In 1964, the World Health Organization (WHO) determined that environmental factors caused 60 to 80 per cent of all cancers. Many scientific bodies have since concurred with WHO's judgment. Recently, the president's Toxic substances Strategy Committee (TSSC) - representing 18 federal agencies - reported that 80 to 90 per cent of all cancers may be environmentally caused (1981:55).

Excluding skin cancer, just over one in three Canadians will develop some form of cancer during their life. Thousands of new cases of cancer are diagnosed every year and cancer now is a major cause of mortality in Canada (National Cancer Institute, 1990). Ozone layer depletion and increased exposure to ultraviolet radiation poses additional health risks to the population; it is especially linked to an increase in melanoma skin cancer, the production of cataracts and depression of the immune system (Environment Canada, 1986; Eitzen and Zinn, 1989:102).

The use of chemicals in some industries, most notably in agriculture, has received considerable attention (Bolaria, 1991, 1992). Use of pesticides and other chemicals not only affects the health of the farmers, farmworkers and their families, but the pesticides also end up in the food chain putting the health of the whole population at risk.

The release of toxic chemical wastes into the waterways is creating a harmful physical environment for aquatic and human life. Mercury poisoning causes neurological damage (Minamata disease), kidney and liver dysfunction, and death (Science Council of Canada, 1977). Elevated levels of mercury in a number of rivers and lakes have led to their closure for commercial fishing (Environment Canada, 1986). Many fish are killed and those that survive may not be safe for human consumption. A study by the United States Environmental Protection Agency found that all fish species in the Great Lakes showed evidence of chemical contamination. The entry of these chemicals into the food chain through contaminated water poses a threat to aquatic and human life (Rogers et al., 1988:286).

Elevated levels of lead, or lead poisoning, pose serious health problems, particularly for children. Child lead poisoning has been a major public health issue for many years (Rabin, 1989). It is important to note that relative to their lower body weight, children will have a proportionately higher lead intake than adults. More generally, Eizten and Zinn note that "exposure to excess lead stunts growth, causes mental retardation, causes birth abnormalities, and is a major source of hypertension, stroke and heart attacks" (1989:103).

An eleven year longitudinal study of students revealed that lead poisoning is linked to poor grades and coordination, high absenteeism from school, difficulty reading (six times higher rate of reading disability), and not finishing high school (seven times higher drop out rate). The effects of lead are permanent and are reflected in poor school performance (*Globe and Mail*, January 12, 1990:A10).

The nuclear industry poses a threat to the environment and health in many respects. Excessive exposure to radiation has been definitively linked to illnesses such as cancer, leukemia, and genetic changes. It is estimated that the release of radiation due to fire at the Windscale plant in 1957 caused several hundred cases of cancer, some fatal (Adkins, 1984:15).

The nuclear accident at Chernobyl in 1986 caused deaths and contamination not only in that country but radiation traveled as far away as Scandinavia and Western Europe. Recent reports by the Soviet news agency indicate that the Chernobyl accident continues to affect human, plant, animal and aquatic life, as well as forests. These findings included: plants with serious abnormalities, genetic defects in wildlife, high concentrations of radioactivity in reservoirs near the accident affecting the aquatic life, and damage to forests (*StarPhoenix*, August 15, 1989:C7). Radioactive waste poses additional hazards. Some waste components remain radioactive, causing harmful health effects for as long as 250,000 years (Freudenberg, 1989; Eitzen and Zinn, 1989).

As the above discussion indicates, there is increasing recognitionof the linkages between environmental conditions and health status. While environmental conditions affect the health of the whole population, socially and economically disadvantaged groups bear a disproportionate burden of environmental degradation.

Social medicine is primarily concerned with the social, economic, and environmental conditions in the society that produce illness and mortality. Epidemiological data clearly demonstrates the differential health status of the population by socio-economic status. The health gap between the rich and the poor continues to exist in Canada, where the principle of universality was a major impetus to the introduction of medical care in the sixties (see for example, National Council of Welfare,

1990). On average, upper-income Canadians live longer, healthier, and more disability-free lives than do poor Canadians. This gap in health status is primarily due to the "debilitating conditions of life that poverty forces upon people" (National Council of Welfare, 1990:6). Social and material conditions of existence, such as poor housing, poor nutrition, personal and social pathologies, all contribute to high morbidity and mortality in the low-income populations. As the following discussion indicates, the negative health consequences of environmental degradation are also differentially experienced by socially and economically disadvantaged groups in the society.

Native people, one of the most disadvantaged groups, bear a disproportionate burden of illness and mortality. They not only have low socio-economic status but are subject to more pollutants than the general population because they frequently live in environmentally unsafe areas. Mercury poisoning of rivers and lakes at some Indian reserves in Ontario has received a great deal of attention (Castrilli, 1982; Smith and Smith, 1975). The Native People of the White Dog and Grassy Narrows reserves had 40 to 150 times more mercury in their blood than the average Canadian (McDonald, 1975; Moore, 1975). Mercury poisoning, as previously noted, causes neurological damage, kidney and liver dysfunction and deaths.

Radiation spills, another source of pollution, in the first instance affect the plant and mine workers and the nearby communities. These spills pose a threat to community water supply and potentially affect the fish catch, a central food and income resource for some Native communities. Native people and their communities in some areas are most severely affected by pollutants (Adam, 1990). In addition, the social and economic environment also affects their health. High mortality, high disability and low health status of Natives are associated with environmental, social and living conditions of this population (Borsellino, 1990; Mao et al., 1992).

Low-income groups face adverse conditions and an unhealthy environment both at the workplace and in their homes, neighborhoods and communities. Low-status and low-income jobs tend to be unsafe, arduous and emotionally less rewarding (Berman, 1978). Studies of occupational health and safety have mostly been concerned with physical sickness. Now it is being recognized that employment conditions are also related to psychological illnesses. In this regard, job-related stress and its implications for health have received most attention. Evidence indicates that low status jobs and jobs where workers have very little control over their work conditions are conducive to job dissatisfaction and stress (Karasek, 1979). Workers in "caring jobs" and service jobs dealing directly with the public, experience most stress and strain in their work (Hochschild, 1983). This affects women in particular, as a disproportionate number of women are in low status and caring and service jobs. In addition, women face additional sources of stress that are related to the social environment at the workplace. For instance, sexual harassment, almost entirely a female experience, is associated with stress and job satisfaction and performance (Gruber and Bjorn, 1982; Working Women, 1984).

Workplace hazards affect not only the workers but also their family members. Evidence suggests that children of workers exposed to certain chemicals are more likely to have some type of malignant brain tumours (Starfield, 1984).

Residents of poor neighborhoods experience higher mortality levels than those living in rich neighborhoods. Poor residential areas are often close to industrial areas exposing residents to higher levels of air and chemical pollution and noise. Evidence indicates that children exposed to constant noisy environments show blood pressure abnormalities and certain cognitive and behavioural difficulties (Starfield, 1984). A study from the United States indicates that lead poisoning is far more common in minority and low income children. These children are more likely to be exposed to chips of lead-based paint and other sources of lead poisoning, such as gasoline (Mahaffey et al., 1982). That lead-blood-levels are associated with place of residence, demographic and environmental factors is supported by evidence from Canada (O'Heany et al., 1988). Based on a study of children aged 2 to 12 years in Murdochville, a community in Quebec near a copper smelter, the researchers concluded that children who lived near the smelter or lived with a smelter worker had the highest levels of lead in their blood (Chenard, Turcotte and Cordier, 1987). The children who lived away from the copper smelter had the lowest levels of lead in their blood. Research also indicates that children living in cities have higher lead in their blood (Duncan et al., 1988). Children with persistent exposure to lead even at low levels may experience developmental difficulties and learning and behavioural problems.

Children's health may also be affected because of parental exposure to radiation, even during the preconception period (*Medical Post*, 1990:8). A study in England found that the risk of a child developing leukemia increased six to eightfold if a child's father was exposed to 100msv dose of radiation, and "the closer the radiation exposure was to conception the greater the risk." In Quebec province, the regional health authorities of Trois Rivieres region were compelled to launch an investigation when they discovered that three babies were born with birth defects - imperforate anuses (Charbonneau, 1990). On further investigation, the authorities found that as many as nine children had been born with congenital defects at birth since 1987. This area is located near two nuclear plants.

Higher mortality levels in low-income neighborhoods are well documented. (Thomson, 1990; National Council of Welfare, 1990). Evidence indicates that the poorer the area, the shorter the life expectancy of both men and women residents. The data on life expectancy of males by neighborhood income, in 1986, indicate that men in the poorest neighborhoods had a life expectancy of 70.4 years as compared to 76.1 years for men in the richest neighborhoods. The life-expectancy gap for women by place of residence was much smaller. The average life span for women in the poorest neighborhood was 79.1 years as compared to 80.9 years in the richest neighborhoods (National Council of Welfare, 1990). Research also shows a link between income levels and infant mortality rates. While infant mortality rates have come down over the years, data for 1986 show that children of parents in the poorest neighborhoods have twice the infant mortality rates of children of parents in the richest neighborhoods — 10.5 and 5.8, respectively. That the health gap exists between the rich and poor is confirmed by other evidence. For instance, mortality for lung and oral cancer for men and lung and cervical cancer for women increases as income decreases (National Cancer Institute, 1990).

Women and racial minority workers in some sectors bear a disproportionate burden of work-related and environmentally produced ill health. Evidence indicates that farm workers, garment workers, and female domestics, chars, and cleaners are exposed to numerous health hazards (for a review of studies, see Bolaria, 1988). In the case of farm labour, with a large number of racial minority workers, unsafe and unsanitary living conditions, exposure to herbicides and pesticides and arduous tasks all contribute to their ill health. Textile and garment workers face numerous health hazards in "sweatshops." As sewing work is being transferred to individual homes, many of the health hazards faced by workers in factories are now being transplanted into households. This directly exposes the whole family to health risks associated with textile work. The textile workforce is primarily composed of racial and ethnic minority women, as are the domestics and cleaners. The conditions in which women domestics, chars, and cleaners work are damaging to their physical and psychological well-being.

The above discussion provides evidence of the linkage between environmental degradation and certain illnesses. While the whole population is at risk, certain groups bear a disproportionate burden of hazardous industries and environmental degradation.

Conclusion

The evidence presented in this chapter indicates that many industries provide hazardous work environments and contribute to environmental degradation. The discussion of chemical, air, water, and radiation pollution has provided a glimpse of the extent and the severity of the problem.

While environmental degradation places the whole population at risk, the effects of carcinogens and toxins are even more acute for workers directly involved in the production and handling of toxic chemicals and hazardous substances. It is primarily at the point of production that employees are exposed to excessive levels of certain contaminants. Workers in certain industries are more at risk than others. To be sure, sooner or later, workplace health hazards become community and environmental health problems.

While communities and whole populations face health risks because of pollutants in the environment, the socially and economically disadvantaged, women and racial minority workers, those living near the hazardous industries and families and children of workers who are employed in those industries, bear a disproportionate burden of illnesses associated with hazardous work environments and environmental degradation.

The discussion presented here also brings into question the individualistic-clinical and individual lifestyles and consumption patterns paradigms that tend to downgrade the importance of social and environmental factors in the production of health, illness and disease.

A version of this paper appeared in *Social Issues and Contradictions in Canadian Society*, B. Singh Bolaria (ed.). Toronto: Harcourt Brace Jovanovich, 1991.

References

Adkins, J. 1984. "Trouble at the World's Nuclear Dustbin." *Multinational Monitor* 5(July):15.
Adam, Betty. 1990. "90,000-Litre Collins Bay Spill Quickly Contained." *StarPhoenix* January 10:3.
Berman, Daniel M. 1978. *Death on the Job: Occupational Health and Safety Struggles in the United States*. New York: Monthly Review Press.

Berman, Daniel M. 1986. "Asbestos and Health in the Third World: The Case of Brazil." *International Journal of Health Services* 16:253-263.

Bird, Peter M. and David J. Rapport. 1986. *State of the Environment Report for Canada.* Ottawa: Ministry of Supply and Services Canada.

Bolaria, B. Singh. 1988. "The Health Effects of Powerlessness: Women and Racial Minority Immigrant Workers." pp. 439-459 in B. Singh Bolaria and Harley D. Dickinson (eds.), *Sociology of Health Care in Canada.* Toronto: Harcourt Brace Jovanovich.

Bolaria, B. Singh. 1991. "Environment, Work and Illness." pp. 222-246 in B. Singh Bolaria (ed.). *Social Issues and Contradictions in Canadian Society.* Toronto: Harcourt Brace Jovanovich.

Bolaria, B. Singh. 1992. "Farm Labour, Work Conditions and Health." pp. 228-245 in David Hay and Gurcharn S. Basran (eds.) *Rural Sociology in Canada.* Toronto: Oxford University Press.

Borsellino, Matt. 1990. "Poor Health Care, Housing Blamed for Natives' High Disability Rate." *Medical Post* March 27:20.

Bueckert, Dennis. 1989. "Ozone Pollution Level High in Many Canadian Cities." *Times Colonist* July 18:B11.

Cassels, Derek. 1975. "Minamata." *Medical Post* September:30.

Castrilli, J. 1982. "Control of Toxic Chemicals in Canada: An Analysis of Law and Policy." *Osgoode Hall Law Journal* 2(June):322-401.

Charbonneau, Leo. 1990. "Birth Defects in Quebec Linked to Nuclear Power Plant." *Medical Post* March 27:8.

Chenard, L., F. Turcotte and S. Sordier. 1987. "Lead Absorption by Children Living Near a Primary Copper Smelter." *Canadian Journal of Public Health* 78:295-298.

Duncan, C.E. et al. 1988. "Blood Lead and Associated Risk Factors in Ontario Children." *Science of the Total Environment* 71(3): 477-83.

Eitzen, Stanley and Maxine Baca Zinn. 1989. *Social Problems.* 4th ed. Toronto: Allyn and Bacon.

Environment Canada. 1986. *Canada's Environment: An Overview.* Ottawa: Supply and Services Canada.

Environment Canada. 1988. *Public Opinion and the Environment.* Ottawa: Supply and Services Canada.

Freudenberg, Nicolas. 1989. "The Corporate Assault on Health." *Perspectives in Medical Sociology.* Phil Brown (ed.). Belmont, California: Wadsworth Publishing Company.

Globe and Mail. 1990. "Lead Damage Long-Term, Study Says." January 12:A10.

Gruber, James and Lars Bjorn. 1982. "Blue Collar Blues: The Sexual Harassment of Women Autoworkers." *Work and Occupation* 9:271-298.

Health and Welfare Canada. 1992. *A Vital Link: Health and the Environment in Canada.* Ottawa: Minister of Supply and Services.

Hochschild, Arlie. 1983. *The Managed Heart: Commercialization of Human Feeling.* San Francisco: University of California Press.

Karasek, Robert. 1979. "Job Demands, Job. Decision Latitude and Mental Strain: Implications for Job Redesign." *Administrative Science Quarterly* 24:285-308.

Kazis, Richard and Richard L. Grossman. 1982. *Fear at Work: Job Blackmail, Labor and the Environment.* New York: The Pilgrim Press.

Mahaffey, Kathryn R., Joseph L. Annest, Jean Roberts and Robert S. Murphy. 1982. "National Estimates of Blood Lead Levels: United States, 1976-1980. *New England Journal of Medicine* 307(10):573-579.

Mao, Yang, Brent Moloughney, Robert M. Semenciw and Howard Morrison. 1992. "Indian Reserve and Registered Indian Mortality in Canada." *Canadian Journal of Public Health* 83:350-353.

McDonald, Marie. 1975. "The Massacre at Grassy Narrows." *Maclean's* October 20.

Medical Post. March 27, 1990.

Moore, Steve. 1975. Mercury Poisoning, Native People and Reed Paper Company. Toronto: Alliance Against Racism and Political Repression. Pamphlet No. 1.

National Cancer Institute of Canada. 1990. *Canadian Cancer Statistics 1990.* Toronto.

National Council of Welfare. 1990. *Health, Health Care and Medicare.* Ottawa: Minister of Supply and Services.

Navarro, Vincente. 1986. *Crisis, Health and Medicine.* New York: Tavistock Publications.

New York Times. 1981. July 28:B4; September 13:48. cited in Nicholas Freudenberg, 1989, "The Corporate Assault on Health." *Perspectives in Medical Sociology.* Phil Brown (ed.). Belmont, California: Wadsworth Publishing Company.

Newsweek. 1981. "Pesticides' Global Fallout." August 17:53-55.

Norris, R. 1982. *Pills, Pesticides and Profits: The International Trade in Toxic Substances.* New York: North River Press.

O'Heany, J., R. Kusiak, C.E. Duncan, J.R. Smith, and L. Spielberg. 1988. "Blood Lead and Associated Risk Factors in Ontario Children." *The Science of the Total Environment* 71:477-483.

Parenti, Michael. 1978. *Power and the Powerless.* 2nd ed. New York: St. Martin's Press.

Parenti, Michael. 1988. *Democracy for the Few.* 5th ed. New York: St. Martin's Press.

Porterfield, Andrew and David Weir. 1987. "The Export of U.S. Toxic Wastes." *Nation* (October 3):325-343.

Rabin, Richard. 1989. "Warnings Unheeded: A History of Child Lead Poisoning." *American Journal of Public Health* 79:1668-1674.

Rogers, Everett M., R.J. Burge, Peter F. Horsching, and Joseph F. Donnermeyer. 1988. *Social Change in Rural Societies.* Englewood Cliffs, New Jersey: Prentice Hall.

Science Council of Canada. 1977. *Policies and Poisons: The Containment of Long-Term Hazards to Human Health in the Environment and in the Work Place.* Ottawa: Supply and Services Canada.

Smith, E.W and A. Smith. 1975. *Minamata.* New York: Holt, Rinehart and Winston.

Starfield, Barbara. 1984. "Social Factors in Child Health." *Ambulatory Paediatrics.* Morris Green and Robert J. Haggerty (Eds.). Philadelphia: W.B. Saunders: 12-18.

Synergistics Consulting Ltd. and Environics Research Group. 1990. "Fall Tabular Results." *Environmental Monitor* December 5.

Thomson, Molly. 1990. "Association Between Mortality and Poverty." *B.C. Medical Journal* 32(8):337-338.

Waitzkin, Howard. 1983. *The Second Sickness: Contradictions of Capitalist Health Care.* New York: The Free Press.

Working Women. 1984. *9 to 5 Stress Survey.* Cleveland: Working Women's Education Fund.

Yanko, David. 1989. "Uranium Mine Spills Total 153: Most Spills Radioactive." *StarPhoenix*, November 10:A7.

5

Globalization of Environmental and Industrial Health Hazards

B. Singh Bolaria and Rosemary Bolaria

Introduction

There is an increasing awareness of environmental pollution and hazardous work environment and the linkages between environmental degradation and illness. While the general population is exposed to illness-producing substances in the environment, the effects of these substances are even more acute for workers at the point of production. It is often argued that these problems are the result of contradictions between the corporate drive for profits and the costs associated with maintaining occupational health and safety standards and a healthy environment. Furthermore, the global reach of the multinational corporations and the dispersion of industrial production have ensured that these issues are not confined to any single country. The dispersed location of events such as the Chernobyl nuclear plant accident in the former USSR and the Union Carbide plant in Bhopal, India, point to their global significance. Some of these industries and plants pose hazards not only to the work force and the population in the community and surrounding area, but also to populations living far away. For instance, the fall-out from the nuclear accident in Chernobyl was detected in agricultural products throughout much of Europe. Acid rain and nuclear accidents know no national boundaries.

This chapter focuses on the environmental consequences of globalization of production.

Capital Flight and Globalization of Production

Monopoly capital, primarily in the form of multinationals, in the search for profits and capital accumulation does not stop at national boundaries, and capital investments are no longer confined to domestic sources, raw materials, or labour. Sustained corporate profits generally require expansion, low production costs, cheap labour, diversification, access to cheap resources, and new markets. Areas of low-cost labour, mostly Third World countries, are being invaded increasingly by profit-motivated corporations because the business climate in these countries is most favourable for profits and capital accumulation. In addition to saving labour costs, costs are reduced even further by avoiding rigid environmental standards and health and safety regulations regarding hazardous industries (Bolaria, 1988).

For instance, foreign investments by American-based corporations have increased considerably. While this investment amounted to $16 billion in 1950 and $192 billion in 1980, by 1984 the direct investments by American-based corporations in foreign countries amounted to $233.4 billion (Vernon, 1986). Millions of workers in the Third World work for multinationals for poor wages and are exposed to hazardous work conditions (Bolaria, 1988). Fuentes and Ehrenreich (1983:111) state: "There are over one million people employed in industrial free trade zones in the Third World. Millions more work outside the zones in multinational-controlled plants and domestically-owned subcontracting factories." In light-assembly work 80 to 90 percent of the workers are women. In addition to working for low wages, women are preferred over men as assembly workers for other reasons. Fuentes and Ehrenreich (1983:11) state: "Multinationals want a workforce that is docile, easily manipulated and willing to do boring, repetitive assembly work. Women, they claim, are the perfect employees, with their 'natural patience' and 'manual dexterity.'"

Governments of poor countries who want to attract foreign capital "advertise their attractive low-paid women with their 'nimble fingers'" (Mies, 1986). This is illustrated by an advertisement by the Government of Malaysia:

> The manual dexterity of the oriental female is famous the world over. Her hands are small and she works fast with extreme care. Who, therefore, could be better qualified by nature and inheritance to contribute to the efficiency of a bench-assembly production line than the oriental girl? (Grossman, 1979:8).

The personnel officer of an American-based corporation in Malaysia said: "We have girls because they have less energy, are more disciplined and are easier to control" (Grossman, 1979:2). The racist and sexist overtones of these statements are quite apparent. Labour in these countries is also weak, open to accepting low wages, and less likely to present an organized challenge to working conditions. For example, the enormous wage differential in the textile industry is one of the reasons for the United States Capital Company to locate production in Asia and other countries (Chossudovsky, 1981). Third World workers are additionally exploited by long working hours and compulsory overtime work without overtime pay. There is also a more frequent use of labour of women and children, who are generally paid low wages (Mies, 1986, 1988; Morokvasic, 1984). As Parenti (1980) has observed, the ultimate purpose of corporate investments is to extract wealth from poor nations.

Suffice it to say that the access of capital to cheap labour and the threat of multinationals to locate in these areas puts downward pressure on wages in the advanced country. Capital, of course, is also moved within the same country as corporations shut down operations in one community and start up elsewhere.

This mobility of capital strengthens its position and power over the workers and weakens the position of labour in any one community, state, or country. Workers are forced to make wage concessions to labour in unhealthy work environments and live in polluted environments to keep their jobs and compete for investors.

Globalization of Health Hazards

As hazardous industries come under increasing scrutiny in the advanced industrial nations, some corporations are locating their production in Third World countries (Castleman, 1979, 1981; Elling, 1977; Myers, 1981; Laporte, 1978; Berman, 1986). Legislative action regarding environmental standards and occupational health and safety regulations in hazardous industries potentially threatens corporate profits. Rather than complying with costly workplace safety and health standards and environmental pollution-control regulations, dangerous industries move to locations where such standards are either inadequate or nonexistent and where cheap, unorganized, and uninformed labour is plentiful.

The governments of underdeveloped countries are often willing to provide tax shelters, relaxed environmental, health, and safety standards, and other "incentives" to attract these industries and jobs (Castleman,

1979, 1981, 1983; Butler et al., 1978; Elling, 1977; Hassan et al., 1981). They try to outbid each other to provide "pollution havens" for industrial polluters (Barnett and Muller, 1974). For example, one advertisement by the government of Mexico read:

> Relax. We've already prepared the ground for you. If you are thinking of fleeing from the Capital because of the new laws for the prevention and control of the environmental pollution affect your plant, you can count on us (cited in Elling, 1977:218).

Workers and their communities in poor countries are exposed to health hazards not acceptable in the advanced countries. When a hazardous product is banned in one country and not in others, this creates what Castleman (1983,5) calls "the double standard in industry hazards," that is, a situation where workers and communities in Third World countries are exposed to dangers that would not be tolerated in the advanced countries.

Many multinationals have moved their operations to areas of low-cost non-unionized work forces and where production costs can be reduced further by favourable tax exemptions, loans at reduced rates of interest, and lax health and safety standards and environmental regulations (Elson and Pearson, 1981; Mitter, 1986; Hovell et al., 1988; Rebhan, 1980, 1985). Maquiladora Plants, near the Mexican-American border, have received considerable attention in recent years. Maquiladoras are foreign-owned enterprises that enjoy special tariff benefits and use Mexican workers in their labour-intensive operations (Hovell et al., 1988). Women constitute a significant proportion of the labour force in these industries. A number of studies point to the inadequate health and safety standards, long and arduous work hours, unsafe and noisy machinery, exposure to many carcinogens, job insecurity, and generally stressful work environment. Health problems among the workers vary from eye problems and musculoskeletal disorders to hand injuries, and electronic workers report loss of visual acuity (see, for example, Rebhan, 1985; Fernandez-Kelly, 1983; Dilman, 1976). In addition, Maquiladoras have very little by way of environmental controls.

Other studies point to the exploitation of women in the Third World. Women workers continue to be concentrated in service-sector jobs and in selected areas of manufacturing, such as clothing, textiles, and electronics.

Women have been entering the textile industry in increasing numbers in Third World countries as many multinationals have located their production there in search of cheap and submissive labour force (Chapkis and Enloe, 1983; Phizacklea, 1990). The textile industry poses many health risks such as *byssinosis orii* or "brown lung." These workers are also at risk from chemicals used in the processing and dyeing of fabrics. The electronics industry is another major employer of women. Despite its image as a "clean" industry, it also poses many health risks (Baker and Woodrow, 1984). Health problems such as dizziness, nausea, and headaches are often the result of chemicals used in the electronics industry. A study of female electronic workers in Hong Kong revealed that 48 percent suffered from constant headaches, 36 percent had frequent sore throats, and 39 percent reported frequent drowsiness. Vision problems are also common in the electronics industry. Many workers require glasses to continue working and many others are forced to leave their employment because of bad eyesight (Grossman 1979; Lim, 1978). Textile workers are also affected by excessive noise in the workplace, sore backs caused by long hours of sitting at sewing machines, injuries from broken needles, skin, nose, and eye irritation; and psychological stress.

The asbestos industry is another example of exported health hazards. Historically, most of the world's asbestos manufacturing has been done in the advanced industrial nations. But now that these nations are applying increasingly costly health and safety production standards, a significant proportion of manufacturing has shifted to countries without adequate standards. For instance, while the United States did most of its own asbestos manufacturing up to 1970, since then its imports of asbestos textiles have increased significantly, particularly from Mexico, South Korea, Taiwan, and Brazil (Elling, 1981; Castleman, 1979). Health and safety regulations to protect workers from asbestos in these countries are not enforced, are inadequate, or do not exist at all. While workers in the Third World suffer from ill health, the manufactured asbestos is profitably exported to the markets of the advanced countries.

In Mexico, for example, there are no specific regulations to protect workers from asbestos or to control asbestos pollution of air and water. An American-based company, Amatex, operates two asbestos textile plants in Mexico. The asbestos fibre used in these mills comes from Canada. In one of these plants, as described by Castleman (1979), the workers had no respirators to protect them from dust, there was a lack of dust control, and asbestos waste was strewn across the dirt road behind the plant. Taiwan and South Korea, like Mexico, lack health and safety standards. Castleman (1979, 578) notes that "there were no specific health regulations for asbestos in South Korea. Taiwan's ceiling limit of 2 milligrams per cubic meter of air amounts to classifying asbestos as little more than a nuisance dust."

Data from asbestos plants in other Third World countries provide additional evidence of the double standard in health and safety protection. Sluis-Cremer (1970) reported a high incidence of asbestosis among South African asbestos miners. In an article entitled, "Double Standards: Asbestos in India," Castleman (1981) reports on two asbestos plants — the Shree Digvijay Cement Company in Ahmedabad and Hindustan Ferodo in Bombay. Both these plants are associated with Western multinationals. Workers and others in and around these plants are exposed to health hazards that would not be permitted in the West. Untreated wastes litter the areas surrounding the plants.

These two Indian asbestos plants, according to Castleman, illustrate a fundamental point; that is, that "life-saving medical and engineering technology that should be exported along with dangerous technology is often left behind." He concludes, "It is time for responsible members of the business world to step forward and make a commitment not to profit by such abuses" (Castleman, 1981, 523).

Numerous other industries that are required by health and safety standards and environmental regulation to implement costly methods to reduce their workers' and the community's exposure to hazardous materials are also locating their plants in the poorer countries. For instance, a significant proportion of benzidine dye industries, mercury chloride, pesticide, textile, and microelectronics industries are either moving their production there or are exporting banned products to these countries (Castleman, 1979, 1983; Castleman and Vera Vera, 1980; Laporte, 1978; Geiser, 1986; Elling, 1981).

The Seveso catastrophe in northern Italy in 1976 received worldwide attention (Laporte, 1978). The plant, owned by the Swiss-based Givaudan Corporation (a subsidiary of Hoffman-LaRoche), manufactured trichlorophenol. On July 10, 1976, this plant emitted into the atmosphere one of the most toxic substances extant, TCDD, a dioxin, which was "accidentally produced during trichlorophenol synthesis" (Laporte, 1978, 619).

There have been such accidents in a number of countries since 1949. However, this was the first accident where the contamination was not confined to the plant, and where people in the neighbourhood of the plant were exposed to TCDD and the surrounding soil was contaminated. The Seveso plant did not have a heat-control mechanism or holding tank backup, standard safety features without which excessive buildup of heat in the reactor will cause an explosion. The workers were not made aware of potential dioxin hazards. It is doubtful that under these circumstances this plant would have been allowed to operate in Switzerland.

An even more scandalous disaster took place in Bhopal, India in 1984, where over 2,800 people were killed and over 200,000 injured when poisonous methyl isocyanate gas was emitted from a Union Carbide plant (Everest 1985; Kurzman, 1987; Shrivastava, 1987; Jones, 1988).

Some hazardous products are exported with the assistance of government agencies. For instance, the U.S. Agency for International Development (AID), as part of the U.S. assistance program, exported the pesticide leptophos, known to have caused serious nerve damage among workers in Texas. It is important to note that leptophos was not registered for use in the United States "because the manufacturers withdrew the application for registration after reports of delayed neurotoxicity became widely publicized. However, it was exported to many Third World countries" (Shaikh and Reich, 1981, 740). In Egypt, during the early, 1970s, leptophos was considered to have caused the death of one farmworker, the poisoning of several other fieldworkers, and numerous deaths among water buffalo. The export of this product was halted in 1976, when it was known that the health of the American workers who produced the pesticide was seriously damaged (Shaikh and Reich, 1981). Heptachlor, Chlordane, and DDT are other pesticides, banned or in the process of being banned in the United States, that AID shipped to Third World countries (Milius, 1976, cited in Castleman, 1979). Since 1957, the shipment of pesticides under the AID program has amounted to over $500,000 million (Castleman, 1979). It is important to note that U.S. law allowed the export of pesticides that are banned in the United States to other countries (Weir, Schapiro, and Jacobs, 1979; Norris, 1982; Eckholm and Scherr, 1978).

Because of the awareness and concern in the advanced countries about the dangers of toxic chemical wastes, the Third World countries are also increasingly becoming dumping grounds for hazardous wastes (Castleman, 1983). The United States alone sent over four hundred shipments of hazardous substances for dumping in other countries in 1986 (Porterfield and Weir, 1987). Typically, these shipments are sent to the Caribbean and Central America, and sometimes to Africa and the Philippines.

The Third World is a rapidly expanding market for the multinational pharmaceutical companies to dump inappropriate, dangerous, and potentially toxic drugs. Silverman, Lee, and Lydecker in *Prescription for Death: The Drugging of the Third World* (1982) indicate that products that are banned or never approved in the industrialized countries are widely promoted in the poor nations, with exaggerated claims of their effectiveness and minimal warning of the dangers of serious or lethal side-effects. These practices are also documented by Yudkin (1978, 1980). The activities of some food industries are much like those of the pharmaceuticals. The promotion of infant formula has led to "commerciogenic malnutrition," which has contributed to increased infant morbidity and mortality in the poor nations. In their search for new markets and sustained corporate profitability, multinationals are the most powerful promoters of infant formula.

Advanced countries also contribute to environmental degradation in poor countries by their indiscriminate exploitation of the natural resources of the Third World. Gigantic multinationals control the world economy and impose upon those countries in which they invest and operate the resource use and development policies that are in their own best interest (Barnett and Muller, 1974; Parenti, 1980; Eitzen and Zinn, 1989:55-88). Rich countries continue to have a disproportionate consumption of world resources while poor countries, where most of the people live, bear a disproportionate burden of environmental degradation.

Living in a poor country is in itself a liability. Large populations already live in unhealthy environments. The struggle to survive is a constant threat to rapidly depleting resources. For instance, the burning of forests to clear land for agriculture and cutting down the forest for fuel are depleting forest resources with additional negative environmental consequences, such as floods and climatic changes. Social and economic conditions of existence pose an additional threat to people's health. Material poverty, unsanitary conditions, and low nutritional levels all lower resistance to disease, contributing to ill health and high morbidity and mortality. In this context, the impact of additional imported hazards is likely to be even more serious. However, the full impact of exposure to some industrial hazards may not be statistically evident. Workers may succumb to other "natural" causes of death before they die of diseases with long latency periods, such as asbestosis and cancer. We mostly learn of dangerous industries when accidents occur, as in Bhopal, India, where the death and destruction are immediately evident. The long-range health and environmental consequences may be more devastating.

Export of industrial hazards and double standards in health and safety, thus, worsen the already degraded environmental and public health in poor countries.

Boomerang: The Third World Comes Home

What happens in the Third World has important consequences for occupational health and safety standards and for environmental conditions and people's health in advanced countries. While chemical production poses a global threat (about 14,000 deaths and 750,000 cases of poisoning per year), the Third World bears the brunt of pesticides (Bull, 1982; Weir, 1985). Someone in these countries is poisoned by pesticides every minute of the day (Weir and Schapiro, 1981) and "while developing countries use only one-sixth of pesticides manufactured globally, they suffer about two-thirds of all pesticide related deaths" (Weir, 1985:9). Third World people are also the victims of pesticides banned in advanced countries. This, however, does not protect the workers and consumers in advanced countries from these pesticides. The "circle of poison" and the "circle of victims" starts at the point of production. The production workers are the "very first victims of the circle of poison" (Weir and Schapiro, 1981:8-9). These pesticides move from the point of production to fieldworkers in the Third World and are then returned to the advanced countries in imported food, thus completing the circle. Pesticides end up on breakfast and dinner tables in imported food and other commodities. Pesticides are primarily used on crops produced for export. Food and other commodities such as bananas, coffee, sugar, tomatoes, tea, cocoa, tapioca, strawberries, peppers, and olives are sprayed with pesticides banned in the countries to which these products are exported (Weir and Schapiro, 1981:82). Well-to-do and well-fed people eat the food produced in poor countries where health and lives of the poor and hungry are endangered by poisonous pesticides (Weir and Schapiro, 1981).

What happens in the Third World with regard to occupational health and safety standards affects workers and consumers in the advanced countries in other ways. The ability of the multinationals to relocate their production from the advanced to the poor countries may discourage the workers from demanding higher wages and pushing for more stringent health and safety standards at the workplace. Similarly, the single industry communities may be reluctant to push for strict pollution emission and waste-disposal standards for fear of loss of industry. The threat of loss of jobs and industry may compel workers to accept low wages, an unsafe and unhealthy workplace, and a polluted environment, very similar to the poor countries. What is suggested here is that low wages and an unhealthy environment do not remain confined to the Third World. In some sectors, where predominantly women and a legally and politically vulnerable racial minority immigrant work force are employed, working conditions approximate those in the developing countries. Commenting on the clothing industry in Britain, Harrison (1983) makes reference to "creeping underdevelopment" and "creation of a Third World country in our midst" (Harrison, 1983). Though Harrison was referring to the clothing industry, his comments also apply to conditions in agriculture (Bolaria, 1992) and electronics (Baker and Woodrow, 1984) in many countries. Therefore, occupational health and safety and environmental health in the advanced countries cannot be divorced from occupational health and safety and environmental standards in the poor countries. Because of this, health is a global rather than a national issue.

Conclusion

This chapter has explored the linkages between the corporate drive for profits and the social production of illness, drawing primarily upon the literature dealing with multinationals involved in the production of hazardous products. The health, safety, and environment of people in the Third World are being threatened constantly by profit-motivated multinationals (World Commission on Environment and Development, 1987).

Because of double standards in industrial hazards and in health and safety practised by multinationals, workers and communities in the poor nations are being exposed to dangers not tolerated or situations that are illegal in the advanced countries. These double standards are manifested in a number of ways, including export of hazardous industries, export of hazardous products, and dumping of toxic waste. However, export of health hazards to the poor countries does not protect the people in the rich countries. Many of the toxic chemicals are returned to the rich countries in food products. Mobility of capital and the ability of multinationals to relocate their production from the rich to the poor countries has enabled corporations to avoid compliance with occupational health and safety and environmental standards in the advanced countries. Thus, what happens in the Third World with respect to the environment and to occupational health affects the working conditions and environmental health of the people in the advanced countries.

Globalization of production, on the one hand, weakens the position of labour in any one country, and on the other, strengthens the economic and ideological position of capital. The capitalist ideology of progress and development (the growth ethic) has often been successful in portraying environmental concern as antiprogress and antilabour, which threatens the capital investments and standard of living. Transnational corporations, through their control of capital and investments and with the assistance of local elites, have been able to impose development policies that are contributing to further degradation of the environment and health in poor countries.

It should be noted, however, that the "proletarian ethics" in the

Eastern bloc countries have not done any better in protecting the health and safety of the workers and the environment than have the capitalist profit and growth ethics. Recently emerging evidence indicates that pollution in the workplace and environmental degradation pose threats to the health of the proletariat and the public. For instance, a 1988 report of the Polish Academy of Sciences estimated that one-third of the Polish people are living in an "ecological disaster area." Air and water pollution daily threaten the health of many Polish people (Simmons, 1988). Evidence indicates that major water systems and rivers in many Eastern bloc countries are polluted due to chemical and raw municipal and industrial sewage dumping (Schapiro, 1990; Schwarz, 1988). Industrial pollution in cities such as Chernivitse, in Ukraine, is rampant (Kudla, 1990). Children in this city were struck with a mysterious illness leading to loss of hair and baldness. Hundreds of children have been affected since it first emerged in August 1988. In addition to hair loss, symptoms include gastrointestinal and liver problems, and behavioural problems, such as apathy, agitation, and nightmares (Kudla, 1990). While the cause of this disease still eludes the experts, Ukrainian doctors consider it an environmental disease. Environmental degradation, according to a member of the national coordinating council of Zelenij Svit ("Green World"), has damaged water and soil in Ukraine. "There are more than 1,000 chemical plants in the Ukraine. About 20,000 small streams have disappeared and 60% of the Chernozem, the renowned black earth that made the Ukraine the Breadbasket of Europe has been destroyed" (Kudla, 1990:10).

In the Baltic port city of Ventspils, Latvia, two out of five babies born have birth defects (Swift, 1990). These defects include blindness, neurological problems, and skull deformities and are blamed on the vast quantities of toxic chemicals and "toxic damaged parents." Chemicals have also affected women's reproductive health. Fifty percent of the women are sterile and young couples without children are advised by doctors to leave the town.

Thus, environmental pollution and degradation and industrial production of health hazards are not confined to a single country or a single region. Nuclear accidents and oil spills all clearly demonstrate that these incidents have an ecological impact far beyond the borders of a particular nation. Globalization of production has led to globalization of health hazards.

Parts of this chapter were published previously.

References

Baker, Robin and Sharon Woodrow. 1984. "The Clear, Light Image of the Electronics Industry: Miracle or Mirage?" Pp. 21-36 in Wendy Chavkin (ed.) *Double Exposure: Women's Health Hazards on the Job and at Home*. New York: Monthly Review Press.

Barnett, R.J. and R. E. Muller. 1974. *Global Reach: The Power of the Multinational Corporations*. New York: Simon and Schuster.

Berman, Daniel M. 1986. "Asbestos and Health in the Third World: The Case of Brazil." *International Journal of Health Services* 16: 253-263.

Bolaria, B. Singh. 1988. "Profits and Illness: Exporting Health Hazards to the Third World." Pp. 477-496 in B. Singh Bolaria and Harley D. Dickinson (eds.) *Sociology of Health Care in Canada*. Toronto: Harcourt Brace Jovanovich.

Bolaria, B. Singh. 1992. "Farm Labour, Work Conditions and Health." Pp. 228-245 in David Hay and Gurcharn Basran (eds.) *Rural Sociology in Canada*. Toronto: Oxford University Press.

Bull, David. 1982. *A Growing Problem: Pesticides and the Third World*. Oxford: Oxfam.

Butler, J., D. Giovannetti, M. Harner and H. Shapiro. 1978. "Dying for Work: Occupational Health and Asbestos." *NACLA Report on the Americas* 12: 1039.

Castleman, Barry I. 1979. "The Export of Hazardous Factories to Developing Nations." *International Journal of Health Services* 9: 569-606.

Castelman, Barry I. 1981. "Double Standards: Asbestos in India." *New Scientist* (February 26): 522-523.

Castlelman, Barry I. 1983. "The Double Standards in Industrial Hazards." *International Journal of Health Services* 13: 5-14.

Castleman, B. I. and M.J. Vera Vera. 1980. "Impending Proliferation of Asbestos." *International Journal of Health Services* 10, 3: 389-403; also in *Health and Work Under Capitalism: An International Perspective*. V. Navarro and D.M. Berman (eds.). Farmingdale, N.Y.: Baywood Publishing. Pp. 123-37.

Chapkis, Wendy and Cynthia Enloe. 1983. *Of Common Cloth: Women in the Global Textile Industry*. Amsterdam: Transnational Institute.

Chossudovsky, Michael. 1981. "Human Rights, Health and Capital Accumulation in Third World." Pp. 37-52 in Vincente Navarro (ed.) *Imperialism in Health and Medicine*. Farmingdale, N.Y.: Baywood Publishing Company.

Dilman, C.D. 1976. "Maquiladoras in Mexico's Northern Border Communities and the Border Industrialization Program." *Journal of Economic and Social Geography* 67(3): 138-150.

Eckholm, E. and S.J. Scherr. 1978. "Double Standards and the Pesticide Trade." *New Scientist* 16.

Eitzen, S. and M.B. Zinn. 1989. *Social Problems*, 4th ed. New York: Allyn and Bacon.

Elling, Ray H. 1977. "Industrialization and Occupational Health in Underdeveloped Countries." *International Journal of Health Services* 7: 209-235.

Elling, Ray H.. 1981. "The Capitalist World System and International Health." *International Journal of Health Services* 11: 21-51.

Elling, Ray H. 1989. "The Political Economy of Workers' Health and Safety." *Social Science and Medicine* 28: 1171-1182.

Elson, Diane and Ruth Pearson. 1981. "Nimble Fingers Make Cheap Workers: An Analysis of Women's Employment in the Third-World." *Feminist Review* 7: 87-107.

Everest, Larry. 1985. *Behind the Poison Cloud: Union Carbide's Bhopal Massacre*. Chicago: Banner Press.

Fernandez-Kelly, M.P. 1983. *For We Are Sold, I and My People: Women and Industry in Mexico's Frontier*. Albany: State University of New York.

Fuentes, Annette and Barbara Ehrenreich. 1983. *Women in the Global Factory*. New York: South End Press.

Geiser, K. 1986. "Health Hazards in the Microelectronics Industry." *International Journal of Health Services* 16, 1: 105-20.

Grossman, R. 1979. "Women's Place in the Integrated Circuit." in "Changing Role of South East Asian Women" (Special Issue) *South East Asian Chronicle and Pacific Research*, 9: 2-17.

Harrison, P. 1983. *Inside the Inner City: Life Under the Cutting Edge*. London: Penguin Books.

Hassan, A. et al. 1981. "Mercury Poisoning in Nicaragua: A Case Study of the Export of Environmental and Occupational Health Hazards by a Multinational Corporation." *International Journal of Health Services* 11: 221-226.

Health and Welfare Canada. 1992. *A Vital Link: Health and the Environment in Canada*. Ottawa: Minister of Supply and Services.

Hovell, Melbourne F., Carol Sipan, C. Richard Hofstetter, Barbara C. DuBois, Andrew Krefft, John Conway, Monica Jasis and Hope L. Isaacs. 1988. "Occupational Health Risks for Mexican Women: The Case of the Maquiladora Along the Mexican-United States Border." *International Journal of Health Services* 18: 617-627.

Jones, T. 1988. *Corporate Killing: Bhopal's Will Happen*. London: Free Association Books.

Kudla, Lida. 1990. "Are We Killing the Children?" *Medical Post*, March 20: 9-10.

Kurzman, D. 1987. *A Killing Wind*. New York: McGraw-Hill Book Company.

Laporte, Joan-Ramon. 1978. "Multinationals and Health Reflections on the Seveso Catastrophe." *International Journal of Health Services* 8: 619-632.

Lifton, Robert Jay. 1986. "Seize the Opportunity." *Nuclear Times* 4(July/August): 23-29.

Lim, Linda. 1978. "Women Workers in Multinational Corporations: The Case of Electronic Industry in Malaysia and Singapore." Michigan University Occasional Papers, N. IX, Fall.

Mies, Maria. 1986. *Patriarchy and Accumulation in a World Scale*. London: Zed Books Ltd.

Mies, Maria. 1988. *Women: The Last Colony*. London: Zed Books Ltd. *Common Fate, Common Bond: Women in the Global Economy*. London: Pluto Press.

Milius, P. 1976. Various articles, *Washington Post* 1-26 December, cited in Castleman 1979.

Mitter, Seasti. 1986. *Common Fate, Common Bond: Women in the Global Economy*. London: Pluto Press.

Morokvasic, Mirjana. 1984. "Birds of Passage Are Also Women. . ." *International Migration Review* 18: 886-907.

Myers, Johnny. 1981. "The Social Context of Occupational Disease: Asbestos and South Africa." *International Journal of Health Services* 11, No. 2.

Norris, R. 1982. *Pills, Pesticides and Profits: The International Trade in Toxic Substances*. New York: North River Press.

Parenti, Michael. 1980. *Democracy for the Few* (3rd. ed.). New York: St. Martin's Press.

Phizacklea, Annie. 1990. *Unpacking the Fashion Industry: Gender, Racism and Class in Production*. London: Routledge.

Porterfield, A. and D. Weir. 1987. "The Export of U.S. Toxic Wastes." *Nation* 3 October: 325-43.

Rebhan, H. 1980. "Labour Battles Hazard Export." *Multinational Monitor* 3: 6-7.

Rebhan, H. 1985. "Economic Development and Occupational Health in Latin America: New Directions for Public Health in Less Developed Countries." *American Journal of Public Health* 75: 536-542.

Schapiro, M. 1990. "The New Danube." *Mother Jones*, April/May: 50-52, 72,74-75.

Schwarz, W. 1988. "Green Issues Rise in the East." *Manchester Guardian Weekly*, December 11:88.

Shaikh, R. and M.R. Reich. 1981. "Haphazard Policy on Hazardous Exports." *The Lancet* 3 October: 740-42.

Shrivastava, P. 1987. *Bhopal: Anatomy of a Crisis.* Cambridge, Ma.: Ballinger Publishing Company.

Silverman, M., Phillip Lee and M. Lydecker. 1982. *Prescriptions for Death: The Drugging of the Third World.* Berkeley: University of California Press.

Simmons, M. 1988. "Pollution Threat to 12 Million Poles." *Manchester Guardian Weekly,* December 11:22.

Sluis-Cremer, G.K. 1970. "Asbestos in South African Asbestos Miners." *Environment Research* 3 (November): 310-19.

Swift, Diana. 1990. "Defect Rate Hits 40% in Latvian City." *Medical Post* March 20:10.

Vernon, Raymond. 1986. "Multinationals Are Mushrooming." *Challenge* 29 (May-June).

Weir, D. 1985. "The Global Pesticide Threat." *Multinational Monitor* 6 (September): 8-9.

Weir, David and Mark Schapiro. 1981. *Circle of Poison: Pesticides and People in a Hungry World.* San Francisco: Institute for Food and Development Policy.

Weir, D., M. Schapiro and T. Jacobs. 1979. "The Boomerang Crime: It Comes Home in Your Coffee, Your Bananas . . ." *Mother Jones* 4: 40-48.

World Commission on Environment and Development. 1987. *Our Common Future.* Oxford University Press.

Yudkin, J.S. 1978. "Wider World: Provision of Medicines in a Developing Country." *The Lancet* 15 April: 810-12.

Yudkin, J.S. 1980. "The Economics of Pharmaceutical Supply in Tanzania." *International Journal of Health Services* 10, 3: 455-77.

6

Different Cultures or Unequal Life Chances: A Comparative Analysis of Race and Health

Li Zong and Peter S. Li

Introduction

Much research on race and health in North America tends to focus on comparisons of vital statistics and health indicators between the white majority and marginalized minorities such as the Aboriginal peoples. The findings thus far overwhelmingly confirm that among the Aboriginal peoples, life expectancy is lower, infant mortality is higher, and certain illnesses are more frequent (Brady, 1983; Bobet, 1990; Frideres, 1993). In short, the status of health is poorer among certain non-white populations than the white majority.

While the disparity of health status between Aboriginal peoples and those of European origin is indisputable, the interpretation of how "race" may have contributed to this difference is not clear. On the one hand, race, as measured by those of Aboriginal origin versus others of European origin, represents differences of cultural values, heritage and lifestyles that may affect the health status. For example, it can be argued that unfamiliarity with modern medicine and suspicion of European physicians and medical technology may discourage Aboriginal peoples from seeking medical services. Together with poorer living conditions, the apprehension towards modern medicine and an adherence to a traditional lifestyle would contribute to poor health and higher mortality. Hence, the essence of the argument is that while poor living conditions may have contributed to higher rates of illness and lower life expectancy, the traditional lifestyle and values of the Aboriginal peoples deter them from fully benefiting from the scientific and medical advancements of modern society. On the other hand, race is often confounded with unequal material conditions of life such that Aboriginal peoples are more deprived than those of European origins in almost every aspect of life. Consequently, racial differences in health status and life expectancy may simply reflect unequal life chances that result from material deprivation. Accordingly, the effects of race on health reflect differences in economic conditions and not culture.

The difficulty in resolving these competing explanations lies in the simple fact that marginalized racial minorities are also economically deprived such that the effect of material conditions and cultural origins cannot be practically separated. The purpose of this paper is to provide an empirical test to the problem of race and health by comparing 118 countries to assess the effects of racial origins on health status. If it can be shown that the effects of race on life expectancy and mortality persist despite controlling for differences in wealth and nutritional levels, then the comparison would at least provide some empirical grounds for claiming that race has a direct effect on health independent of material conditions, and therefore racial differences in health status may reflect cultural variations. Conversely, if it can be shown that the effects of race disappear after adjusting for variations in wealth and nutritional levels, then it would suggest that material conditions of life override the possible effects of culture in accounting for differences in health.

Race, Economic Conditions and Health Status

Studies examining health status and economic conditions in North America have systematically shown that mortality rates are strongly related to economic conditions, with the lowest socioeconomic status group suffering from the highest mortality rates (Adamchak, 1979; Markides and Barnes, 1977). This relationship is most evident when comparisons are made between Native Indians and non-Indians. Using standardized rates, Brady (1983) found that the mortality rate for registered Indians in Saskatchewan rose from 9.9 per 1,000 in 1966 to 11.5 in 1978, whereas that for the non-Indian population declined from 6.6 in 1966 to 5.9 in 1978. He also found that from 1959 to 1978, registered Indians suffered from higher death rates for accidents, suicide, homicide, and congenital anomalies than non-Indians; as well the frequency of pneumonia was 3.3 times higher and that of tuberculosis 9.4 times higher among registered Indians. In his analysis of health conditions among Indians in Northwestern Ontario, Young

(1987) showed that despite a declining trend in the infant mortality rate among Indians since the 1970s, it remained twice as high as the national average. The national statistics in Canada further confirm the precarious health conditions among Indians. The age-standardized death rates per 100,000 people were 950 for Indians in 1987 and 650 for Canada as a whole; by the early 1990s, despite a dramatic decline in the infant mortality rate among Natives, it stood at 17.5 per 1,000 for Natives and 7.9 for Canada (Bobet, 1990; Frideres, 1993: 204-7).

The data on death and illness clearly indicate that there is a strong statistical relationship between health status and race. However, exactly how race may have contributed to health conditions is not entirely clear. Frideres (1988, 1993) attributes the poor health status of Natives to what he calls the "environmental conditions" which include overcrowding, poor nutrition, chronic unemployment and community and family violence. He further argues that these conditions create the health problem to begin with, and that medical treatments may be useful in treating an ailment, but ineffective in changing social and economic conditions (Frideres, 1988, 1993: 207). Brady (1983) contends that poor health status of Indians is a natural consequence of colonial domination that has been imposed upon the Aboriginal peoples. Thus, he implies that colonial domination brings about undesirable social and economic conditions for Natives that inevitably lead to poor health. Others have drawn attention to the potential influence of culture on health. Commenting on major differences between Indians and non-Indians in rates of psychiatric disorders and rates of using medical services, Fritz and D'Arcy (1983) suggest the possibility that biological and cultural factors may influence the formation of psychiatric disorders, and that attitudinal and organizational factors may affect the use of treatment services. However, the authors only advocate a need to better understand Indian cultural values without clarifying how such values would affect the development of illnesses.

The difficulty in unraveling the meaning of race on health has to do with the fact that cultural effects subsumed under race are confounded with social and economic conditions which are also associated with race. Simply put, Indians suffering from poor health also suffer from poor economic conditions. In order to entertain whether cultural effects subsumed under race may play a part in the development of poor health, it is necessary to expand the comparison to an international scale where there is greater variability in health and economic conditions. In the analysis to follow, we will first compare the health status of 118 countries to see whether variations in life expectancy and infant mortality rates are related to the racial composition of countries, which is measured in terms of whether a country's population is mainly white or non-white. Then we will introduce per capita Gross National Product and per capita protein level as controls of economic and nutritional conditions to see whether racial effects, or the implied cultural influences, persist. To the extent that race remains important in accounting for health conditions after controlling for economic and nutritional levels, then one can claim that there are grounds to suggest a possible effect of culture on health. Conversely, if the effects of race on health disappear after adjusting for differences among countries in economic and nutritional levels, then it would suggest that whatever cultural effects race may exert on health, they are accounted for or mediated by material conditions of life.

Source of Data

The data on health status for this study are based on statistics from *Compendium of Social Statistics and Indicators* (United Nations, 1991). These statistics were originally prepared by the Population Division of the United Nations Secretariat, based on a review of all available sources. Some countries do not have complete and reliable data on births and deaths based on civil registration, and the Population Division of the United Nations used various estimation techniques to calculate life expectancy and infant mortality rates, based primarily upon population surveys of households.

Three dependent variables are used to indicate the health status of a country: life expectancy at birth for males (X_1), life expectancy at birth for females (X_2), and infant mortality rate per 1,000 (X_3), as measured by the number of babies born alive who die within a year of birth. These data are based on 1990 statistics.

The independent variables used are Gross National Product per capita (X_4), protein per day per capita (X_5), and the racial composition of a country (X_6). Gross National Product (GNP) measures the total domestic and foreign value added claimed by residents; it comprises Gross Domestic Product (GDP) plus net factor income from abroad, which is the income residents receive from abroad for factor services (labour and capital) less similar payments made to nonresidents who contributed to the domestic economy. Data on GNP per capita, also based on 1990 statistics, are mainly compiled from *World Development Report 1992* (World Bank, 1992). Currency differences have been standardized by the World Bank using U.S. dollars to calculate GNP figures. In 11 cases, the 1990 figures are not available, and the most current figures, mainly from 1987 to 1989, are used (World Bank, 1991).

The average supply of protein per day per capita (X_5) is used as an indicator of the nutritional level of a country; this figure does not show the actual level consumed by individuals. Data for this variable also come from *Compendium of Social Statistics and Indicators* (United Nations, 1991). Since the data for 1990 are not available, the 1988 figures are used instead.

Finally, the variable on "racial composition" (X_6) is a dummy variable, constructed on the basis of whether is country is composed of a mainly white (coded as 1) or non-white population (coded as 0).

Complete data on the foregoing variables are available for 118 countries, with 85 "non-white" countries.

Variations on Health Status

When gender-specific life expectancy rate and infant mortality rate are used as indicators of general health status, data on 118 countries show wide variations, especially when the racial composition of countries is taken into account. For the 118 countries, the average life expectancy at birth is 64 years for men, and 68.6 years for women (Table 1). However, when the racial composition of countries is being considered, the data show that life expectancy is higher among countries of mainly white populations than those of mainly non-white populations: 71.6 years for males and 77.9 years for females among countries of white populations, and 61.1 for males and 65 years for females among countries of non-white populations. The data clearly indicate that people in mainly "white" countries live 10 years longer for men and 13 years longer for women than people in mainly "non-white" countries.

The data on infant mortality rates show a similar pattern. The overall death rate for infants for the 118 countries is 48 per 1,000, but it drops to 12.7 per 1,000 among countries of mainly white populations, and rises to 61.7 per 1,000 among countries of mainly non-white populations. In other words, the infant mortality rate is about five times higher among "non-white" countries than "white" ones.

The data in Table 1 clearly show that there is a strong relationship between health status and racial composition. However, the variable "racial composition" is also correlated with economic level in that "non-white" countries are in general poorer countries, such that it is not clear whether it is the "racial composition" or material condition which is responsible for the variation in health status. To separate the effects of these two potential causes, it is necessary to develop a multivariate model which would permit isolating the influence of one from the other.

Table 1. Gender-Specific Life Expectancy Rates And Infant Mortality Rates Of Countries By Racial Composition, For 118 Countries

	ALL COUNTRIES		COUNTRIES OF MAINLY WHITE POPULATIONS		COUNTRIES OF MAINLY NON-WHITE POPULATIONS	
	MEAN	SD	MEAN	SD	MEAN	SD
AVERAGE MALE LIFE EXPECTANCY AT BIRTH	64.0	9.0	71.6	2.8	61.1	8.8
AVERAGE FEMALE LIFE EXPECTANCY AT BIRTH	68.6	10.2	77.9	2.6	65.0	9.7
INFANT MORTALITY RATE PER 1,000	48.0	40.8	12.7	9.9	61.7	40.1
NO. OF COUNTRIES	118		33		85	

Sources: Data on life expectancy for male and female and infant mortality rate (per 1,000) are compiled from United Nations, *Compendium of Social Statistics and Indicators*, 1988, New York: United Nations, 1991, Series No. 9, Table 15, pp. 340-358.

The Effects of Race and Economic Conditions

The influence of race on health status can be gauged more precisely by examining the bivariate correlations between race and indicators of health status. The correlation coefficients in Table 2 show that the relationship between "male life expectancy" and "race" is 0.531, thus indicating that 28 percent (r^2) of the variation in male life expectancy can be accounted for by the racial composition of countries. Similarly, "race" accounts for 33 percent of the variation in "female life expectancy" (0.572^2) and 29 percent of the variation in "infant mortality" (-0.541^2). In short, about one-third of the differences among countries in life expectancy and infant mortality can be attributed to whether a country is made up of a mainly white or non-white population.

Table 2 also provides information on how much the variable "race" overlaps with economic levels. The correlation between "race" and "GNP per capita" is 0.630, which means that about 40 percent of the variation in one variable is related to that of the other; and the

Table 2. Bivariate Correlations Among Health Status Variables and Independent Variables for 118 Countries

VARIABLES		X_1	X_2	X_3	X_4	X_5	X_6
LIFE EXPECTANCY AT BIRTH FOR MALE, 1990	X_1	—	.989	-.962	.612	.755	.531
LIFE EXPECTANCY AT BIRTH FOR FEMALE, 1990	X_2		—	-.971	.634	.780	.572
INFANT MORTALITY RATE (PER 1,000), 1990	X_3			—	-.593	-.741	-.541
GNP PER CAPITA, 1990 (US$)	X_4				—	.671	.630
PROTEIN PER CAPITA, GRAMS PER DAY, 1988	X_5					—	.778
RACIAL COMPOSITION	X_6						—
MEAN		64.020	68.606	48.000	5,152.900	74.509	0.280
SD		8.964	10.156	40.824	7,648.930	22.029	0.451
NUMBER OF COUNTRIES		118	118	118	100	116	118

Sources: Data on life expectancy for male and female for 1990, infant mortality rate (per 1,000) for 1990, and protein per capita, grams per day for 1988 come from United Nations, *Compendium of Social Statistics and Indicators*, 1988, New York: United Nations, 1991, Series No. 9, Table 15, pp. 340-358; Table 19, pp. 392-398. Data on GNP per capita (US$) for 1990 mainly from the World Bank, *World Development Report 1992: Development and the Environment*, New York: Oxford University Press, 1992, Table 1, pp. 218-219.

correlation between "race" and "protein per capita" is 0.778, or an overlap of 60 percent. Thus, these correlations confirm what is already known: "non-white" countries are also more likely to have lower income levels and poorer nutritional conditions.

The results of the multivariate analysis are presented in Table 3. Each indicator of health status is treated as a dependent variable, and the effects of "race," "GNP per capita" and "protein per capita" are simultaneously considered. As noted above, differences in racial composition account for 28 percent of the variation in the life expectancy for men (equation 1). When the variables "GNP per capita" and "protein per capita" are also considered along with "race," the three variables account for 61 percent of the variation in male life expectancy (equation 2), 64 percent of the variation in female life expectancy (equation 5), and 57 percent of the variation in infant mortality (equation 8). These equations indicate that when the per capita GNP and the per capita protein level of each country are taken into account, the ability of the independent variables to explain the variation in the dependent variable is greatly improved. However, equations 2, 5, and 8 also show that when the effects of per capita GNP and per capita protein level are considered simultaneously with that of "racial composition," the influence of "racial composition," as measured by the beta coefficient of "race" in each equation, turns out to be statistically insignificant. These findings suggest that the correct model to use is to remove "race" from the equations, since its effects on health status are essentially taken care of by other independent variables in the equation.

Equations 3, 6, and 9 show the final model without the variable "race." In equation 3 for example, it can be seen that even without the influence of "race," "GNP per capita" and "protein per capita" still account for 59 percent of the variation in "male life expectancy." In other words, the unique contribution of "race" in equation 2, in terms of its ability to explain any additional variation in "male life expectancy," is only about 1 percent. Comparisons of equations 5 and 6, and equations 8 and 9 also show that the unique effect of "race" tends to be less than 1 percent. In other words, the removal of the variable "race" in these equations do not bring about a reduction in the percentage of variation accounted for by the remaining variables in the model. Equations 8 and 9 also indicate that effect of "GNP per capita" on infant mortality is not statistically significant, although its unique contribution is about 2 percent.

The above analysis suggest that although "racial composition" as a variable alone accounts for about one-third of the variations in the health status of countries, the effect of "racial composition" disappears

Table 3. Standardized Regression Coefficients of Per Capita GNP, Per Capita Protein and Racial Composition on Life Expectancy and Infant Mortality

			Racial composition	GNP per capita, 1990 (US$)	Protein per capita, grams per day, 1988	R^2
Life expectancy at birth for male, 1990	X_1	(1)	0.5308*			0.2817
		(2)	-0.2077	0.2320*		0.6067
		(3)		0.1913*	0.7612*	0.5906
					0.6269*	
Life expectancy at birth for female, 1990	X_2	(4)	0.5717*			0.3268
		(5)	-0.1519	0.2310*		0.6389
		(6)		0.2012*	0.7430*	0.6303
					0.6448*	
Infant mortality rate (per 1,000), 1990	X_3	(7)	-0.5411*			0.2928
		(8)	-0.1446	-0.2022*		0.5731
		(9)		-0.1738	-0.7176*	0.5653
					-0.6241*	

* $p <$ or $= 0.05$

Sources: Data on life expectancy for male and female for 1990, infant mortality rate (per 1,000) for 1990, and protein per capita, grams per day for 1988 come from United Nations, *Compendium of Social Statistics and Indicators*, 1988, New York: United Nations, 1991, Series No. 9, Table 15, pp. 340-358; Table 19, pp. 392-398. Data on GNP per capita (US$) for 1990 mainly come from the World Bank, *World Development Report 1992: Development and the Environment*, New York: Oxford University Press, 1992, Table 1, pp. 218-219.

when "GNP per capita" and "protein per capita" are taken into account. Thus, the data show that differences in economic conditions and nutritional levels among the 118 countries, and not a presumed cultural influence subsumed under "race," are responsible for the fluctuations in life expectancy and infant mortality rates. In other words, if cultural influence is important in explaining variations in health status of countries, its effect is at best mediated by material conditions of life.

Summary and Conclusions

Studies of race and health status in North America show that racial minorities such as Aboriginal peoples suffer from poor health and high mortality, and that the relationship of race on health status seems to be well established. However, the literature has not provided a definitive explanation as to how race may affect health status.

Two interpretations have been suggested to explain why various racial groups in North America are associated with unequal health status. On the one hand, health status is believed to be an outcome of different lifestyles which are influenced by cultures and values, and the effects of race are considered mainly primordial. On the other hand, health status is seen as a consequence of unequal life chances, and race amounts to a surrogate measure of unequal opportunities and conditions of life. Using health data from 118 countries around the world, this paper tests the effects of material conditions and racial composition on health status. The findings show that racial effects on health disappear when the material conditions of life have been taken into account. The comparative study fails to provide the empirical basis to support the suggestion that culture as subsumed under race is directly responsible for health status.

The study confirms the importance of economic conditions in accounting for differences in health status. The World Health Organization has emphatically stated that "the state of economic development is a strong determinant of the health situation of a country" (World Health Organization, 1992: 28). Data from a cross-section of countries have systematically shown that the income level of a country is positively correlated with the health of a country, usually measured by life expectancy at birth. In addition to confirming this relationship, the present study also shows that when variations in economic conditions are taken into account, cultural effects subsumed under race have no influence on health. On the basis of this finding, it would be logical to claim that the cultural factor at best serves as one of many forces which advance or impede the economic development of a country.

Even if this may be the case, the burden of proof is on those who support the cultural argument to show how specific cultural elements are at work in this process.

References

Adamchak, Donald. 1979. "Emerging Trends in the Relationships Between Infant Mortality and Socioeconomic Status." *Social Biology* 26: 16-29.

Bobet, Ellen. 1990. *Inequalities in Health: A Comparison of Indian and Canadian Mortality Trends.* Ottawa: Health and Welfare Canada.

Brady, Paul D. 1983. "The Underdevelopment of the Health Status of Treaty Indians." Pp. 39-55 in Peter S. Li and B. Singh Bolaria, (Eds.), *Racial Minorities in Multicultural Canada.* Toronto: Garamond Press.

Frideres, James S. 1988. "Racism and Health: The Case of the Native People." Pp. 135-47 in B. Singh Bolaria and Harley D. Dickinson (Eds.), *Sociology of Health Care in Canada.* Toronto: Harcourt Brace Jovanovich.

Frideres, James S. 1993. *Native Peoples in Canada: Contemporary Conflicts*, Fourth Edition. Scarborough, Ontario: Prentice-Hall Canada.

Fritz, Wayne and Carl D'Arcy. 1983. "Comparisons: Indian and Non-Indian Use of Psychiatric Services." Pp. 68-85 in Peter S. Li and B. Singh Bolaria (Eds.), *Racial Minorities in Multicultural Canada.* Toronto: Garamond Press.

Markides, K.S. and D. Barnes. 1977. "A Methodological Note on the Relationship Between Infant Mortality and Socioeconomic Status with Evidence from San Antonio, Texas." *Social Biology* 24: 38-44.

United Nations. 1991. *Compendium of Social Statistics and Indicators.*, 1988. New York: United Nations.

World Bank. 1991. *World Bank's Tables, 1991.* Baltimore: John Hopkins University Press.

World Bank. 1992. *World Development Report 1992: Development and the Environment.* New York: Oxford University Press.

World Health Organization. 1992. *1991 World Health Statistics Annual.* Geneva: World Health Organization.

Young, T. Kue. 1987. "The Health of Indians in Northwestern Ontario: A Historical Perspective." Pp. 109-26 in David Coburn, Carl D'Arcy, George Torrance, and Peter New (Eds.), *Health and Canadian Society*, Second Edition. Toronto: Fitzhenry and Whiteside.

PART 2:

Immigrants, Race, Gender and Health

7

Mortality Differences Between the Canadian Born and Foreign Born in Canada, 1985-1987

Frank Trovato

Introduction

Migrant studies of mortality can provide valuable insights into the sociological, epidemiologic and demographic dimensions of immigration. In Canada, there is a considerable body of literature which deals with the adaptation and adjustment process of immigrants (Kalbach and Richmond, 1980; Richmond, 1967; Kalbach, 1970); however, limited attention has been directed to other social demographic aspects of foreigners in Canada, particularly their mortality experience. This situation contrasts sharply with that of other receiving nations such as Australia, France, the United States, and England where mortality differences by nationality have been documented extensively (e.g., Young, 1987, 1991; Brahimi, 1980; Marmot et al., 1983, 1984a, 1984b; Kitagawa and Hauser, 1973; Kestenbaum, 1986; Jacobson, 1963).

The few studies based on Canadian data demonstrate that the foreign born tend to have lower or comparable survival probabilities in relation to the Canadian born population (Trovato and Clogg, 1992; Trovato, 1992, 1990, 1985; Sharma, Michalowski and Verma, 1989; Michalowski, 1990; Kliewer, 1979). This observation coincides with much of the documented evidence in other countries where immigrants comprise a significant portion of the total population (i.e., USA, Australia, France, England and Wales).

However, differences by cause of death are not always consistent with their general conclusion, as in some cases the immigrants show higher death rates than the receiving society. In the United States, prior to World War II, foreigners had higher death rates than the American born population from virtually all major causes of death, such as from cancer, cardiovascular disease, accidents, violence and suicide (Jacobson, 1963; Dublin, 1933; Dublin et al., 1949; Dublin and Baker, 1920). According to Kestenbaum (1986) the contemporary situation is reversed: the immigrant population shows better survival probabilities than the American born population from these major cause-of-death groupings.

A similar situation is documented for France by Brahimi (1980). In relation to French born males, foreign born men have reduced odds of death from cardiovascular complications, cancers, alcoholism and suicide, but they have a higher risk of death from accidents and violence. Females born outside France have higher mortality risks from cardiovascular disease, cerebrovascular problems, respiratory ailments, and accidents and violence in relation to French born women.

In Australia, Young (1987, 1991) has recently corroborated previous findings by Burwill and colleagues (1973, 1982), Stenhouse and McCall (1970) and McMichael et al., (1980). With respect to external causes of death (i.e., suicide, violence, accidents), most immigrant groups continue to show higher rates of mortality than the host population. In connection with degenerative and chronic diseases, however, foreigners generally fare better than native born Australians.

Research by Marmot and colleagues in England and Wales (1983, 1984a, 1984b) indicates that, overall, the immigrant population tends to exhibit a lower risk of mortality from major causes of death. Death rates from accidents and violence are higher across all immigrant groups studied, however.

Objectives of this Study

The main objectives of this study are as follows: (1) to document mortality differences between two components of Canada's population, native born and foreign born, in the period 1985-1987, since previous research has generally not covered the time period beyond 1971; (2) to test a number of statistical models describing the level and age pattern of mortality differences between the foreign born and the native born populations; (3) to derive estimates of life expectancy at age zero for these two groups. To the knowledge of this writer, there does not exist any estimate of life expectancy for the Canadian born and foreign born for the period 1985-87.

Demographers in Canada have either implicitly or explicitly assumed that the immigrant population of Canada has the same mortality level and pattern as the Canadian born. We will examine the available data with this point in mind. It will be demonstrated that this assumption is not consistent with what the data reveal.

This study confines itself to general mortality. A detailed analysis of cause-specific death rate is beyond the scope of this investigation and remains a topic for further exploration.

Data Sources

The data are taken from this nation's official data bank, The Mortality Data Base, at Statistics Canada in Ottawa. Statistics Canada receives from the provinces all official death records for all decedents during a given year. The death certificate contains identifying information on the decedent, plus the coroner's assessment of what caused the death of a given person (medical and/or non-medical causes). The population counts for the computation of rates were taken from the 1986 Census (special tabulations from Statistics Canada).

Data Problems

The official records, while containing much valuable medical information, suffer from the limitation that there are few social demographic variables beyond age and sex that get coded on the death certificate.

Although it is possible to cross-classify deaths by cause, year, age, sex, province of birth, province of death, country of birth, and marital status, there is no information, for example, on the decedent's occupation, education, income, lifestyle and additional meaningful social demographic variables. Consequently, it is very difficult to correlate death rates by cause with factors that are presumed to be relevant in the chain of causation that led to the person's death.

A second limitation of official mortality records pertains to the degree of completeness in the reporting of some of these variables on the death certificate (see Trovato, 1985 and Trovato and Clogg, 1992 for a detailed discussion of this). While variables such as cause of death, age, sex and marital status are almost fully coded, the same cannot be claimed for variables such as ethnicity (now discontinued) and country of birth of decedents.

During the early fifties, country of birth was reported in virtually all cases. In subsequent periods (e.g., early sixties and eighties) a significant number of deaths have been coded as "missing" or "unknown" country of birth. The proportion of such cases is exceedingly high for some years. Trovato and Clogg (1992) report, for example, that in 1980-81, 24 percent of all deaths to persons aged 15 and older could not be classified by country of birth. Trovato (1985) has documented the situation for the census periods from 1950 through 1972.

Analysts have resorted to a number of procedures to cope with this problem. When the proportion of cases exceeds five or ten percent, statistical results will contain a nonsignificant degree of error. It is clear that the common practice of confining one's analysis only to the "known" country of birth cases is inadequate when the proportion of "missing" nationality exceeds 10 percent. Trovato (1985) and Trovato and Clogg (1992) have reviewed methods to handle this problem and have suggested appropriate statistical adjustments. Fortunately, the proportion of deaths with an unknown country of birth is only 3.26 percent for the period under investigation. It was therefore decided to apportion the "unknowns" on the basis of the "known" distribution of deaths. The assumption inherent in this procedure is that the "unknowns" are randomly distributed. Given the small proportion of such cases, the degree of error in this procedure is probably very minor.

Another problem, not related to data quality, has to do with methods of analysis. A common approach in the literature involves the computation of basic measures of mortality, from which inferences are drawn on the basis of observed differences. Few analysts have applied new multivariate techniques for mortality analysis to investigate group differences (see Trovato, 1985, 1992; Trovato and Clogg, 1992). As a result of this tendency, little gain has been made in moving beyond a basic understanding of mortality differentials between immigrants and the Canadian born population. In this study, I apply a log-rate model to draw insights about the differences and pattern of mortality between the Canadian born and the foreign born, not readily detectable with conventional demographic techniques.

To the best of my knowledge, we have had no estimates of what is the life expectancy of the foreign born population and how it compares with that of the native born in recent years. Indications from previous research suggests that the foreign born have either higher or comparable life expectations in relation to the native born (Kliewer, 1979; Trovato, 1985). An estimate of differences in life expectancy at age zero is provided in this investigation for the census period 1985-87. This measure will be assessed against an acceptable standard in order to evaluate the degree of error in the obtained estimate. I confine the analysis to three variables: nativity, age and sex.

Preliminary Analysis

The analysis proceeds with an examination of group differences in age and sex composition and death distributions followed by the presentation of basic measures of mortality for the two populations being considered.

Age and Sex Composition

Figures 1 and 2 show the age-sex structures of the Canadian born and foreign born populations in 1986. These two populations show radically different age-sex compositions. The Canadian born is a younger population, with a wider base of the age pyramid than the foreign born. This is understandable since the nature of international migration is inherently characterized by a concentration of migrants in the young adult and adult years. There are, therefore, relatively few immigrants aged 0-4. Although their numbers rise with age, foreigners comprise a smaller proportion in relation to the Canadian born at ages below 35-39. Beyond this age class, the native born are relatively fewer, which means that there are more older people in the immigrant than in the Canadian born population.

Figure 1. Canadian Born Population 1986

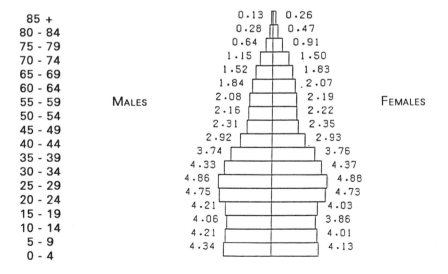

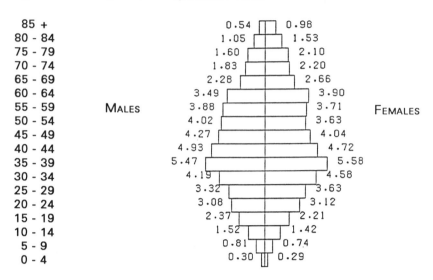

Figure 2. Foreign Born Population 1986

Distribution of Deaths

The shape of death distribution over age should approximate an inverted pyramid. That is, there should be relatively few deaths at the younger ages, and relatively more at advanced ages. This fact is evident in Figures 3 and 4, corresponding to the death distribution of Canadian born and foreign born populations, respectively.

Two differences in these figures are worth noting. While in both cases male deaths outnumber female deaths, there occurs a reversal of this fact at ages 80-84 and 85+ within the Canadian born. In the foreign born population the reversal does not occur until age 85+. Thus, in both cases there are more deaths to women than men at the oldest ages (absolute numbers), which is largely a function of the differential survival experience of the sexes. The sex ratio at advanced ages is grossly distorted in favour of females; and by age 80 or so, there are fewer men alive to eventually die.

The larger proportions of deaths in the older ages within the immigrant population may be indicative of a higher force of mortality in relation to the Canadian born. The opposite indication seems to prevail, however, at ages below 75-79, suggesting more advantaged survival probabilities for foreigners. A more conclusive picture of mortality levels and differences by age and sex can be obtained once death rates are computed.

Mortality Differences

Figure 3. Canadian Born Deaths 1985 - 1987

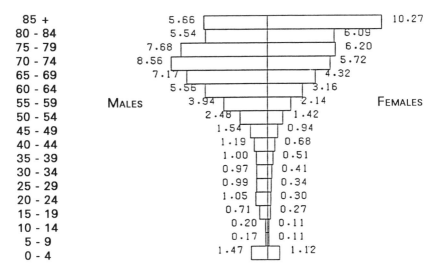

Figure 4. Foreign Born Deaths 1985 - 1987

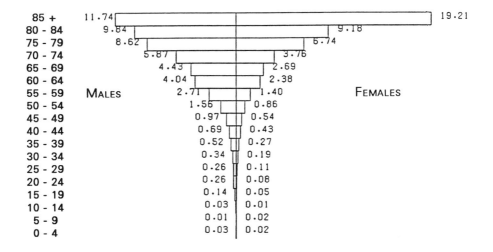

Death Rates

The varying age-sex compositions and mortality distributions of the two populations are radically different, therefore, the crude death rates in Table 1 are of limited value in drawing substantive conclusions about mortality differences. Although the immigrants have very high crude death rates, the age-standardized rates reveal that the Canadian born have higher levels of mortality once differences in age composition between the two populations have been taken into account. The standardized death rates for Canadian born men and women are 7.90 and 6.06 per 1,000, respectively. The corresponding levels for the immigrants are 6.87 and 5.45.

The sex difference in mortality is greater within the native born population. The male rate is 30.4 percent greater than the female rate (7.90 versus 6.06). This differential is only 26.1 percent greater for men in the foreign born population.

Native born men have a higher standardized death rate than their foreign born counterparts. The ratio of the two rates is 1.15 (or 15 percent higher for the Canadian born). This ratio is 1.12 (or 12 percent higher in the case of females). In a relative sense, then, immigrant men have slightly better survival prospects than immigrant females in Canada.

Table 1. Crude and Standardized Death Rates for the Canadian Born and Foreign Born Populations of Canada, 1985 -1987.

	CANADIAN BORN		FOREIGN BORN	
	MALE	FEMALE	MALE	FEMALE
CRUDE DEATH RATES (PER 1000)	7.24	5.59	13.24	11.63
STANDARDIZED RATES (PER 1000)*	7.90	6.06	6.87	5.45

* Directly standardized using the Canadian Population in 1971 as the standard.

Age Pattern of Mortality

In order to explore these differences further, age-sex specific death rates are shown in Figures 5 and 6. These rates were derived from a log-linear rate model and represent smoothed rates based on the expected death rates generated by the model (to be explained later).

Mortality Differences

For both sexes, the age-specific death rates are lower for the immigrant than the native born population. This differential is noticeably wider in the case of males, particularly from age 20 through 64. Notwithstanding these differences, both nativity groups display a similar pattern of mortality: lower rates in infancy for immigrants; higher odds of death in the age group 5-9 among foreigners; and lower mortality risks for immigrants at ages above 10, with a general narrowing of the gap between groups as age rises, particularly pronounced after age 65.

Figure 5. Age-Specific Death Rates Canadian and Foreign Born Males 1985 - 1987.

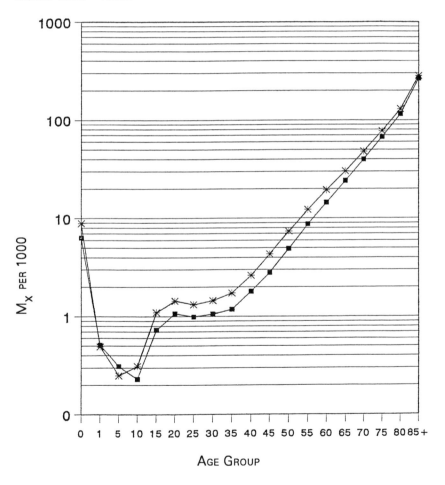

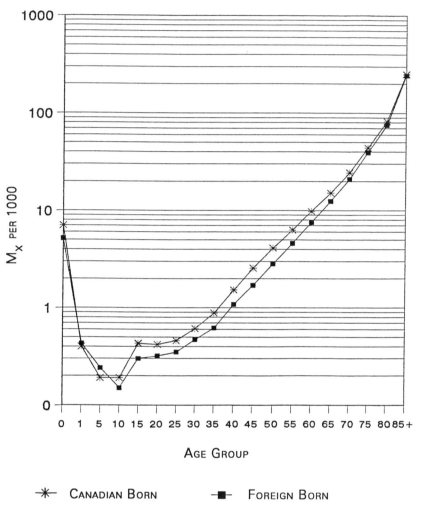

Figure 6. Age-Specific Death Rates Canadian and Foreign Born Females 1985 - 1987.

Model Specification and Parameter Estimation

These observations are useful in that they corroborate the initial results shown in Table 1, that immigrants have a lower level of mortality than their host society, and this differential is also evident over age. Beyond these observations it is important to determine the relative effects of age, sex and nativity in explaining these observed discrepancies and to test for their statistical significance.

A number of log-rate models were fitted to the mortality and population data. A good fitting log-rate model is one which produces the parameters that describe the actual data parsimoniously, that is, without having to consider all possible interaction terms. In Table 2, out of 14 models fitted, number 9 provides the best fit to the data. This model indicates that the death rates can be adequately described by the main effects of nativity (N), age (A), sex (S), and three interaction terms (AS, NA, NS).

This model corresponds to the following log-linear equation for the expected death rate:

$$\log (D_{ijk}/P_{ijk}) = \lambda + \sum_{i=1}^{I=2} \lambda_i^A + \sum_{j=1}^{I=19} \lambda_j^A + \sum_{k=1}^{K=2} \lambda_k^S + \sum \lambda_{jk}^{AS} + \sum \lambda_{ij}^{NA} + \sum \lambda_{ik}^{NS}, \quad (1)$$

i = nativity (1 = Canadian born, 2 = foreign born)
j = age group (1 = 0, 2 = 1 - 4,..., 19 = 85+)
k = sex (1 = male, 2 = female)

where:
D_{ijk} = deaths by nativity, age and sex,
P_{ijk} = the corresponding exposures for D_{ijk},
λ = the intercept term (baseline hazard),
λ_i^N = the parameter for nativity, $\Sigma \lambda_i = 0$,
λ_j^A = the parameter for age, $\Sigma \lambda_j = 0$,
λ_k^S = the parameter for sex, $\Sigma \lambda_k = 0$,
λ_{jk}^{AS} = interaction parameters of age and sex, $\Sigma \lambda_{jk} = 0$,
λ_{ij}^{NA} = interaction parameters of nativity and age, $\Sigma \lambda_{ij} = 0$
λ_{ik}^{NS} = interaction parameters of nativity and sex, $\Sigma \lambda_{ik} = 0$

This model assumes that deaths are Poisson distributed: they occur randomly and are independent with mean and standard deviation = λ; the population exposed to the risk of death is large, and the probability of death is small. The model is inherently multiplicative in that the expected number of deaths (E_{ijk}) is the product of the probability of death (μ_{ijk}) in the population multiplied by the number of people exposed to the risk of death (P_{ijk}); therefore,

$$E(D_{ijk}) = \mu_{ijk} P_{ijk} \quad (2)$$

This multiplicative equation can be expressed in its multivariate form for the expected death rate by taking the exponent of terms in (1):

$$D_{ijk}/P_{ijk} = \gamma \cdot \gamma_i^n \cdot \gamma_j^A \cdot \gamma_k^S \gamma_{jk}^{AS} \cdot \gamma_{ij}^{NA} \cdot \gamma_{ik}^{NS} \quad (3)$$

Equations (1) and (3) are hazard models (Cox, 1972) containing all first order interaction terms. That is, the hazard for the nativity groups is age and sex dependent. The hazard (probability of death) is assumed to be constant within given combinations of categories of covariates (e.g., Canadian born males aged 15-19). This restriction is a function of the log-linear rate model's link to the exponential distribution which assumes a constant hazard (Feller, 1968; Clogg and Eliason, 1987; Laird and Olivier, 1981).

Multivariate Analysis

From panel (B) in Table 2, it is evident that age has the largest effect in reducing the error in the overall death rate (refer to ΔL^2) followed by nativity and the interaction of age and sex. Although nativity's interactions with age and sex are not as impressive, they are statistically significant and must be considered important.

Table 3 presents the additive (log-linear) parameters from model 9. Of main interest are the coefficients involving nativity. The main effect of nativity is positive ($\lambda = .11489$) indicating that Canadian born persons share a disproportionate risk of death in relation to the foreign born. The risk is over 12 times greater for the host population ($\exp(.11489) = 1.122$). This effect is highly significant ($Z = 12.87$, $p \leq .01$).

The interaction of nativity with sex shows that Canadian born men have a slightly higher conditional chance of death than foreign born men. This difference, although small, is also highly significant. Conversely, Canadian born females, in comparison to their foreign born counterparts, possess a slightly lower probability of death, net of main and interaction effects in the model. Thus, while it is true that men have higher death rates than women (by 34 percent as shown by the main effect of sex) the interaction of nativity with sex results in immigrant men sharing a slight advantage in comparison to Canadian born men, while foreign born women experience a slight disadvantage in relation to women born in Canada.

The interaction effects of age with nativity reflect an interesting and unexpected pattern. Even after all main and other interaction terms in the model have been taken into account, some age-by-nativity parameters are statistically significant. These coefficients show that the Canadian born tend to do better than foreigners in terms of survival probabilities at ages 1-4, 5-9, and at ages 65 and older. However, at all other ages immigrants share superior levels of survivorship (see Figure 7).

Figure 7. Differential Risk of Mortality by Age, Canadian Born-Foreign Born (Parameters from Log-Rate Model N, A, S, AS, NS, NA) 1985 - 1987.

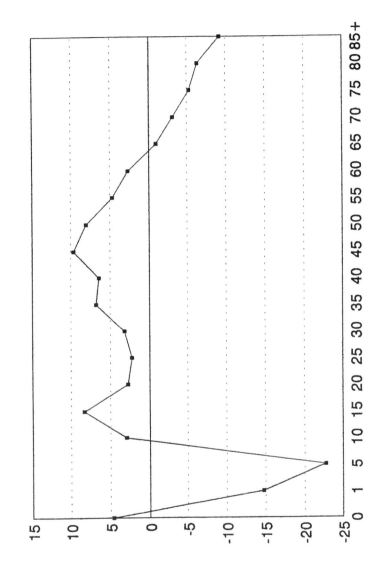

Table 2. Log — Rate models fitted to mortality and population data for the Canadian Born and the Foreign Born Populations of Canada, 1985 - 1987.

(A)

Model Fitted*	L^2	df
1. λ (Baseline)	1,717,188.44	75
2. N	1,676,036.82	74
3. A	45,562.68	57
4. S	1,710,425.73	74
5. N, A, S	8,498.40	55
6. N,A,S,NA	7,376.81	37
7. N,A,S,NS	7,945.03	54
8. N,A,S,NA,NS	6,965.11	36
9. N,A,S,AS,NA,NS	33.15	18
10. N,A,S,AS,NA	53.23	19
11. N,A,S,AS,NS	1,129.19	36
12. N,A	43,221.02	56
13. N,S	1,669,128.68	73
14. A,S	11,201.89	56
15. Saturated Model	0.00	1

(B)

Effect	Decomposition			
	Models Contrasted	ΔL^2	Δdf	Probability
N	2 - 1	41,151.62	1	< .01
A	13 - 5	1,660,630.28	18	< .01
S	13 - 2	6,907.93	1	< .01
NA	6 - 5	1,121.59	1	< .01
NS	8 - 6	411.70	18	< .01
AS	9 - 8	6,931.96	18	< .01
Residual	—	33.15	18	< .01
Total		1,717,188.44	75	

*   N   = Nativity (Canadian Born = 1, Foreign Born = -1)
    A   = Age Group (1 = 0, 2 = 1 - 4, 3 = 5 - 9, . . ., 19 = 85 +. Each group is coded as 1, else = 0, and age 85 + = -1)
    S   = Sex (Male = 1, Female = -1)
    λ   = Intercept Term

It is interesting to compare these results with those presented earlier. In Figures 4 and 5 it was shown that with the exception of the age class 5-9, the foreign born (both sexes) had lower age-specific death rates. However, the parameters from the multivariate model indicate that between the ages of 1 and 9, the foreign born actually possess higher death rates in comparison to the Canadian born. Moreover, at ages 65 and above, people born in Canada show a superior pattern of survivorship than the immigrants. Such an unexpected pattern of differences would have not been detected had we not proceeded beyond the analysis in Table 1 and Figures 4 and 5.

Table 3. Selected parameters from Log — Rate Model [N, A, S, AS, NA, NS]

Effect			Parameter	Z
Intercept			-4.91442	—
Nativity (CB vs. FB)			.11489	12.87
Nativity × Age				
CB vs. FB:		0	.04600	0.55
		1 - 4	-.14761	-1.69
		5 - 9	-.22729	-3.31
		10 - 14	.02956	0.49
		15 - 19	.08322	2.72
		20 - 24	.02771	1.17
		25 - 29	.02255	0.97
		30 - 34	.03189	1.58
		35 - 39	.06822	3.88
		40 - 44	.06447	4.11
		45 - 49	.09641	6.77
		50 - 54	.08049	6.42
		55 - 59	.04668	4.16
		60 - 64	.02691	2.57
		65 - 69	-.00920	-0.89
		70 - 74	-.03136	-3.15
		75 - 79	-.05302	-5.48
		80 - 84	-.06354	-6.61
		85 + (R)	-.09209	—
Nativity × Sex				
CB vs. FB.		Male	.00725	4.48
		Female	-.00725	—

Note: (R) = Reference category
— = Z score not computed
Full equation available on request to the author.

We may speculate on the meaning of the results in Table 3. The main effect of nativity captures a host of factors that are unmeasurable. Perhaps immigrants have lifestyles that are healthier than do the Canadian born (better diets, etc.) and/or they are selected for good health as a consequence of personal selection (i.e., the more qualified, skilled, healthy and adventurous migrate) and mandatory health screening before entry into Canada. Another possibility may be that the foreign born have higher levels of socioeconomic status (e.g., more education, more professional, and higher incomes) than the Canadian born, and that these differences somehow culminate in better health and hence lower death rates for immigrants. It is also likely that immigrants may benefit by a greater level of social supports due to the existence of their ethnic communities which serve to facilitate the adjustment and adaptation of newcomers to the new society (Trovato, 1992; Trovato and Jarvis, 1986; Trovato and Clogg, 1992; Breton, 1964; Reitz, 1980; Darroch and Marston, 1984).

The fact that immigrants' advantage in survivorship is largely concentrated in the working ages (from 20 to 64) lends some credence to the selectivity hypothesis. According to Brahimi (1980), a similar differential for immigrants and the native born prevails in France. He has hypothesized that this age-specific pattern of differences in mortality risk is indicative of selection because the variation is most visible in the working ages. Since most immigration is economically and occupationally (work) driven, it can be expected that only the most healthy and robust will make a permanent change of country.

The reversal at post retirement ages also fits with this hypothesis. The higher conditional likelihood of death among the foreign born at advanced ages may be a reflection of accumulated stresses and/or trauma during the working years, such as due to prolonged exposure to occupational hazards, injuries, and psychological problems arising out of the immigration experience (e.g., adjustment and adaptation to a new culture, etc.). Perhaps the selection process is most intensive within the working ages, but reduces its "protection" against the odds of death in old age. A detailed study of mortality differences by cause of death will shed some light on this pattern of survivorship for immigrants and the host population. It is also possible that the mortality crossover at the advanced ages may reflect a lower degree of health selection among foreigners currently in their 70s and older, who may have migrated to Canada at around the turn of the century, when the point system was less stringent. Health selection may have played a smaller role than is the case for more recent immigrants.

Differences in Life Expectation

Table 4 provides detailed calculations involved in the estimation of life expectancy at age zero for the Canadian born and the foreign born for the period 1985-1987. Deriving a credible estimate of life expectancy is not a straightforward task. It would be relatively easy to construct life tables with the available data, but the results may be difficult to accept unless one has some standard reference with which to gauge the derived results.

Columns (2) and (3) give the computed life expectancies at age zero for the Canadian born and the foreign born, respectively. The difference in life expectancy is denoted in column (4). On average, immigrant men aged zero can expect to live 2.72 more years than native born men at this age. For females, this difference is 1.71 years on average in favour of immigrants.

In order to determine whether these results are of acceptable quality, I computed overall life tables for men (Canadian born plus foreign born) and for women (both groups added together). The life expectancies at age zero from these tables should conform to the official published life table figures for the sexes produced by Statistics Canada (see column (1)). Any discrepancy between the official figures and those derived by using the data in this study would be a function of differences in method of life table construction and data quality.

The computed life table in the present study is based on the Reed-Merril method (Shryock and Siegel, 1975). The official life tables are constructed by a different methodology (Statistics Canada, 1989). They are based on single years of life, while those computed here are abridged. The official tables apply a more refined measure of infant mortality since they take into account infant deaths over age and calendar year by birth cohort. In the computed life tables, it was not possible to refine the infant death rate in this manner; the exposures for the infant mortality rate is the population aged zero instead of births. It is also worth mentioning that for foreign born infants there cannot be any corresponding births, therefore, for this group there is only one possible measure of infant mortality: deaths to infants divided by the population aged zero. A detailed discussion of methodological differences between the official life tables and the ones computed here is beyond the scope of this paper. It suffices to say that important differences exist and that therefore the estimated measures of life expectancy will probably differ from the official ones.

Table 4. Estimated Life Expectancy at Age Zero for the Canadian Born and the Foreign Born, 1985 - 1987.

Age and Sex	(1) Official E_0	(2) Canadian Born E_0	(3) Foreign Born E_0	(4) Observed Difference in $E_0 = (2)-(3)$	(5) CB and FB Combined E_0	(6) Bias=(5)-(1)	(7) W_i^{CB}	(8) W_i^{FB}	(9) Predicted E_0^{CB} $|(6)|\cdot(7)+(2)$	(10) Predicted E_0^{CB} $|(6)|\cdot(8)+(3)$	(11) Predicted Difference in Ex=(9)-(10)
Age Zero											
Males	73.04	71.86	74.58	-2.72	72.44	-0.60	0.845019	0.154981	72.37	74.67	-2.30
Females	79.73	78.01	79.72	-1.71	78.38	-1.35	0.842096	0.157904	79.15	79.93	-0.78

Notes: (1) From Published life tables for 1985 - 1987. Statistics Canada Vital Statistics and Disease Registries Section, 1989. Life Tables, Canada and Provinces, 1985 - 1987.

(2), (3), (5) Computed by the Reed-Merril Method.

All things considered, the discrepancies between the official figures and the ones computed in this study are not large. For example, column (6) shows that the estimated life expectancy for males is lower than the official one by -.60 of a year, while for females it is -1.35 years lower.

These discrepancies suggest that the estimated life expectancies for immigrants and the native born need to be raised by .60 for males and by 1.35 for females. The question is how to allocate these underestimates to the two nativity groups. One may decide to assign all of the underestimates to the Canadian born, or alternatively, to the foreign born, but this seems intuitively unappealing: It is unlikely that all of the differences pertain to either group alone.

It was decided that the sex-specific underestimates would be allocated to the two sex-nativity specific groups on the basis of their relative weight in the total population. These weights are shown in columns (7) and (8) of Table 4. Predicted life expectancies for the two nativity groups were therefore obtained as indicated in columns (9) and (10).

These calculations derived life expectancies at age zero of 72.37 and 79.15 for Canadian born men and women, respectively, and 74.67 and 79.93 for foreign born men and women, respectively. Therefore, the predicted difference in life expectancy for the sexes is -2.30 and -.78. On average, immigrant men at age zero enjoy a better level of survivorship than native born men by 2.3 years. Immigrant women in relation to women born in Canada share .78 of a year longer life expectancy at age zero. Thus, the relative advantage in survivorship is larger for immigrant men than for immigrant women. It was speculated earlier that the selection process associated with immigration may be more pronounced for men than for women. However, the substantive reasons for this fact remain unexplored and warrant further attention in subsequent analysis.

Conclusion

Based on data for the census period 1985-1987, it was shown that immigrants enjoy a relatively lower level of mortality than the Canadian born. This observation is consistent with previous studies in other receiving countries such as France, England-Wales, Australia and the United States. The pattern of mortality differences indicates that the advantage for the immigrants is largely concentrated in the adult working years, from age 20 to age 64. Beyond retirement age, the Canadian born have a higher probability of survival. It was suggested that this pattern of differences in conditional death probabilities is partly a function of health selectivity and other factors such as occupational and lifestyle differences between immigrants and their host population. Another interesting finding is that the relative advantage in survivorship is somewhat greater for immigrant men than for immigrant women.

In future research, emphasis must be placed on uncovering the causes of death that contribute to the observed differences and pattern of differences over age and by sex. More multivariate analysis is needed and should be expanded to include additional predictors of mortality such as marital status and socioeconomic position.

It has been implicitly assumed throughout this analysis that the denominators (the populations at risk) are free of error. Attention was directed solely on problems associated with the death counts. In this study, the problem of "unknown" nationality is minimal, largely due to the fact that such cases represent a very small proportion of all deaths in the period under investigation. Population counts by nativity in the census are subject to some degree of error due to undercoverage, however, in Canada this problem is small. The estimated undercoverage rate is less than two percent (Sharma, Michalowski and Verma, 1989). There is little reason to suspect that there is a disproportionate degree of error in the population counts applied in this analysis, especially since the two groups studied are well defined (born in Canada versus born outside Canada), thus minimizing the potential for classification problems and errors associated with small populations (e.g., if the foreign born had been disaggregated into many nationality groups).

Finally, the results of this analysis suggest that we cannot continue to assume that the mortality pattern and level of the foreign born in this country is the same as the Canadian born. The assumption of homogeneity in death probabilities is often introduced by demographers due to lack of information. A change in thinking about this matter may be warranted.

This research was supported by a Research Grant from the Social Sciences and Humanities Research Council (Grant No. 5567408). I am grateful to Mr. Chuck Humphrey for his computing assistance and to Dr. N. Lalu for his comments on an earlier draft of this paper.

References

Brahimi, M. 1980. "La Mortalite des Etrangers en France." *Population* 35: 603-622.

Breton, R. 1964. "The Institutional Completeness of Ethnic Communities and the Personal Relations of Immigrants." *American Journal of Sociology* 70: 193-205.

Burwill, P.W., M.G. McCall, N.S. Stenhause and T.A. Reid. 1973. "Deaths from Suicide, Motor Vehicle Accidents and All Forms of Violent Deaths Among Migrants in Australia, 1962-66." *Acta Psychiatrica Scandinavica* 49: 208-250.

Clogg, C.C. and S.R. Eliason. 1987. "Some Common Problems in Log-Linear Analysis." *Sociological Methods and Research* 16(1): 8-44.

Cox, D.R. 1972. "Regression Models and Life Tables" (with discussion). *Journal of the Royal Statistical Society* B74: 187-220.

Darroch, G.A. and W.G. Marston. 1984. "Patterns of Urban Ethnicity: Toward a Revised Ecological Model." Pp. 127-159 in *Urbanism and Urbanization: Views, Aspects and Dimensions*, edited by N. Iverson. Leiden, Netherlands: E.J. Brill

Dublin, L.I. 1933. *To Be or Not to Be: A Study of Suicide*. New York, N.Y.: Ronald Press.

Dublin, L.I. and C.W. Baker. 1920. "The Mortality of Race Stocks in Pennsylvania and New York." *Quarterly Publication of the American Statistical Association* 17: 13.

Dublin, L.I., A.J. Lotka and M. Spiegelman. 1949. *Length of Life*. New York, N.Y.: Ronald Press.

Feller, W. 1968. *An Introduction to Probability Theory and Its Application* (3rd Edition). New York: John Wiley.

Jacobson, P.H. 1963. "Mortality of the Native and Foreign-Born Population in the United States." Proceedings, International Population Conference, New York, NY: IUSSP, 1961. Vol. 1: 667-674.

Kalbach, W.E. 1970. *The Impact of Immigration on Canada's Population*. Ottawa, Ontario: Dominion Bureau of Statistics.

Kestenbaum, B. 1986. "Mortality by Nativity." *Demography* 23 (1): 87-90.

Kitagawa, E. and P.M. Hauser. 1973. *Differential Mortality in the United States*. Cambridge, M.A.: Harvard University Press.

Kliewer, E. 1979. *Factors Influencing the Life Expectancy of Immigrants in Canada and Australia*. Ph.D. Dissertation, the University of British Columbia, Vancouver, B.C., Canada.

Laird, N. and D. Olivier. 1981. "Covariance Analysis of Censored Survival Data Using Log-Linear Analysis Techniques." *Journal of the American Statistical Association* 76 (374): 231-240.

Marmot, M.G., A.M. Adelstein and L. Buluso. 1983. "Immigrant Mortality in England and Wales." *Population Trends* 33: 14-17.

Marmot, M.G., A.M. Adelstein and L. Buluso. 1984a. Immigrant Mortality in England and Wales, 1970-1978. Cause of Death by Country of Birth. Studies on Medical and Population Subjects No. 47, London, England: HMSO.

Marmot, M.G., A.M. Adelstein and L. Buluso. 1984b. "Lessons from the Study of Immigrant Mortality." *Lancet* 1: 1455-1457.

McMichael, A.J., M.G. McCall, J.M. Hartshorne and T.W. Woodings. 1980. "Patterns of Gastrointestinal Cancers in European Migrants to Australia: The Role of Dietary Change." *International Journal of Cancer* 25: 431-437.

Michalowski, M. 1990. "Mortality Patterns of Immigrants: Can They Measure the Adaptation?" Paper presented at the XIIth Congress of Sociology, Madrid, Spain, July 9-13, 1990.

Reitz, J.G. 1980. *The Survival of Ethnic Groups*. Toronto: McGraw-Hill.

Richmond, A.H. 1967. *Post War Immigrants in Canada.* Toronto, Ontario: University of Toronto Press.

Richmond, A. and W.E. Kalbach. 1980. *Factors in the Adjustment of Immigrants and Their Descendants.* Ottawa, Ontario: Statistics Canada.

Sharma, R.D., M. Michalowski and R.B.P. Verma. 1989. "Mortality Differentials Among Immigrant Populations in Canada." Paper presented at the 21st IUSSP Meetings in New Delhi, India, September 20-27, 1989.

Shryock, H.S. and J.S. Siegel. 1975. *The Methods and Materials of Demography.* U.S. Bureau of the Census, Washington, D.C.

Statistics Canada. 1989. Life Tables, Canada and Provinces, 1985-1987. Vital Statistics and Diseases Registries Section (Formerly Catalogue 84-532). Ottawa, Ontario.

Stenhause, N.S. and M.G. McCall. 1970. "Differential Mortality from Cardiovascular Disease in Migrants from England and Wales, Scotland, Italy and Native-Born Australians." *Journal of Chronic Diseases* 23: 423-431.

Trovato, Frank. 1992. "Violent and Accidental Mortality Among Four Immigrant Groups in Canada, 1970-72." *Canadian Studies in Population* 19(1): 47-80.

Trovato, Frank. 1990. "Immigrant Mortality Trends and Differentials." Pp. 91-109 in *Ethnic Demography: Canadian Immigrant, Racial and Cultural Variations*, edited by S.S. Halli, F. Trovato and L. Driedger. Ottawa, ON: Carleton University Press.

Trovato, Frank. 1985. "Mortality Differences Among Canada's Indigenous and Foreign-Born Populations." *Canadian Studies in Population* 12 (1): 49-80.

Trovato, Frank and Clifford C. Clogg. 1992. "General and Cause-Specific Adult Mortality Among Immigrants in Canada, 1971 and 1981." *Canadian Studies in Population* 19(1): 47-80.

Trovato, Frank and George K. Jarvis. 1986. "Immigrant Suicide in Canada: 1971 and 1981." *Social Forces* 65 (2): 433-457.

Young, C.M. 1991. "Changes in the Demographic Behaviour of Migrants in Australia and the Transition Between Generations." *Population Studies* 45: 67-89.

Young, C.M. 1987. "Migration and Mortality: The Experience of Birthplace Groups in Australia." *International Migration Review* 21 (3): 531-554.

8

Immigrant Status and Health Status: Women and Racial Minority Immigrant Workers

B. Singh Bolaria and Rosemary Bolaria

Introduction

Foreign workers now constitute a significant part of the labour force in many developed countries. These workers have become a permanent part of the economic structure of many countries, and their labour cannot be relinquished. The volume, composition, and immigrant status of these workers varies, however, depending upon the labour force needs and other structural requirements of the economies of the labour-importing countries. The influx of workers, as well as their immigrant status, is controlled by immigration laws and regulations. Internationally, the direction of flow is from the periphery to the core countries. Canada is one of the major users of "foreign" labour.

These workers, precisely because of their legal-political status as "foreigners," have become an important and perhaps sole source of labour in certain sectors of the Canadian economy. Some workers are imported for specific tasks in specific sectors where, because of low pay, arduous work, and an unsafe and unhealthy environment, indigenous workers are unwilling to work. One of the areas in which foreign workers have become a permanent structural necessity is the agricultural sector, where employers have difficulty in attracting and retaining workers. The effect of immigration regulations and contractual obligations is to make foreign workers reliable, dependable, and docile farm labour. Foreign workers, with very little legal or political status, are, from the employer's point of view, ideal labour. On the other hand, for these workers, this distinctive legal-political status has significant effects on health and other areas. These effects are discussed in this chapter.

Immigrant Status and Foreign Labour

Foreign workers can be broadly classified into landed immigrant settler labour, migrant contract labour and transient workers, and illegal or undocumented workers. It is the immigration laws and regulations which set criteria for admission and determine the legal status of foreign labour.

Landed immigrants are those workers who have "lawful permission to come into Canada to establish permanent residence" (Canada, Employment and Immigration, 1984:100). Landed immigrants are entitled to seek employment and enjoy many legal rights. However, they are not citizens. They are entitled to apply for citizenship after a three-year residency in this country. It is precisely this probationary period which is of significance in the context of this chapter. During this period immigrants are in a vulnerable position because the Immigration Act gives the state the right to impose many restrictions on permanent residents, many of which impinge on their legal and political rights (Immigration Act 1992. See, in particular, R.S., C28 (4th Supp.), S.7(1)). The new arrivals, particularly unskilled, uneducated, racial minority and women workers, may be intimidated by various regulations (Bolaria, 1992).

In addition to immigrant workers, Canada also relies upon migrant workers under the Non-Immigrant Employment Authorization Program. An employment authorization is "a document issued by an immigration officer whereby the person to whom it is issued is authorized to engage or continue employment in Canada" (Canada, Employment and Immigration, 1984:100).

At a broader level, non-immigrant employment authorization regulations were introduced in 1973 to allow admission of non-immigrants for employment. Since the implementation of this programme, thousands of workers have come to Canada to work (Bolaria, 1992).

Temporary work authorizations are given only if the immigration office is satisfied that no Canadian citizen or permanent resident is available for the job in question. This means that, in most cases, jobs will be either menial and low-paying, such as domestic or farm work, or highly skilled and specialized. Also, the work authorization is specific to the job and for a determinate time period (Law Union of Ontario, 1981: 113-14). It is crucial to note that these non-immigrant workers have been allowed to enter Canada even when there is high unemployment.

Canada continues to import migrant contract workers to supplement the labour force in agricultural and service sectors (Bolaria, 1984; Bolaria, 1992; Bolaria and Li, 1988).

Migrant workers are in a vulnerable position. As the Law Union of Ontario states (1981:115): "The bargaining power of temporary workers is practically non-existent, since their presence in Canada is dependent on their continued employment by their employer. Such people often experience deplorable working conditions, long working hours and low wages."

In addition to temporary status in this country, migrant workers have other constraints imposed by restrictive contractual obligations which tie them to a particular job. The vulnerability and, consequently, the compliance of migrant labour is achieved through the control of political boundaries, immigration laws, and contractual obligations (Bolaria and Li, 1988).

Together with landed immigrants and migrant workers, illegal or undocumented workers now constitute a significant part of the labour force in many countries. Officially, these workers do not exist. Illegal status and the threat of deportation assure their compliance, docility, and cheap labour. These workers are in a weaker position than any others.

Thus, a very large segment of the labour force in Canada at any given time is in quite a vulnerable position (Bolaria and Li, 1988). Immigration laws and contractual obligations place all foreign workers in a distinctly disadvantaged position in political and economic relations; racial discrimination places additional specific pressures on non-white workers, which indigenous Canadian workers are not subjected to (Miles, 1982). Though minorities and women are now employed in diverse occupations, in certain areas of the labour market there is still a disproportionately high representation of minority workers and women. For instance, racial minority workers comprise a substantial portion of the agricultural labour force in British Columbia and Southern Ontario. Almost all of these workers are newly arrived immigrants or migrant contract workers. The numbers of women workers are disproportionately high in the service sector, domestic work, and garment work (Arat-Koc, 1992; Seward, 1990; Seward and McDade, 1988). In these sectors, workers are often not adequately protected by labour legislation.

The exploitation of immigrants is repeatedly documented (Berger and Mohr, 1975; Castells, 1975; Bolaria, 1984; Carney, 1976). Contrary to popular assumption, this is not due to some *natural* docility of workers determined by their personality or cultural background: rather, it is dictated by the vulnerable circumstances — legal and political — of immigrants.

Most of these workers would not work or continue to work in undesirable, low-paying jobs if they were at liberty to sell their labour in the open market. However, many of the alternative job opportunities are closed to them, and their subordinate status is unreasonably prolonged through immigration regulations and contractual obligations (Arnopoulos, 1979; Law Union of Ontario, 1981; Task Force on Domestic Workers, 1981; Task Force on Immigration Practices and Procedures, 1981:26).

When people need jobs, they have to take what is available to them. For many workers, coming to Canada is a chance to escape the poverty and unemployment of home and to earn a regular wage, however menial and low-paying the available jobs might be. Their economic needs thus make them susceptible to exploitation. A labour force composed mostly of women and racial minority workers can be hired cheaply (Brown, 1983:106).

The vulnerability of these workers also results from the absence of union organization in the workplace. Many work in isolation from other workers; this is particularly true, of course, of domestic workers and in-home textile workers (Task Force on Domestic Workers, 1981; Johnson and Johnson, 1982).

In summary, immigration laws, contractual obligations, inadequate protection by labour legislation, lack of alternative job opportunities, poverty and unemployment in the country of emigration, and the absence of union organization place many foreign workers in a vulnerable position and render them powerless vis-a-vis the employer.

Immigrant Status and Health Status

The Canadian labour market is characterized by occupational, gender, and racial stratification and segmentation (Royal Commission, 1984). Often foreign workers either end up in, or are specifically brought in to fill, positions in sectors where there is a shortage of Canadian labour or where Canadian workers are unwilling to work. For example, migrant workers are specifically imported for seasonal work in agriculture. Another area where there is a disproportionately high concentration of women and racial minorities is domestic and textile work.

In some sectors, all workers, whether foreign or Canadian, are in a disadvantaged and powerless position vis-a-vis their employers because of lack of union organization, lack of minimum wage coverage, lack of health and safety legislation and Workers' Compensation Board regulations, and so forth. Foreign workers (recently arrived immigrants and migrant workers on work authorizations, for example), because of their tenuous legal-political status are even more disadvantaged and powerless than are indigenous workers. Therefore, immigrant labour assumes special significance for the employers. As Sassen-Koob

(1980:27) states: "Immigrant workers can then be seen as one basic factor in the reproduction of low-wage, powerless labour supply, and not simply as a quantitative addition to cheap workers."

The interest of the employer lies in procuring labour that is not only cheap, but also can be consumed under specific conditions. These conditions have to do with the organization of work and the control of the production process, which is primarily a product of the outcome of the historical struggle between labour and capital. Labour has had some victories, but the production process under capitalism is still characterized by the primacy of management control. The institutionalization of this control varies with the nature of the production process. In the case of low-cost labour, management's control rests primarily on the powerlessness of the workers (Sassen-Koob, 1980).

In the following section, the health effects of this powerlessness are discussed, with a primary focus on farm labour, domestic workers, and garment workers both in factories and in the household.

Farm Labour: A Bitter Harvest

Workers are exposed to unsafe and unhealthy working conditions not only in industrial-sector production but also in the agricultural sector (Bolaria, 1994; Denis, 1988). Farming in North America is the third most dangerous industry (Reasons et al., 1981), and possibly the least protected in terms of acceptable labour standards. The agricultural sector in Canada, as in many other countries, makes extensive use of the low-cost labour provided by racial or ethnic minorities (Martin, 1985; Burawoy, 1985; Waitzkin, 1983; Sharma, 1982; Sharma, 1983; B.C. Human Rights Commission, 1983; Bolaria, 1994).

The agricultural labour force is supplemented by migrant labour under the Non-Immigrant Work Authorization Program (initiated in 1973) and the Seasonal Agricultural Workers' Program (initiated in 1966). These workers provide a valuable labour force for many producers and "meet identifiable shortfalls in the available supply of Canadian workers for the harvesting of fresh fruit and vegetable crops and the processing of these same commodities" (Canada Employment and Immigration Commission, 1981:2).

Long before the introduction of non-immigrant work authorizations, foreign workers had been admitted to meet the seasonal labour demand in agriculture. The Seasonal Agricultural Workers' Program helps to create a versatile labour pool for farmers harvesting highly perishable fruit and vegetable crops. In light of the experience with the Caribbean countries, a similar bilateral programme was established with Mexico in 1974. In 1976 the Caribbean programme was extended to include the Eastern Caribbean Islands.

The deplorable working conditions of both the domestic transient farm labour and migrant imported workers are well documented (Sanderson, 1974; Labonte, 1980, 1982; Sandborn, 1983; Canada Department of Manpower and Immigration, 1973; Report of the Special Committee on Visible Minorities in Canadian Society, 1984; Sharma, 1982; Kelly, 1983; B.C. Human Rights Commission, 1983). Workers and their families are often exposed to harmful substances on the farms. There is inadequate or no enforcement of the Health Act regulations concerning physical danger, occupational diseases, pesticides, and a high risk of injury. Farm workers are also not adequately protected in terms of minimum wage legislation, working hours, and overtime wages (Report of the Special Committee on Visible Minorities in Canada, 1984).

Both the living and working conditions of farm workers contribute to their ill health. A 1973 federal task force report on the seasonal migrant farm workers in Ontario uncovered instances of "child labour, sick, pregnant, and otherwise unfit adults working in the fields; and of entire families working with only the head of the family being paid" (Sanderson, 1974:405). The task force was "shocked, alarmed, and sickened" by the working conditions, wage levels, malnutrition, non-existent health facilities, and the "indescribable squalor" of living conditions which migrant farm workers had to endure (Canada, Department of Manpower and Immigration, 1973:17; Sanderson, 1974). There were many cases discovered of violations of the Immigration Act, Child Labour Act, human rights, and minimum sanitation standards. Employers, of course, benefited from family labour and were "delighted" to have foreign workers with large families (Canada, Manpower and Immigration, 1973).

The working and living conditions of farm workers in British Columbia are similar to the conditions which minority workers face in Ontario. Farm workers in British Columbia, exploited by the labour contracting system, face long hours of work, low wages with no overtime pay or benefits, unhealthy working conditions, lack of toilet or drinking water facilities on many farms, crowded and dangerous housing, and exposure to chemicals and pesticides in the field (Sharma, 1982; Canadian Farm workers' Union, 1980; Labonte, 1980, 1982-83; Kelly, 1983).

Due to the lack of day-care facilities, incidents of children's deaths due to drowning in buckets of drinking water in the shacks, or in unfenced ponds, have been reported (Sharma, 1982; Sharma, 1983). There are a number of other examples during the past few years that illustrate the continuous high risks and mortality faced by children (MacQueen, 1990; Heyer et al., 1992).

The agricultural labour force is composed primarily of racial minority workers, "marginal" domestic workers, newly arrived immigrants, and migrant contract workers, all of which are low-paid, seasonally employed, and transitory. In the case of families, subsistence wages can be earned only through the labour of the whole family. Not only parents, but children and very old members of the family also work in the field and are exposed to all the health hazards. Because families need work to survive, and complaints or resistance to intimidation or abuse means loss of jobs, these workers are less likely to report cases of violation of the Labour Relations Act. Union organization has been difficult in the case of farm workers due to racial, cultural, and linguistic barriers and divisions and the abundant availability of foreign labour brought in with the support of the state. The formation of the Canadian Farm Workers' Union in 1980 was the first serious attempt to organize farm workers.

Entire families work and in effect live in the fields, in crowded, unhealthy, and unsanitary accommodations — without clean drinking water or proper wash-up facilities. In some cases workers have to pay high rents for "housing accommodations" provided by the farmers. These are usually small, overcrowded, and insalubrious firetraps without in-unit bathrooms or running water (Sharma, 1982:13). A survey of 270 farm workers in 1982 revealed that a large proportion of the accommodations (about 80 percent) had no proper wash-up facilities, and 44 percent had no access at all to shower facilities (Matsqui, Abbotsford Community Services, 1982). This study also revealed that farm workers are exposed to dangerous pesticides, either through direct contact with pesticides or through spraying. Many of the workers spend long hours in the fields and therefore have prolonged periods of exposure to pesticides. As many of the pesticides are carcinogenic, farm workers suffer from many ill effects of exposure to spraying. The Matsqui study revealed that 90 percent of the workers had experienced one or more symptoms of pesticide spraying, such as rashes, itching, headaches, dizziness, gastrointestinal problems, and central nervous system disorders.

The majority of the workers did not speak English and many of them did not receive information or instructions on health hazards of pesticides. A vast majority (over 80 percent) ate their lunches in the sprayed field areas. One writer has commented that "the living and working conditions of Canadian farm labourers (especially in B.C.'s Fraser Valley) bear a closer resemblance to those of Third World peasants than to those of the average Canadian worker" (Labonte, 1982-83:6).

Also, pesticide safety regulations are either not enforced, or non-existent altogether. There is continued use of pesticides that have never been adequately tested for safety, and cases of severe pesticide poisoning and death are not uncommon (Labonte, 1982:6-7).

In the face of all the ill effects of pesticides, the "agrichem" business flourishes, and continued use of many pesticides is allowed despite the fact that they have not been properly tested and, in some cases, are known to be carcinogenic (Goff and Reasons, 1986; B.C. Human Rights Commission, 1983).

As noted above, agricultural workers fare very badly in regards to general living conditions, being housed in labour compounds — typically unsanitary, unsafe, and overcrowded accommodations; this, combined with long hours of arduous work tend to produce ill health. Working conditions are equally stressful: the misery of the material, social, and environmental deprivations, racial subordination, long-distance migrations and uprooting from stable traditional cultures and disruption of community ties, all contribute toward psychological distress and mental disorders (Doyal and Pennell, 1979; Eyer, 1984; Waldron et al., 1982; Kuo and Tsai, 1986).

In summary, workers are exposed to health hazards not just in the industrial workplace, but also in agriculture. Both the living and working conditions of farm labour are "dangerous to their health." Unsafe and unsanitary living conditions and exposure to dangerous pesticides and other detrimental agents contribute to excessive physical health problems, injuries, and premature death. These circumstances also damage workers' psychological health. Insecure and depressing working conditions, social isolation, and racial subordination all contribute toward psychological distress and mental disorders.

Women Workers: Home Sewing and Domestic Servants

Because of increased employment of women, there is considerable interest in the effects of employment on women's health. They face many chemical, biological, and physical health hazards in the workplace (Hinch and DeKeseredy, 1994). Even apparently safe female-dominated occupations, such as service, clerical, sales, teaching, and health, are associated with significant hazards (George, 1976; Waldron, 1983). For instance, women health workers face many health hazards, such as an increased risk of viral hepatitis, back strain, and exposure to anesthetic gases which can cause spontaneous abortions (Waldron, 1983). Women workers are exposed to chemicals in dry-cleaning and laundry establishments, and hairdressers and beauticians have increased risk of respiratory disease due to extended exposure to hairsprays (Blair et al., 1978). Dental hygienists, technicians, and assistants are exposed to anesthetics, radiation, and mercury (George, 1976). Sales clerks, constantly on their feet, suffer from varicose veins and run an increased risk of contagious diseases because of constant contact with the public. Teachers are susceptible to mumps, measles, influenzas, and performance stress. Pregnant women face special problems at the workplace, as many substances are dangerous to the baby (Waldron, 1983; Messing, 1983; George, 1976). In manufacturing industries, female workers are exposed to occupational carcinogens. In the garment industry, where a very high proportion of workers are women, exposure to cotton fibres and dust puts workers at a high risk of developing brown lung, or byssinosis (Harris et al., 1972; Merchant et al., 1973). Eye irritation and strain are common health problems in a number of industries, including textiles and electronics (Hricko and Brunt, 1976). Due to the dual responsibility of job and care of the family and the home, many employed women experience stress (Johnson and Johnson, 1977).

The above brief account covers only some of the health hazards faced by employed women; there are many additional physical, chemical, and biological health hazards which women workers face in these and other work settings (Stellman and Dawn, 1973; Stellman, 1977; Hricko and Brunt, 1976; Newhouse, 1967; Newhouse et al., 1972; Miller, 1975).

Attention has been focused primarily on the paid work force; however, women also face numerous health hazards in their own homes (Hinch and DeKeseredy, 1994). Many of these hazards are the same as at the outside workplace: accidents, stress, and exposure to chemicals, laundry detergents, and solvents. The risk of accidents may be as high for homemakers as for women in the labour force (Krute and Burdette, 1978). Like the latter, homemakers experience stress, though for different reasons: social isolation and the monotonous and unrewarding nature of housework are primary contributors (Ferree, 1976; Oakley, 1974). Homemakers are more likely than employed women to report such health problems as asthma, allergies, heart disease, and restricted activity and bed rest due to illness and psychiatric impairment (Waldron, 1983). One study indicates higher suicide rates for homemakers than for employed women (Cumming et al., 1975).

Besides homemaking, women also engage in paid labour in their own households. Because of economic necessity to supplement family income and lack of day-care facilities, and to combine their family responsibilities with work, many women are now engaged in such contract work and employed labour. Home work appeals to women housebound by child care and other responsibilities; it is attractive to the employers as a means of lowering their labour and other overhead costs, particularly in enterprises which are threatened by unions and international competition. Home work is being promoted "with the ideology of liberation through self-employment. Touted as a way of escaping the ills of modern 9-to-5 work, it is promoted as a way for women to 'have it all' — children, family and job" (Berch, 1985:41). Households have become little cottage industries and all the health hazards faced by workers at the workplace are now transplanted into the households. The garment industry illustrates this point.

In an attempt to lower the labour costs and improve competitive advantages, there has been a restructuring and reorganization of garment production in several countries (Lipsig-Mumme, 1987; Morokvasic et al., 1986; Johnson and Johnson, 1982), specifically in those where the garment industry is faced with shortages of low-cost labour and higher labour costs. To preserve the rate of profit against labour shortages and higher labour costs, two basic strategies are used: increasing the intensity of labour exploitation (i.e., increasing workers' productivity), and/or resorting to low-cost labour (Portes, 1979). The search for low-cost labour takes two primary forms: (1) establishing firms where such labour is available, and (2) importing such labour to replace or supplement the local labour force. Not all enterprises can take advantage of these strategies. The first option is available only to the monopolistic firms. It is evident that the corporations which have the ability to move elsewhere are doing so (NACL, 1979), and the ability of transnational corporations to relocate in cheap labour areas (or their threats to do so) is being used to impose wage cuts, harsher working conditions, and undervaluation of labour power on employees (Dixon et al., 1982). On the other hand, there are the small, competitive firms, which lack capital and resources, and are therefore mostly dependent upon the availability of low-cost labour in the local market. This labour force consists largely of immigrant and migrant women.

To reduce labour costs, one common strategy used by employers is restructuring of garment production, in effect achieving de-industrialization and de-unionization by shifting work to individual households. There has been a renaissance of home sewing. In the home, as in the factories, it is usually women who do this work, because they are the ones who have sewing skills. The textile and garment industries are characterized by gender-typed low-wage jobs and are major employers of minority and immigrant women (Reasons et al., 1981; Johnson and Johnson, 1982; Lipsig-Mumme, 1987; Morokvasic et al., 1986; George, 1976).

Workers in the textile industry face numerous health hazards. Numerous chemicals used in this industry for dyeing, shrinking, and waterproofing fabrics have known health hazards (George, 1976); many are teratogenic and carcinogenic. Textile workers are affected by excessive noise in the workplace, sore backs caused by long hours of sitting at sewing machines, injuries from broken needles, skin, nose, and eye irritations, headaches and dizziness, and even psychological changes because of certain chemicals and liquids used in the industry (George, 1976).

Workers are also exposed to large quantities of lint, dust, and fabric scraps (Reasons et al., 1981; Johnson and Johnson, 1982; George, 1976). Inhalation of cotton fibres and cotton dust presents the risk of developing brown lung, or byssinosis. The common symptoms of this respiratory problem are shortness of breath, cough, and chest tightness (George, 1976). Textile workers may also face risk of asbestosis, now commonly recognized among workers exposed to asbestos, which may be used in the production of curtains and rugs. Scarring of lungs, reduction in size and elasticity of lungs, lowered lung capacity, coughing, and breathlessness are common signs of asbestosis (George, 1976)- Asbestosis may also cause certain cancers — lung cancer, mesothelioma, and gastrointestinal cancers (Stellman and Daum, 1973; Newhouse et al., 1972).

The above overview should give some indications of the working conditions and health hazards faced by workers in the garment industry. A British Columbia Ministry of Labour study of the garment industry observed that "the very fact that the industry cannot recruit personnel from the mainstream of the labour force raises some questions regarding working conditions in the industry." Other studies on the working conditions of the immigrant women employed in the garment industry point to poor working conditions, job hazards, low wages, and high stress for the workers (Arnopoulos, 1979; White, 1979).

Unsatisfactory as the work environment and working conditions are for the factory workers, the working conditions for workers in their households are even worse — loose piecework rates, low overall wages, irregularity of work, irregular and unpredictable working hours, and uncertain income (Johnson and Johnson, 1982). As Morokvasic et al., (1986:406) state, "sewing is often considered only as an extension of women's 'natural' and unpaid domestic tasks, so that women can be expected to do the work for nothing or for extremely low wages." Immigrant women, because of cultural, linguistic, and legal barriers, may not be able to sell their labour in the open labour market. They also have fewer options because of domestic responsibilities (family and child care). For some there may be other structural barriers: gender discrimination combined with racism increases their vulnerability (Morokvasic et al., 1986).

Home workers are exposed to health risks similar to those faced by factory workers. However, in this case, the whole family suffers the hazards of fabric dust, lint, and accompanying allergic symptoms. Home workers, like their counterparts in the factories, suffer from back problems from sitting and sewing for long hours without breaks (Johnson and Johnson, 1982). Economic necessity and the lack of paid sick leave forces many to work even when they are not well. As Johnson and Johnson (1982:81) state: "If she wants to earn money, she must keep working. This means that many home workers continue to do their sewing even when they are ill." Pressure to meet the deadlines and fulfill the quotas creates severe stress for the home workers. These women must also balance the competing demands of two roles of homemaker and home worker. As home sewing is messy work, it adds to existing cleaning and housework pressures and thus constitutes an additional source of stress (Johnson and Johnson, 1982).

Home workers constitute an individually isolated (working alone in their own homes) and vulnerable labour force. These workers are characterized as "invisible segments of production," "captive and underpaid labour force," "invisible labour force," and "clandestine employment" (Lipsig-Mumme, 1987; Morokvasic et al., 1986). These conditions contribute to home workers' powerlessness. Their vulnerability is primarily due to their status as immigrants, and to inadequate legal protection in the workplace (Johnson and Johnson, 1982). Home workers are usually considered as "sub-contractors" and not workers. This situation permits the evasion of health and safety regulations, if indeed any regulations exist at all. It also allows the employers to evade labour regulations, if any.

In summary, while attention has been focused primarily on the paid work force, women also face numerous health hazards in their own homes. To supplement household income while meeting other domestic responsibilities, numerous homemakers engage in employed labour in their homes, into which many of the health hazards faced by workers at the workplace are now transplanted. In this case, not only the worker, but the worker's whole family is exposed to health risks.

Women Domestics, Chars, and Cleaners

Women continue to be concentrated in traditional gender-typed occupations. Many women also work in low-paid, low-status, arduous service sector jobs. Many foreign workers on non-immigrant work authorizations are being admitted to Canada to supplement the service sector's labour force. The presence of these workers is particularly crucial in some occupations. For example, due to undesirable working conditions, low wages, and low value placed upon domestic work, Canadian workers and landed immigrants are unwilling to accept and keep jobs as live-in domestics (Arat-Koc, 1992; Estable, 1986; Buckley and Nielsen, 1976; Hook, 1978; Ballantyne, 1980; Arnopoulos, 1979; Law Union of Ontario, 1981). There is a chronic shortage of Canadians for these jobs. Landed immigrants admitted for employment in household service occupations invariably leave these jobs soon after their entry into Canada (Task Force on Immigration Practices and Procedures, 1981). Consequently, it is foreign workers on non-immigrant work authorizations who constitute the chief segment of this labour force. For instance, in 1980, 11,555 "domestic" employment authorizations were issued: 6,160 for "domestic occupations," such as maid domestic, housekeeper, personal attendant; the remaining were child-care occupations, such as babysitter, child nurse, parent's helper (Task Force on Immigration Practices and Procedures, 1981:48). Visible minorities are heavily represented in paid domestic work (Arat-Koc, 1992; Royal Commission on Equality in Employment, 1984).

Domestic workers confined to individual households are an "invisible" work force. Live-in domestic workers face almost all conceivable employment problems — low wages, long working hours, stress and loneliness, work while being ill, and sexual abuse (B.C. Human Rights Commission, 1983; Law Union of Ontario, 1981; Hendleman, 1964; Boldon, 1971). In most instances, live-in domestics were paid less than the minimum wage (Hook, 1978; B.C. Human Rights Commission, 1983). Even if they are paid minimum wage, one third of their income is deducted for room and board (*Star Phoenix*, 2 April 1987).

These conditions for domestics prevail and are partially due to the deficiency of labour legislation and the gap between regulations and enforcement, and partially due to the general attitude toward domestic work. As a representative of an organization set up to advance the rights of domestic and other workers in Ontario states: "It all stems from the general feeling that it's OK to pay people less because what happens in the house is not really work" (*Star Phoenix*, 2 April 1987). A brief submitted to the B.C. Human Rights Commission (1983:26) by the Committee for the Advancement of the Rights of Domestic Workers (CARDWO), reflects similar attitudes experienced by workers.

> People look upon us as nothing. They ask us why we leave our country to come and clean someone else's house. They don't look on it as the same job as working in a hospital, hotel or nurses' home, cleaning and making beds. The only difference with it is that those of us who are domestics live in the home where we work. We have long working hours. Some don't get any holidays. That's because we are not covered by the Labour Act. It's up to the goodwill of our employer to pay us.

Many workers must continue working even when they are ill or pregnant because of inadequate legal provision for sick leave or maternity leave (B.C. Human Rights Commission, 1983). Besides becoming domestic workers, women end up as chars, janitorial helpers, chambermaids, nurses' aides, and in restaurants as dish washers and cook's helpers (Sharma, 1982). All these jobs are low-status, low-paid, and unhealthy. Chars may not have the stigma of a live-in domestic, but they face similar disadvantages and exclusion from labour legislation. Long hours of work can lead to many health problems, and the insecurity of the job is worrisome (B.C. Human Rights Commission, 1983:30). Women must endure personal humiliation in silence at the hands of the employers. As a woman in the CARDWO brief states (B.C. Human Rights Commission, 1983:31): "We are considered dumb, incompetent and untrustworthy . . . and every day in smaller ways, I'm treated as if I'm not a real person, with a mind, feelings and dreams of my own. That kind of attitude really makes me angry, but I have to keep my mouth shut unless I want to risk losing my job."

It is evident that the working conditions of women domestics, chars, and cleaners are damaging to physical and psychological health. Long working hours, stress and loneliness, low social status, and the ever-present threat of unemployment all contribute toward physical illness and psychological distress. Domestics and chars suffer from sore feet, aching backs, and varicose veins. Job insecurity creates anxiety and worries about the future. Interpersonal subordination and humiliation — being considered stupid, incompetent, and untrustworthy — may produce additional "psychosocial injuries."

Summary and Conclusions

The discussion presented in this chapter shows that farm workers, garment workers, women domestics, chars, and cleaners are exposed to numerous health hazards. Their living and working conditions are "dangerous to their health." In the case of farm workers, unsafe and unsanitary living conditions, exposure to pesticides and herbicides, lack of job security, arduous tasks, and interpersonal subordination each contribute to their physical and psychological ill health. Our discussion of garment workers indicates that many of the health hazards faced by them in factories are also now transplanted to the households. This directly exposes the whole family to health risks associated with textile work. It is also clear that the conditions in which women domestics, chars, and cleaners work are damaging to their physical and psychological wellbeing.

Under such conditions, the high accident and illness rates among immigrant workers from the Third World are often attributed to "accident-proneness" due to their cultural background and their inability to function in an industrial setting. However, evidence suggests that "immigrants and indigenous workers tend to fall into separate categories with immigrant workers consistently filling the most dangerous jobs" (Lee and Wrench, 1980:563). Their job-related accidents have "less to do with immigrants themselves than the tasks they perform and the environment in which they find themselves" (Lee and Wrench, 1980:563). For instance, the health problems of farm workers, garment workers, domestics chars, and cleaners have essentially nothing to do with their ability to function in an industrial setting. Almost all of these workers are engaged in manual labour.

In many sectors, all workers, foreign or Canadian, are in a disadvantaged and powerless position vis-a-vis their employers because of the absence of union organization, inadequate labour legislation, insufficient health and safety regulations, and so forth. Foreign workers, however, because of their particular legal-political status, are even more disadvantaged than the indigenous labour force.

These workers are a low-cost labour force whose vulnerability stems from various economic, social, legal, and political considerations, and not from some natural docility of their gender or racial and cultural background. Among farm workers, garment workers, domestics, chars, and cleaners, a failure of legal protection seriously affects women, racial minorities, and immigrant workers.

This lack of protection might seem surprising at first glance, even if only because good health and physical fitness are important to maintain high worker productivity and a stable labour force. As Marx wrote: "When capitalist production lengthens the hours of work, it shortens the lives of the workers." However, employers' concern about workers' health depends upon the production costs, and availability and replacability of the work force. Workers who become ill are sent home, and quickly replaced by healthy workers at little or no cost to the employers or the state. When labour is plentiful and can be easily replaced, employers will be less concerned about the health of employees (Schatzkin, 1978). Access to foreign workers assures an almost infinite supply of labour. The workers on non-immigrant work authorizations may be characterized as a "bonded forced rotational" system of labour procurement (Bohning, 1974; North, 1980). Health screening tests assure the supply of physically fit immigrant labour.

In conclusion, the greater exploitation of immigrant labour must be understood in the objective context of workers' legal-political vulnerability. The health, health care, and safety of workers must be analyzed in the context of the organization of labour process. Evidence from selected cases, namely agricultural workers and textile workers, suggests that immigrant workers, because of their vulnerability, are subjected to harsher working conditions than is the indigenous labour force. Gender and race compound workers' disadvantages — minority workers and women are exposed to an even more hazardous working environment.

A revised version of the chapter which first appeared in *Sociology of Health Care in Canada*, B. Singh Bolaria and Harley Dickinson (eds.). Toronto: Harcourt Brace Jovanovich, 1988.

References

Arat-Koc, Sedef. 1992. "Immigration Policies, Migrant Domestic Workers and the Definition of Citizenship in Canada." Pp. 229-242 in Vic Satzewich (Ed.), *Deconstructing a Nation: Immigration, Multiculturalism and Racism in 90's Canada*. Halifax, N.S.: Fernwood Publishing.

Arnopoulos, S.M. 1979. Problems of Immigrant Women in the Canadian Labour Force. Ottawa: Canadian Advisory Council on the Status of Women.

Ballantyne, Susan. 1980. Domestic Workers: Proposals for Change. Toronto: University of Toronto, Faculty of Law.

Berch, Bettina. 1985. "The Resurrection of Out Work." *Monthly Review* 37(6):37-46.

Berger, John, and Jean Mohr. 1975. *A Seventh Man: Migrant Workers in Europe*. New York: Viking Press.

Blair, A., P. Decoufle, and D. Grauman. 1978. "Mortality Among Laundry and Dry Cleaning Workers." *American Journal of Epidemiology* 108:238.

Bohning, W.R. 1974. "Immigration Policies of Western European Countries." *International Migration Review* 8(2): 155-63.

Bolaria, B. Singh. 1984. "Migrants, Immigrants, and the Canadian Labour Force." In *Contradictions in Canadian Society*. Edited by John A. Fry, 130-39. Toronto: John Wiley and Sons.

Bolaria, B. Singh. 1988. "The Health Effects of Powerlessness: Women and Racial Minority Immigrant Workers." Pp. 439-459 in B. Singh Bolaria and Harley Dickinson (Eds.), *Sociology of Health Care in Canada*. Toronto: Harcourt Brace Jovanovich.

Bolaria, B. Singh. 1992. "From Immigrant Settlers to Migrant Transients: Foreign Professionals in Canada." Pp. 211-228 in Vic Satzewich (Ed.), *Deconstructing a Nation: Immigration, Multiculturalism and Racism in 90's Canada*. Halifax, N.S.: Fernwood Publishing.

Bolaria, B. Singh. 1994. "Agricultural Production, Work and Health." Pp. 684-697 in B. Singh Bolaria and Harley Dickinson (Eds.), *Health, Illness and Health Care in Canada*. Toronto: Harcourt Brace.

Bolaria, B. Singh and Peter Li. 1988. *Racial Oppression in Canada*. Toronto: Garamond Press (2nd edition).

Boldon, Bertram. 1971. "Black Immigrants in a Foreign Land." In *Let the Niggers Burn!* Edited by Dennis Forsythe, 22-40. Montreal: Black Rose Books.

British Columbia Human Rights Commission. 1983. "What This Country Did to Us, It Did to Itself." A Report of the B.C. Human Rights Commission on Farm Workers and Domestic Workers. February.

British Columbia Ministry of Labour. 1974. "Manpower Analysis of the Garment Industry." Victoria, B.C.

Brown, Carol A. 1983. "Women Workers in the Health Service Industry." In *Women and Health: The Politics of Sex in Medicine.* Edited by Elizabeth Fee, 105-16. Farmingdale, New York: Baywood Publishing Co.

Buckley, Helen and Soren T. Nielsen. 1976. "Immigration and the Canadian Labour Market. Research Project Group." Strategic Planning and Research, Manpower and Immigration.

Burawoy, Michael. 1976. "The Functions and Reproduction of Migrant Labour: Comparative Material from Southern Africa and the United States." 181: 1050-87.

CAREDWO (Committee for the Advancement of Rights of Domestic Workers). 1982. Submission to B.C. Human Rights Commission, June 17.

Canada. Department of Manpower and Immigration. 1973. "The Seasonal Farm Labour Situation in Southwestern Ontario — A Report." Photocopy.

Canada. Employment and Immigration. *Annual Report* 1982-83. 1983. Ottawa.

Canada. Employment and Immigration. 1984. *Immigration Statistics.* Ottawa.

Canada. Employment and Immigration. 1989. *Immigration Statistics.* Ottawa.

Canada. Employment and Immigration. 1990. *Immigration Statistics.* Ottawa.

Canada Employment and Immigration Commission. 1981. Commonwealth Caribbean and Jamaican Seasonal Agricultural Workers' Program: Review of 1979 Payroll Records. Labour Market Planning and Adjustment Branch. Hull, Quebec. Photocopy.

Canada Employment and Immigration Commission. 1981. 1980 Review of Agricultural Manpower Programs. Labour Market Planning and Adjustment (June). Photocopy.

Canada Department of Manpower and Immigration. 1974. The Immigration Program: 2. (Green Paper).

Canada House of Commons. 1984. Equality Now! Report of the Special Committee on Visible Minorities in Canadian Society. Ottawa.

Canada Royal Commission. 1984. Equality in Employment. Ottawa Minister of Supply and Services.

Canada. Task Force of Immigration Practices and Procedures. 1981. Domestic Workers on Employment Authorizations — A Report. Ottawa Supply and Services.

Canadian Civil Liberties Association. 1977. Brief to the House of Commons Standing Committee on Labour, Manpower and Immigration, June 2, regarding Immigration Bill C-24.

Canadian Farm workers' Union. Support British Columbia Farm Workers. 1980. Carney, John. "Capital Accumulation and Uneven Development in Europe: Notes on Migrant Labour." *Antipode* 8(1): 30-36.

Castells, Manud. 1975. "Immigrant Workers and Class Struggles in Advanced Capitalism: The Western European Experience." *Politics and Society* 5: 33-66.

Cumming. E., C. Lazer, and L. Chisholm. 1975. "Suicide as an Index of Role Strain Among Employed and Non-Employed Married Women in British Columbia." *Canadian Review of Sociology and Anthropology* 12:462-70.

Denis, Wilfred. 1988. "Causes of Health and Safety Hazards in Canadian Agriculture." *International Journal of Health Services* 18(3): 419-436.

Dixon, Marlene, S. Jonas, and Ed McCaughan. 1982. "Reindustrialization and the Transnational Labour Force in the United States Today." In *The New Nomads*. Edited by Marlene Dixon and S. Jonas, 105-15. San Francisco: Synthesis Publications.

Dosman, J. (Ed.). 1985. *Health and Safety in Agriculture*. Saskatoon: University of Saskatchewan.

Doyal, Lesley and Imogen Pennell. 1979. *The Political Economy of Health*. London: Pluto Press.

Economic Council of Canada. 1978. For a Better Future. Ottawa. Joseph Eyer. "Capitalism, Health and Illness." In *Issues in the Political Economy of Health Care*. Edited by John B. McKinlay. New York: Tavistock Publications.

Estable, Alma. 1986. "Immigrant Women in Canada — Current Issues." Background Paper. Ottawa: Canadian Advisory Council on the Status of Women.

"Farm Safety Rules Scrapped." 1983. *Victoria Times Colonist*, 12 March: A8.

"A Fatal Mistake." 1978. *Vancouver Sun*, 18 March: A4.

Ferree, M.M. 1976. "Working Class Jobs: Housework and Paid Work as Sources of Satisfaction." *Social Problems* 23: 431-41.

George, Anne. 1976. Occupational Health Hazards to Women. Ottawa: Advisory Council on the Status of Women. October.

Glasbeek, H. 1982. "The Work Place As A Killing Ground." *This Magazine* 16(2): 24-27.

Glavin, Terry. 1980. "Breaking the Back of Back Breaking Labour." *Canadian Dimension* (August).

Goff, Colin H. and Charles E. Reasons. 1986. "Organizational Crimes Against Employees, Consumers, and the Public." In *The Political Economy of Crime*. Edited by Brian D. MacLean. Scarborough, Ontario: Prentice-Hall.

Goff, Colin H. and Charles E. Reasons. 1987. "Group Threatens to Sue Ontario For Domestic Rights." *StarPhoenix* 2 April: 9B.

Halliday, Fred. 1977. "Migration and the Labour Force in the Oil Producing States of the Middle East." *Development and Change* 8: 263-91.

Harris, T.R., J.A. Merchante, K.H. Kilburn et al. 1972. "Byssinosis and Respiratory Disease of Cotton Mill Workers." *Journal of Occupational Medicine* 14: 199-206.

Hendleman, Dan. 1964. "West Indian Association in Montreal." Unpublished M.A. thesis, Department of Sociology and Anthropology, McGill University.

Heyer, N.J. et al. 1992. "Occupational Injuries Among Minors Doing Farm Work in Washington State: 1986-1989." *American Journal of Public Health* 82: 557-560.

Hinch, Ronald and Walter DeKeseredy. 1994. "Corporate Violence and Women's Health at Home and in the Workplace." Pp. 326-344 in B. Singh Bolaria and Harley Dickinson (Eds.) *Health, Illness and Health Care in Canada*. Toronto: Harcourt Brace.

Hook, Nancy C. 1978. Domestic Service Occupation Study. Department of Family Studies, University of Manitoba.

Hricko, A. and M. Brunt. 1976. Working for your Life: A Woman's Guide to Job Health Hazards. Berkeley: Labour Occupational Health Program.

Hull, Diana. 1979. "Migration, Adaptation, and Illness: A Review." *Social Science and Medicine* 13A: 25-36.

Immigration Act, 1992. 1993. Ottawa: Queen's Printer.

INTERCEDE (International Coalition to End Domestic Exploitation). 1981. The Status of Domestic Workers on Temporary Employment Authorization. A Brief Submitted to the Task Force on Immigration Practices and Procedures.

Johnson, C.L. and F.A. Johnson. 1977. "Attitudes Toward Parenting in Dual-Career Families." *American Journal of Psychiatry* 134: 391-95.

Johnson, Laura C. and Robert E. Johnson. 1982. *The Seam Allowance*. Toronto: Women's Education Press.

Kelly, Russell. 1983. "Bitter Harvest." *New West Review* November.

Koch, Tom. 1983. "Farm Poison Death Government's Fault, Jury Says." *Vancouver Province* 17 March: Bl.

Kreckel, Reinhard. 1980. "Unequal Opportunity Structure and Labour Market Segmentation." *Sociology* 14(4): 525-50.

Krute, A. and M.E. Burdette. 1980. "1972 Survey of Disabled and Non-disabled Adults: Chronic Disease, Injury and Work Disability." *Social Science Bulletin* April: 3-16.

Kuo, W.H. and Y. Tsai. 1986. "Social Networking, Hardiness and Immigrants' Mental Health." *Journal of Health and Social Behavior* 27: 133-49.

Labonte, Ron. 1982-83. "Of Cockroaches and Berry Blight." *This Magazine* 15(6), December 1982-January 1983: 4-9.

Labonte, Ron. 1980. "The Plight of the Farm Workers." *Vancouver Sun*, 25 August 1980.

Labonte, Ron. 1982. "Racism and Labour: The Struggle of British Columbia's Farm Workers." *Canadian Forum* June-July.

Law Union of Ontario. 1981. *The Immigrant's Handbook*. Montreal: Black Rose Books.

Lee, Gloria and John Wrench. 1980. "Accident Prone Immigrants: An Assumption Challenged." *Sociology* 14(4): 551-56.

Lipsig-Mumme, Carla. 1987. "Organizing Women in the Clothing Trades: Homework and the 1983 Garment Strike in Canada." *Studies in Political Economy* 22 : 41-71.

MacQueen, K. 1990. "Slim Pickings." *Vancouver Sun*. September 22: B1.

Majka, L.C. and T.J. Majka. 1982. *Farm Workers, Agribusiness and the State*. Philadelphia: Temple University Press.

Martin, P.L. 1985. "Migrant Labour in Agriculture: An International Comparison." *International Migration Review* 19(1): 135-143.

Matsqui, Abbotsford Community Services. 1982. "Agricultural Pesticide and Health Survey Results." A Project of the Matsqui, Abbotsford Community Services. October.

Merchant, J.A. et al. 1973. "Dose Response Studies in Cotton Textile Workers." *Journal of Occupational Medicine* 15 : 222-30.

Messing, Karen. 1983. "Do Men and Women Have Different Jobs Because of Their Biological Differences?" In *Women and Health: The Politics of Sex in Medicine*. Edited by Elizabeth Fee, 139-48. Farmingdale, New York: Baywood Publishing Co.

Miles, Robert. 1982. *Racism and Migrant Labour*. London: Routledge and Kegan Paul.

Miller, A. 1975. "The Wages of Neglect: Death and Disease in the American Work Place." *American Journal of Public Health* 65(11): 1217-20.

Morokvasic, Mirjana, Annie Phizacklea, and Hedwig Rudolph. 1986. "Small Firms and Minority Groups: Contradictory Trends in the French, German, and British Clothing Industry." *International Sociology* 1(4): 397-420.

NACL (North American Congress on Latin America). 1979. "Undocumented Immigrant Workers in New York City." *Latin America and Empire Report* 12(6) Special Issue.

Navarro, Vicente. 1986. *Crisis, Health and Medicine*. New York: Tavistock Publications.

Newhouse, Muriel. 1967. "The Medical Risks of Exposure to Asbestos." *The Practitioner* 199.

Newhouse, Muriel et al. 1972. "A Study of Mortality of Female Asbestos Workers." *British Journal of Industrial Medicine* 29: 134-41.

North, D.S. 1986. "Non-immigrant Workers: Visiting Labor Force Participants." *Monthly Labor Review* 103(10): 26-30.

Oakley, A. 1974. *The Sociology of Housework*. New York: Random House.

Portes, Alejandro. 1979. "Labour Functions of Illegal Aliens." *Society* 14(September-October): 31-37.

Pynn, Larry. 1983. "Exempting Farmers From Safety Rules Attacked." *Vancouver Sun* 11 March.

Pynn, Larry. 1983. "Coroner Urges Pesticide Laws." *Vancouver Sun* 16 March: A1.

Reasons, Charles E., Lois Ross, and Craig Peterson. 1981. *Assault on the Workers.* Toronto: Butterworths.

Sandborn, Calvin. 1983. "Equality for Farm Workers — A Question of Social Conscience." A Submission to the Legislative Caucus of the Provincial New Democratic Party.

Sanderson, G. 1974. "The Sweatshop Legacy: Still With Us in 1974." *Labour Gazette* 74: 400 17.

Sassen-Koob, Saskia. 1980. "Immigrant and Minority Workers in the Organization of the Labour Process." *Journal of Ethnic Studies* 8(1): 1-34.

Sassen-Koob, Saskia. 1981. "Towards a Conceptualization of Immigrant Labour." *Social Problems* 29(1): 65-85.

Schatzkin, Arthur. 1978. "Health and Labour Power: A Theoretical Investigation." *International Journal of Health Services* 8(2): 213-34.

Seward, Shirley B. 1990. "Immigrant Women in the Clothing Industry." Pp. 343-362 in Shiva S. Halli, Frank Trovato and Leo Driedger (Eds.) *Ethnic Demography.* Ottawa: Carleton University Press.

Seward, Shirley and Kathryn McDade. 1988. "Immigrant Women in Canada: A Policy Perspective." Background paper. Ottawa: Canadian Advisory Council on the Status of Women.

Sharma, Hari. 1983. "Race and Class in British Columbia: The Case of B.C.'s Farm workers." *South Asian Bulletin* 3: 53-69.

Sharma, Shalendra. 1982. "East Indians and the Canadian Ethnic Mosaic: An Overview." *South Asian Bulletin* 1: 6-18.

Statistics Canada. 1984. "Canadian Women in the Workplace." Canada Update, from the 1981 Census, Vol. 2(3) January.

Stellman, J.M. 1977. *Women's Work, Women's Health.* New York: Pantheon Books.

Stellman, J.M. and S.M. Daum. 1973. *Work Is Dangerous to Your Health.* New York: Pantheon Books.

U.S. Congress. 1983. Hearings on Migratory Labor. Washington, D.C.: U.S. Government Printing Office.

Waitzkin, Howard. 1972. *The Second Sickness.* New York: Free Press.

Waldron, Ingrid. 1983. "Employment and Women's Health: An Analysis of Causal Relationships." In *Women and Health: The Politics of Sex in Medicine.* Edited by Elizabeth Fee, 119-38. Farmingdale, New York: Baywood Publishing Co.

Waldron, Ingrid, M. Nawotarski, M. Freimer, J. Henry, N. Post, and C. Wittin. 1982. "Cross-Cultural Variation in Blood Pressure: A Quantitative Analysis of the Relationships of Blood Pressure to Cultural Characteristics, Salt Consumption and Body Weight." *Social Science and Medicine* 16: 419-30.

Wall, Ellen. 1992. "Personal Labour Relations and Ethnicity in Ontario Agriculture." Pp. 261-275 in Vic Satzewich (Ed.), *Deconstructing a Nation: Immigration, Multiculturalism and Racism in 90's Canada.* Halifax, N.S.: Fernwood Publishing.

White, Julie. 1979. *Women and Unions.* Ottawa: Ministry of Supply and Services.

9

Health Status and Illness Patterns Among Asian Adolescents in Scotland

Manfusa Shams

Introduction

The voluminous literature on health inequalities in Britain is mainly based on linking the national mortality and morbidity statistics to the decennial census. Research in this area extends as far back as the 1860s with Farr's work on mortality patterns amongst industrial workers in England (Farr, 1864) to the latest publications of the Office of the Population Censuses and Surveys (OPCS) (1990) longitudinal study. There are also occasional national surveys such as the Health and Lifestyle Survey (Cox et al., 1987). However, national data on mortality and morbidity as indicators of health have dominated the literature for a considerable period of time and it is only more recently that other aspects of health such as self-reported symptoms, illness and disease, mental health, height, weight, blood pressure and lung function, smoking and drinking behaviour have been investigated (OPCS, 1980; Macintyre, 1987).

As the mortality rate is an indirect indicator of health and illness patterns of the population and also is believed to aid in the understanding of the etiology of diseases, a brief summary of the immigrant mortality rates and literature related to this will be presented in the following section.

Regional and Ethnic Variations in Mortality in England and Wales

In Britain, a review of the mortality rate is carried out through the

Office of Population Censuses and Surveys at approximately ten-year intervals when census denominators become available, and is presented in terms of the standardized mortality ratio (SMR), which in the present case is a measure of relative mortality in a study population compared to that in the country as a whole, while standardizing for age.

The most recent regional mortality data covered the period of 1979-83 and confirmed the continuation of the familiar regional gradient in mortality from high in the North and West to low in the South and East for both males and females. Areas with significantly high mortality levels relative to the rest of the country also turn out to be predominantly urban areas (OPCS, 1990).

The 1971 census provided denominator data in terms of country of birth and place of father's or mother's birth, the 1981 census provided such data in terms of own country of birth and the latest 1991 census recorded population denominators according to ethnic origin for the first time in Britain. However, this latest census data is still not available. Deaths are recorded by country of birth and the findings are available only in England and Wales, not for Scotland. It is thus difficult to obtain a total picture of the mortality rates of the people originating from the Indian subcontinent as the people who are born in Britain (referred to as British Asian in this paper) have not been separately identified in the available censuses. Also, people of the Indian subcontinent origin who were born in countries other than the Indian subcontinent are identified by their country of birth only. The mortality rates for people born on the Indian subcontinent are available only for England and Wales, providing a partial picture of the mortality rates for this ethnic group, and the comparison of mortality rates for this ethnic minority group across different regions is also not available. Only the mortality rates for people from the Indian subcontinent in England and Wales are given here.

An overview of mortality rates of selected immigrants for all causes is given in Table 1. The mortality rates presented here are based on the denominators from the population census in 1971 and refer only to country of birth.

Table 1 shows that rates for males born on the Indian sub-continent were a little lower, controlling for age, than those for males in England and Wales; in females the rates were higher. This finding for males, repeated more strongly in the OPCS Longitudinal Study (Fox and Goldblatt, 1982) is consistent with the concept of a healthy migration effect; the males who make the effort to migrate are likely to be healthier than the population at large. By 1979-83, however, any male advantage had disappeared, and a significant difference between groups in the rate of mortality decline was observed; compared to other immigrant groups in England and Wales such as African and Caribbean men and women (among whom mortality levels declined sharply), the mortality of immigrants born on the Indian subcontinent declined relatively slowly (Balarajan and Bulusu,1990).

Table 1. Mortality of Selected Immigrants From All Causes by Age, Sex and Country of Birth, 1970-78

Country of Birth		SMR (Age 20 and over)
Indian Sub-Continent	M	98
	F	106
Caribbean Commonwealth	M	94
	F	117
African Commonwealth	M	129
	F	124
All Countries Including England & Wales	M	100
	F	100

Source: M.G. Marmot, A.M. Adelstein, L. Bulusu, *Immigrant Mortality in England and Wales*, 1977-78, (London: HMSO) 1984.

While mortality rates for males born on the Indian subcontinent were low in the earlier studies compared to Britain as a whole, perinatal mortality gives an opposite picture. Stillbirth, neonatal and postneonatal mortality rates are higher for children of mothers born on the Indian subcontinent, African commonwealth countries and the West Indies, than for children of mothers born in the UK (Adelstein et al., 1980). Higher perinatal mortality was also observed among the group whose mothers were born on the Indian subcontinent in a survey in Bradford during 1975-1981 (Gillies et al., 1984).

The contribution to adult mortality of returning migrants with British names has been examined. Table 2 shows mortality of those aged 20-64 born on the Indian subcontinent, distinguishing Indian type names from British type names and based on a one percent sample of the 1971 census.

Mortality for specific causes of death for those born on the Indian subcontinent with Indian-type names has been studied in deaths from 1970-78 through proportional mortality ratios (PMR: a measure of the proportion of all deaths in that population group due to a specific cause, adjusting for age). In a number of cases, distinctive SMRs for those born on the Indian subcontinent were accompanied by similar

PMRs for those with Indian-type names. Of significance was the low proportion of deaths attributed to cancer among the Indian population (detected by name) in both sexes, and the high proportion of deaths from circulatory diseases. Cancers of the lung and trachea (smoking related cancers) are relatively low, and other 'common' cancers of the breast, stomach and colon are also low among people with Indian-type names from the Indian subcontinent, but high rates for cancers of the mouth, liver and esophagus are reported in one or both sexes in this group (Marmot et al., 1984). PMRs for TB mortality are high among people with Indian-type names from the Indian subcontinent and among migrants from Ireland. PMRs for diabetes are above average among those from the Caribbean and for Indian-type names from the Indian subcontinent. SMRs for maternal mortality (no PMRs given) are relatively high among women from the Caribbean and Africa and to a lesser extent among women born on the Indian subcontinent. Except for cancer of the esophagus, these patterns were still apparent among adults from the Indian sub-continent in 1979-83 (OPCS, 1990, Appendix 2). Deaths from coronary heart disease are reported to be high among men and women from the Indian subcontinent (Marmot et al., 1984; McKeigue et al., 1992).

Table 2. Mortality From All Causes, of Immigrants Aged 20-64 Born in the Indian Sub-Continent by Ethnic Group (Selected by Names)

	'Indian Type' Name		'British Type' Name	
	Deaths	SMR	Deaths	SMR
Males	1,506	99	952	114
Females	478	121	664	112

Source: M.G. Marmot, A.M. Adelstein, L. Bulusu, *Immigrant Mortality in England and Wales*, 1977-78, (London: HMSO) 1984.

Notwithstanding these differences, the causes of deaths for men born on the Indian subcontinent and all men in England and Wales were broadly similar in 1971 (Bhopal, 1988). The ten commonest causes of death in Asian men (identified by name) and British men are given in Table 3.

Table 3. Ten Most Common Causes of Death in Asian (Born Indian Sub-Continent) and Non-Asian Men in England and Wales in 1971 (20 and Over).

ASIAN MEN 1970-72		ALL MEN (ENGLAND & WALES 1971)	
CAUSE OF DEATH	NUMBER OF DEATHS	CAUSE OF DEATH	NUMBER OF DEATHS
ISCHAEMIC HEART DISEASE	1533	ISCHAEMIC HEART DISEASE	77,521
CEREBROVASCULAR ACCIDENT	438	CEREBROVASCULAR ACCIDENT	29,005
BRONCHITIS, EMPHYSEMA, & ASTHMA	223	CARCINOMA OF THE LUNG	23,891
CARCINOMA OF THE LUNG & BRONCHUS AND TRACHEA	218	BRONCHITIS & EMPHYSEMA	19,242
PNEUMONIA	214	PNEUMONIA	16,477
MOTOR-VEHICLE ACCIDENT	134	CARCINOMA OF THE STOMACH	6733
ARTERIAL DISEASE	101	MOTOR-VEHICLE ACCIDENTS	4489
HYPERTENSIVE HEART DISEASE	85	ALL OTHER (NON-MOTOR VEHICLE ACCIDENTS)	4915
LEUKAEMIA AND OTHER NEOPLASMS OF LYMPHATIC AND HAEMATOPIOETIC SYSTEM	74	HYPERTENSIVE HEART DISEASE	3795
SUICIDE	69	DIABETES	2905

Source: R.B. McAvoy, J.L. Donaldson, *Health Care for Asians*, (Oxford University), 1990.

Variations in cause of death by religion and ethnic subgroup have also been reported among those born on the Indian subcontinent. Proportional mortality ratios for cancer were lower for Hindus than for Muslims, and were lowest for Punjabis. Mortality due to ischaemic heart disease, high in all groups, was highest among Muslims (Balarajan et al., 1984). Cerebrovascular disease and cirrhosis are highest amongst Punjabi males and diabetes is highest amongst Gujaratis.

Ethnic Patterns of Morbidity

Morbidity measures the amount of disease or illness in a population. It comprises a spectrum of physical states from minor, for which no medical and surgical intervention is required, to major illnesses. The prevalence of these illnesses is not routinely recorded and published data are mainly confined to hospital morbidity (usually only for in-patients rather than out-patients), where country of birth is often recorded but only occasionally analyzed in particular areas, supplemented to some extent by data from community health services and local surveys.

Morbidity statistics in general practice are collected at approximately 10-year intervals (which coincides with decennial censuses for denominators). In 1981, the sample included around 100 practices and country of birth has been recorded in recent surveys.

The disease and illness patterns for ethnic groups are thus not extensively investigated. The last two national morbidity surveys of consultations in primary care suggest that age-standardized consultation ratios for those born on the Indian subcontinent are relatively high, especially for respiratory, musculoskeletal and skin diseases, though in the most recent survey fewer than average women consulted for mental disorders (OPCS, 1982,1990). Two national studies in 1971 and 1981 show lower age-standardized rates of admission to mental hospitals among those born in India or Pakistan compared with those born in England (Cochrane,1977a; Cochrane and Bal, 1989), and community surveys have shown similar findings in regard to psychological symptoms (Cochrane and Stopes-Roe, 1977b, 1981) though other studies of admissions conflict (Rack, 1990).

The incidence of low birthweight is high among children of mothers born on the Indian subcontinent (Macfarlane and Mugford, 1984). Other national data by ethnic group on indicators of health and functioning (height, weight, blood pressure) are virtually lacking (Macintyre, 1986).

The discussion so far is mainly limited to different ethnic minority groups living in England and Wales but it is important to know the mortality rates and morbidity patterns of these groups living in other parts of Britain, for any similarity or differences identified might enrich our knowledge of the epidemiology of diseases of ethnic minority groups. This will also serve as a theoretical framework for the present study.

Mortality Rates in Scotland

Mortality levels in Scotland exceed those in England and Wales and these differentials have persisted over many years (Carstairs and Morris, 1991). Table 4 shows data for 1979 to 1983.

The higher mortality in Scotland compared with England and Wales is also seen in the age/sex specific rates, for both males and females. High levels of mortality are found for some regions in Scotland compared to others, e.g., in the West with premature mortality being particularly high in Glasgow city (Carstairs and Morris, 1991). A report by the Greater Glasgow Health Board (1990) shows that the age-standardized mortality rate in Glasgow is seven percent above the average for Scotland. For the younger group (0-64), the standardized mortality ratio (SMR) is 209 above the Scottish average, and this mortality level for the younger group is expected to persist in coming years. From a United Kingdom perspective the situation is of even greater concern. Standardized mortality ratios for younger men and women are about 25 percent higher in Scotland than in England and Wales, and Glasgow contributes a large proportion of this mortality. The distribution of this mortality according to different ethnic groups living in Scotland is not known. The present study was conducted in the West of Scotland (Glasgow), therefore, a brief account of the mortality and morbidity patterns is of interest here.

Table 4. Standardized Mortality Ratios (SMRs) for Regions of England, Wales and Scotland 1979-80, 1982-83.

REGIONS	MALES (20-64)	FEMALES (20-59)
GREAT BRITAIN	100	100
ENGLAND & WALES	97	97
WALES	105	105
SCOTLAND	124	130
CLYDESIDE	138	145
NORTH	115	112
NORTH WEST	114	113
YORK & HUMBERSIDE	105	104
WEST MIDLANDS	103	101
EAST MIDLANDS	95	96
SOUTH EAST	87	88
SOUTH WEST	87	87
EAST ANGLIA	78	80

Source: V. Carstairs and R. Morris, *Deprivation and Health in Scotland*, (Aberdeen University Press), 1991.

Mortality Rates in Glasgow

Glasgow is one of the larger cities in the United Kingdom with an estimated population of around 933,200 (Scottish Health Statistics, 1990). In socio-economic terms, Glasgow is a disadvantaged area. There are approximately 13,200 deaths each year among the population in the Greater Glasgow Health Board area (Director of Public Health, 1990). Almost 80 percent of total mortality is attributable to four major causes: cancer, heart disease, stroke and respiratory disease (excluding lung cancer). The distribution of death rates for these diseases for the younger group (0-64 years) is above Scottish levels; the age standardized mortality rate for lung cancer and respiratory disease is 45 to 60 percent higher than for Scotland.

Morbidity Patterns in Glasgow

A partial picture of the morbidity patterns for the population in the Greater Glasgow Health Board area (Director of Public Health, 1990) is presented in Figure 1.

Figure 1. Use of Beds in Acute-Care Hospitals by Patients Resident in GGHB Area.

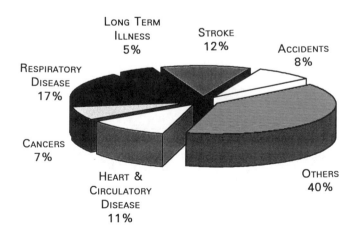

As Figure 1 shows, for the use of beds in acute hospitals, use by patients for respiratory disease (17 percent) is highest followed by heart and circulatory disease (11 percent). Evidence for hospitalization for different ethnic groups, specifically, the people from the Indian subcontinent is not known. However, an attempt will be made to summarize the types of diseases and onset of illness at various stages of life for this ethnic group from various sources.

Literature on Morbidity Patterns for Asians (People from the Indian Subcontinent) in Scotland

Data for Scotland are not separately available from the national morbidity surveys (Greater Glasgow Health Board, 1990). Routinely available morbidity data within the health service, which collect information on morbidity or illness, are relatively limited, as there is no systematic recording of data by ethnic group (Donaldson and Parsons,1990).

A few Scottish studies show differences in illness patterns at a particular age. Between 1971-85, there was a significant rise in the hospital discharge rates of acute appendicitis in Asian boys (whose parents were born in South Asia, including Sri Lanka) sampled by names, aged 10-19 years compared to the indigenous age group (Matheson et al., 1988). Dietary adaptation to indigenous culture was thought responsible for this disease. The paper did not show the rates of this disease among the affected boys according to their country of origin in South Asia. The heterogeneity of the sample in terms of country of origin posed a question of how far dietary adaptation has taken place as diverse dietary practices among the countries in South Asia are prevalent. It is also difficult to determine whether the trend of this disease is higher in one South Asian group than others. Dunnigan et al. (1985) in a review of hospital admissions and surveys over a number of years, reported a high incidence of admissions of children with rickets whose parents were born on the Indian subcontinent. A preventive measure in the form of issuing free vitamin D supplements was launched in 1979. Subsequent evaluation of the program showed its effectiveness (Dunnigan et al., 1985). Higher rates of osteomalacia in women originating from the Indian subcontinent were also reported (Dunnigan et al., l962; Ford et al., 1972; Holmes et al., 1973).

An analysis of the registered cancer patients in the West of Scotland over a 21-year period 1961-1981 shows that the Asian population aged

45-64 years (those whose ethnic origin was in India, Sri Lanka, Pakistan or Bangladesh) experienced significantly lower rates of colo-rectal, breast and lung cancer than the indigenous population and significantly higher rates of cervical cancer (Matheson et al., 1985).

Donaldson and Parsons caution about drawing conclusions from such data, because of potential ethnic differences in selection of hospital admissions. Moreover, there are no valid data on the age and sex-distribution of this ethnic minority group in hospital catchment areas, and there is a resulting difficulty in constructing denominators for the cases of hospital admissions to construct rates.

In 1987, Williams conducted a community study in Glasgow on health and illness issues among 30-40 year-old men and women whose ancestry derives from the Indian subcontinent. The sample was derived from an equal numbers of Muslims and non-Muslims, reflecting national proportions in Britain, and was statistically weighted to represent both concentrated and scattered members of the South Asian community in Glasgow (Ecob and Williams, 1991). I refer to them as Asian Scottish in this paper. The study showed significant differences in blood pressure, in several indices of physical and mental health, and in social and economic background between the Asian Scottish at different densities of settlement. This study furthermore showed that compared with the general Glasgow population of similar age, Asian Scottish men and women were shorter and broader, had smaller lung capacity and faster pulse; more of the women were clinically overweight and reported psychosomatic symptoms; and Asian Scottish men had higher diastolic blood pressure. On the other hand fewer Asian Scottish men had long-standing illness or digestive and other symptoms. Fewer Asian Scottish had had accidents, wore glasses or had lost teeth (Williams, 1992a). This study also suggested that length of immigration is negatively associated with health status, with long-established residents having a worse state of health (Williams, 1992b).

This finding is similar to the evidence of length of immigration being significantly negatively associated with psychological well-being among a sample of unemployed Asian men who originated from the Indian subcontinent (Shams, 1990).

Further inquiry is being made to examine three tentative hypotheses: that a healthy migrant effect is wearing off, that the UK health environment generally is unfavourable in certain respects, or that the economic and social situation of the minority is unfavourable. These questions will also be addressed in the present study. The need for empirical research for Asian Scottish can also be justified by the factual data on their level of concentration in the West of Scotland. Therefore, a socio-demographic sketch is drawn in the next section.

Ethnic Minorities in Scotland

The size of the ethnic minority population by country of birth has been steadily increasing. For example, comparison of 1971 and 1981 census statistics show a 40 percent increase in the numbers of people living in Scotland born on the Indian subcontinent or in the Far East. A survey by the Central Research Unit of the Scottish Office suggests that the increase is the result of both net inward migration from other parts of Britain, and of ethnic minority people having on average more children than white people (CRU, 1991).

Significant Features of Ethnic Minorities in Scotland

The samples of ethnic minority households obtained by the Central Research Unit of the Scottish Office between October, 1988 and September 1989 were screened by name on the electoral register and by reported family country of origin to effect two dominant ethnic minorities in Scotland (Asian and Chinese), in four major cities (Glasgow, Edinburgh, Dundee and Aberdeen). A white comparison group was also sampled. Among individuals in ethnic minority households, Pakistanis are the largest in three main cities, Glasgow (54 percent), Edinburgh (47 percent) and Dundee (46 percent). Sixty-one percent of the ethnic minority individuals were Muslim, 13 percent were Sikhs and 11 percent had no religion. More than half (51 percent) of the ethnic minority individuals were born in Britain. Peak immigration years for all ethnic groups were 1961-1970 for males and 1966-1980 for females. Ethnic minority individuals were younger for both sexes than in the white population. Among males, over half (54 percent) of the ethnic minority adults are aged under 35 compared to 37 percent of white adults. Fifty-eight percent of female adults from ethnic minorities are under age 35 compared to 36 percent of white females. A similar picture is obtained for younger groups: 38 percent of ethnic minority individuals were aged 15 or less compared with 22 percent of the white group. Employment status of ethnic minority groups is varied: 71 percent of ethnic minority males over 16 compared to 69 percent of white males were in the labour market. Contrary to this, females over 16 from ethnic minority groups were less likely to be in the labour market (26 percent) compared to their white counterparts (45 percent). Among those in work, a higher proportion of ethnic minority male householders were self employed (50 percent) than comparable white males (9 percent). Among the working age population (16+), 19 percent of ethnic minority males were unemployed compared to 14 percent of whites (it is worth mentioning here that white includes not only individuals from Scottish origin but anyone from European and other western white communities).

This descriptive account of ethnic minority groups reveals a growing number of young people of Asian Scottish origin with the highest concentration in Glasgow. In particular, the highest proportion of children aged 10-15 years in the population subgroups is in the Asian population (14 percent of Asian individuals sampled) compared to white (7 percent) and Chinese (12 percent).

With such a large proportion of Asian Scottish adolescents in Scotland, surprisingly little research has been carried out either to find out the health and illness patterns of this group or to inquire of the social and psychological processes that are regulating their life styles. There is also little empirical evidence regarding the inequalities of health amongst this ethnic minority age group, although there is sporadic evidence of specific diagnostic or physical measures (Peach, 1984; Ramaiya et al., 1990; Giovanni et al., 1983), and one or two dimensions of health-related behaviours are also examined in some studies, but a holistic approach encompassing qualitative and quantitative methods to investigate these issues is still lacking. The evidence of morbidity patterns for British Asians is mainly concentrated either on middle-aged or on preschool children with hardly any attention to the adolescents. Thus, there is a gap in the understanding of disease patterns and causative factors, and development of relevant preventive strategies on disease and illness for this ethnic minority age group is also not widely undertaken.

The Glasgow Study of Asian Scottish Adolescents

There is an increasing demand from the academic community, social policy makers and from the community itself to deepen the knowledge of health and illness patterns among the British Asian ethnic group whose contribution to every spectrum of British life is substantial.

Implicit in the fabric of British life is the growing need for research on the health of this group in order to balance the level of knowledge about majority and minority groups in different spheres of life. Theoretical and academic debate on racial equality is focused mainly on social services, employment and education. Surprisingly, inequality in health among different ethnic groups has not received that much attention. Thus, the paucity of research serves as a strong impetus to initiate an empirical study on health and illness issues for this ethnic group.

The discussion so far shows a dearth of research materials on morbidity patterns for this ethnic group not only in Scotland but in other regional divisions of Britain as well. There is a lack of coherent understanding of psychosocial aspects of health and illness amongst Asians living in different parts of Britain. It is believed that a study of this kind will enhance the understanding of the etiology of diseases and illnesses among adolescents in general irrespective of their ethnic status. The need to initiate this study is also strengthened by the fact that Glasgow and Clydeside generally have the highest age-standardized morality rates in Britain. It is essential to explore to what extent this environment has a direct or indirect impact on the health state and onset of diseases and illnesses of the major ethnic minority groups in Glasgow, specifically people from the Indian subcontinent (Asian Scottish).

In order to understand the relative contribution of psychosocial and environmental factors to the health and well-being of Asian Scottish adolescents whose parents originated from the Indian subcontinent, it is essential to adopt a comparative approach, focusing on health in the general population. The present study therefore, includes Scottish adolescents from the general population (referred to as general Scottish here) as a comparison group, although the main focus will be the adolescent Asian Scottish. This paper gives some preliminary evidence on various health issues. The findings deriving from a pilot study will serve as a starting point to the inquiry in this area.

Objectives of the Study

The major aims of this study are: first, to compare systematically levels of psychological and physical development and health, and health-related behaviours, between Asian Scottish and general Scottish adolescents (14 and 15 years); second, to elucidate the health-related behaviour of this age group, and to examine the interwoven relationships amongst a number of psychosocial variables that determine health status and are predictive of health behaviour; third, to identify crucial environmental and physical variables as determinants of health and compare these two adolescent groups on these variables; and fourth, to compare the direction and magnitude of differences in health between Asian Scottish and general Scottish adolescents with those already found for the 30-40 year-old groups.

The main aims of the pilot study were to explore the feasibility of a wide-range of self-reported physical and psychosocial measures on these two ethnic adolescent groups, to examine the participant's reactions to height and weight measures taken by a trained nurse and to include other relevant issues arising in the questionnaire session in developing the main study. This pilot study will also give a brief descriptive comparative account of their anthropometric features in order to make an early detection of any suggestive differences in these features and their associations with morbidity indicators.

Design

The study has both cross-sectional and longitudinal components, and the cross-sectional study conducted during March and April, 1992 will be treated as a baseline study. The aim of this baseline study is to give a descriptive account of health, illness and well-being of Asian Scottish adolescents and to make different cross-sectional comparisons (by gender, social class, area of residence, ethnic background and religious affiliation). In the second part of the study, at the beginning of 1993 (March/April, 1993), only the 15 year-olds (who were in their 14th year in 1992) will be followed up. The aim of this stage is to trace any changes in health and well-being of this group and also to examine to what extent these changes are related to the changes on the scores of any predictor variables (such as age, heights and weights, educational experience) if any, on the second occasion.

Method

The main cross-sectional study (conducted in March-April, 1992) consists of 824 boys and girls in their 14th and 15th years randomly selected from nine Secondary Schools, containing high proportions of Asian Scottish pupils. Analysis of data is in preparation. The present data are drawn from a pilot study, a sample of 33 boys and girls in their 14th (n=20) and 15th years (n=13) who were selected from two separate Secondary Schools in the South East of Glasgow city in January, 1992. All Asian Scottish in these two years were approached and an equal number of general Scottish pupils were selected following a random technique. The total number participating for 14 years old were 20 (Asian Scottish=6, general Scottish=14) and the total number for 15 years old were 13 (Asian Scottish=5, general Scottish=8). Seventeen boys and 16 girls (both Asian Scottish and general Scottish combined) comprised the sample.

Measures and Procedures

A wide range of self-reported physical and psychosocial measures was taken to detect the health state and health status of the sample. Sociodemographic measures were taken from the West of Scotland (youth cohort), National Child Development Study, and the General Household Survey. A few were developed by the author. Psychological well-being is measured by the GHQ (Goldberg, 1972), anxiety and depression (Zung, 1965) and self-esteem (Rosenberg, 1965) scales. All these scales are widely used and reported to have high validity and reliability. Moreover, some of the scales' validity and applicability for Asians originating from the Indian subcontinent is also established (Cochrane et al., 1977c; Shams, 1990). Two significant indicators of physical health, height and weight, were measured by a trained nurse in each session.

The self-administered questionnaire session took place in a separate class room provided by the school authority. A brief introduction of the purpose of the study was given by the author prior to the main session, any difficulties and queries being answered during the session. Voluntary participation as well as confidentiality of the answers were emphasized. Height was measured using standard stadiometers, weight (clothed, without shoes and heavy clothes such as jackets/coats) by portable electronic scales. Both of these were taken simultaneously with the questionnaire session.

Some Selected Results

The analysis of the age/sex subgroups on anthropometric features show that there is no consistent difference between these ethnic two groups on heights. Among Asian Scottish, 14 year-old boys and 15 year-old girls were taller than their general Scottish counterparts; while 15 year-old boys and 14 year-old girls were shorter. With weights, however, Asian Scottish were heavier in three of the age/sex groups, only being lighter among 15 year-old boys.

Regarding perceived health, illness and reported long-standing illness, a high percentage of general Scottish adolescents (64 percent) reported good health in the last 12 months compared to the Asian Scottish group (36 percent). Similar to this pattern, more Asian Scottish (44 percent) reported having long-standing illness than their Scottish comparison group (19 percent). Perceived level of fitness was broadly similar.

In order to examine how physical health is being regulated by the frequency and duration of physical exercise, a self-reported exercise schedule was obtained. The results show that in general, Scottish adolescents are taking more frequent physical exercise (32 percent, everyday) compared to Asian Scottish adolescents (9 percent, everyday). The total time spent on physical exercise is also more often high for the general Scottish sample.

Discussion

The findings in this pilot study suggest both similarity and differences in physical and psychological health among these two adolescent groups. First, no consistent differences in heights of these two groups were obtained although 14 year-old Asian Scottish boys show a tendency to be taller than their comparison group. This finding is interesting as the literature in this area suggests that taller individuals are in an advantaged health state (Macintyre, 1988). Only a large sample could verify this trend for a younger age group among the Asian Scottish sample. Lack of normative data on age and spurt of growth makes it difficult to assess the relative position of this group. However, this result contrasts with the findings on 30-40 year-olds where Asian Scottish were markedly shorter than their Scottish counterparts (Williams, 1992a). This possible difference with the middle-aged group needs to be unfolded further since a result like this would suggest rapid assimilation in the second generation.

It is also important to detect the extent of differences in heights between the adolescents and 30-40 year-olds within Asian Scottish and general Scottish groups. If the difference between these two age groups for Asian Scottish is larger than between the age groups from the indigenous population, then it can be hypothesized that environmental factors are influencing the health and well-being of Asian Scottish adolescents more strongly than that of general Scottish adolescents. Further inquiries will be made along this line in the main study.

Height is also a strong predictor of mortality rates, reported in Britain (Marmot et al., 1984) and Norway (Waaler, 1984 quoted in Floud, 1985). Empirical support to generalize this association for this ethnic group is required with a longitudinal design and a large sample. Associations between height with some other variables such as social class, parental occupation, nutrition, area of living, condition at birth, and birth order are reported in some studies (See, Macintyre, 1988). The impact of these variables on heights and weights need to be ascertained for this ethnic group.

Weight is associated with height and is an important indicator of health as well. A greater weight for three of the four age/sex groups of Asian Scottish could be due to the level of physical exercise; presumably they are doing less than normal requirements. This hypothesis can also be tested from the evidence obtained in the 30-40 year-old group, where overweight is a common feature among middle-aged Asian sample study and also in a recent London study (McKeigue et al., 1991). If confirmed, this finding would suggest continued lack of assimilation to general population norms. Overweight can be a potential risk factor to various illnesses including coronary heart disease which, as noted earlier, is an above-average factor in Asian mortality. It may also serve as a vulnerability factor for self-reported health measures. This was confirmed when Asian Scottish adolescents reported a low level of fitness and more long-standing illness. Further exploration of these associations will be made in the main study.

In summary, this pilot study, despite low statistical power associated with the small sizes, highlights the anthropometric features and health status of a small group of 14 and 15 year old Asian Scottish and general Scottish boys and girls living in the West of Scotland. The findings suggest ways in which Asian assimilation to Scottish health norms may be occurring only selectively, and indicate the way to the analysis of the main sample of over 800 cases.

The author expresses her gratitude to all the respondents, for taking part in this important survey. The author is grateful to Professor Sally Macintyre, Dr. Rory Williams and Dr. Patrick West for their valuable comments on this paper. Thanks to Jacqui Irwin for her assistance in typing and Patricia Fisher for preparing the data. The author is grateful to Dr. Rafiq Gardee and two head-teachers for their valued help. Sincere thanks to Ms. Linda Marsh, Head of research, Education department, Glasgow and Mr. Kenneth Corsar, Education officer, Glasgow for their supports and negotiations with selected schools in this study. The author is a research scientist in the Medical Research Council in Glasgow.

References

Adelstein, A.M., D.I. MacDonald, and J. Weatherall. 1980. "Perinatal and Infant Mortality: Social and Biological Factors, 1975-77." *Studies on Medical and Population Subjects*, No.41, OPCS, London, HMSO.

Balarajan, R., A.M. Adelstein, L. Bulusu, and V. Shukla. 1984. "Patterns of Mortality Among Migrants to England and Wales from the Indian Subcontinent." *British Medical Journal* 289:1185-1187.

Balarajan, R. and L. Bulusu. 1990. "Mortality Among Immigrants in England and Wales, 1979-83." In Britton, M (Ed.), *Mortality and Geography*. Office of the Population Censuses and Surveys, London.

Bhopal, R.S. 1988. "Health Care for Asians: Conflict in Need, Demand and Provision." In Equity: *A Prerequisite for Health, Proceedings of the 1987 Summer Scientific Conference*, pp. 52-5. London: Faculty of Community Medicine and WHO.

Carstairs, V. and R. Morris. 1991. *Deprivation and Health in Scotland*. Aberdeen University Press.

Central Research Unit Papers. 1991. *Ethnic Minorities in Scotland*. Edinburgh: The Scottish Office.

Cochrane, R. 1977a. "Mental Illness in Immigrants to England and Wales: An Analysis of Mental Hospital Admissions." *Social Psychiatry* 12:25-35.

Cochrane, R. and M. Stopes-Roe. 1977b. "Psychological and Social Adjustment of Asian Immigrants to Britain: A Community Survey." *Social Psychiatry* 12:195-206.

Cochrane, R., F. Hashmi and M. Stopes-Roe. 1977c. "Measuring Psychological Disturbance in Asian Immigrants to Britain." *Social Science and Medicine* 11:165-173.

Cochrane, R. and M. Stopes-Roe. 1981. "Psychological Symptom Levels in Indian Immigrants to England: A Comparison with Native English." *Psychological Medicine* 11:319-327.

Cochrane, R, S.S. Bal. 1989. "Mental Hospital Admission Rates of Immigrants to England: A Comparison of 1971 and 1981." *Social Psychiatry and Psychiatric Epidemiology* 24:2-11.

Cox, BD., M. Baxter, A.L.J. Buckle., N.P. Fenner, J.F. Golding, M. Gore, F.A. Hupport, J. Nickson, M. Rod, J. Stork, M. Wadsworth and M. Whichelow. 1987. *The Health and Lifestyle Survey*. London: Health Promotion Trust.

Director of Public Health. 1990. *The Annual Report*. Glasgow: Greater Glasgow Health Board.

Donaldson and Parsons. 1990. "Asians in Britain: The Population and Its Characteristics." In McAvoy and Donaldson (Eds.) *Health Care for Asians*, pp.72-89.

Dunnigan, M.G., B.M. Glekin, J.B. Henderson, W.B. Mcintosh, D. Sumner and G.R. Sutherland. 1985. "Prevention of Rickets in Asian Children: Assessment of the Glasgow Campaign." *British Medical Journal* 291:239-242.

Dunnigan, M.G., J.P.J. Paton, S. Haase, G.M. McNicol, M.D. Gardner and C.M. Smith. 1962. "Late Rickets and Osteomalacia in the Pakistani Community in Glasgow." *Scottish Medical Journal* 7:159-167.

Ecob, R. and R. Williams. 1991. "Sampling Asian Minorities to Assess Health and Welfare." *Journal of Epidemiology and Community Health* 45:93-101.

Farr, W. 1864. *Annual Reports of the Registrar General for England and Wales*, 1837-1920.

Ford, J.A., E.M. Colhom, W.B. McIntosh and M.G. Dunnigan. 1972. "Rickets and Osteomalacia in the Glasgow Pakistani Community, 1961-71." *British Medical Journal* 11:677-680.

Fox, J.A. and O.P. Goldblatt. 1982. *Office of the Population Censuses and Surveys. Socio-Demographical Mortality Differentials, Longitudinal Study*. HMSO: London.

Floud, R..1984. "Measuring the Transformation of the European Economies: Income, Health and Welfare." Discussion paper 33. London: Center for Economic Policy Research.

Giovanni, V.J., G.D. Beevers, D.H.S. Jackson, L.V. Osbourne, L.B. Pentecost, M. Beevers, T.L. Bannan and K. Mathews. 1983. "The Birmingham Blood Pressure School Study." *Postgraduate Medical Journal* 59:627-629.

Gillies, D.R.N., G.T. Lealman, K.M. Lumb and P. Longdon. 1984. "Analysis of Ethnic Influence on Stillbirths and Infant Mortality in Bradford, 1975-81." *Journal of Epidemiology and Community Health* 38:214-217.

Goldberg, D.P. 1972. *The Detection of Psychiatric Illness by Questionnaire.* London: Oxford University Press.

Greater Glasgow Health Board. 1990. *The Annual Report of the Director of Public Health.* Health Information Unit.

Holmes, A.M., B.A. Enoch, J.L. Taylor and M.E. Jones. 1973. "Occult Rickets and Osteomalacia Amongst the Asian Immigrant Population." *Quarterly Journal of Medicine* 51:838-843.

Macfarlane, A. and M. Mugford. 1984. "Birth Counts: Statistics of Pregnancy and Childbirth." National Perinatal Epidemiology Unit in collaboration with OPCS. London: HMSO.

Macintyre, S. 1986. "Physical Measures of Health. Development or Functioning: Their Use in the Three Cohort and Related Studies." Glasgow: MRC Medical Sociology Unit Working Paper No.3.

Macintyre, S. 1987. "West of Scotland Twenty-07 Study. Health in the Community. The Survey's Background and Rationale." Glasgow: MRC Medical Sociology Unit Working Paper No. 7.

Macintyre, S. 1988. "Social Correlates of Human Height." Oxford: *Science in Progress* 72:493-510.

Marmot, M.G., A.M. Adelstein and L. Bulusu. 1984. *Immigrant Mortality in England and Wales,* 1977-78. London: HMSO.

Matheson, L.M., J.B. Henderson, D. Hole and M.G. Dunnigan. 1988. "Changes in the Incidence of Acute Appendicitis in Glasgow Asian and White Children Between 1971 and 1985." *Journal of Epidemiology and Community Health* 42:290-293.

Matheson, L.M., G.M. Dunnigan, D. Hole and R.C. Gillis. 1985. "Incidence of Colorectal, Breast and Lung Cancer in a Scottish Asian Population." *Health Bulletin*:245-249.

McAvoy, R.B. and J.L. Donaldson. 1990. *Health Care for Asians.* Oxford University.

McKeigue, P.M., E.J. Ferrie, T. Pierpoint and G.M. Marmot. 1992. "Association of Early-Onset Coronary Heart Disease in South Asian Men with Glucose Intolerance and Hyperinsulinemia: Project-Report." London: Department of Epidemiology and Population Sciences, London School of Hygiene and Tropical Medicine.

McKeigue, P.M., B. Shah and M.G. Marmot. 1991. "Relation of Central Obesity and Insulin Resistance with High Diabetes Prevalence and Cardiovascular Risk in South Asians." *Lancet* 337:382-386.

Office of the Population Censuses and Surveys 1991. *General Household Surveys.* London: HMSO.

Office of the Population Censuses and Surveys 1990. *Longitudinal Study: Mortality and Social Organization.* Longitudinal Study No. 6. London: HMSO.

Office of the Population Censuses and Surveys 1982. *Socio-Demographical Mortality Differentials.* Longitudinal Study. London: HMSO.

Office of the Population Censuses and Surveys 1980. *Mortality and Geography.* London: HMSO.

Peach, H. 1984. "A Critique of Survey Methods Used to Measure the Occurrence of Osteomalacia and Rickets in the United Kingdom." *Community Medicine* 6:20-28.

Rack, P. 1990. Psychological and Psychiatric Disorders. In R.B. McAvoy and J.L. Donaldson (Eds), *Health care for Asians.* Pp.290-303. London: Oxford University Press.

Ramaiya, K.L., V.R.R. Kodali and K.G.M. Alberti. 1990. "Epidemiology of Diabetes in Asians of the Indian Sub-Continent." *Diabetes Metabolism Reviews.*

Rosenberg, D. 1965. *Society and the Adolescent Self-Image.* Princeton: Princeton University Press.

Scottish Health Statistics. 1990. Information and Statistics Division, Edinburgh.

Shams, M. 1990. "Unemployment and Psychological Well-Being Among British Asians." Unpublished Ph.D thesis. Sheffield, England: MRC/ESRC Social and Applied Psychology Unit.

Williams, R., R. Bhopal and K. Hunt. 1992a. "The Health of a Punjabi Ethnic Minority in Glasgow: A Comparison with the General Population." *Journal of Epidemiology and Community Health*, forthcoming.

Williams, R. 1992b. "Health and Length of Residence Among South Asians in Glasgow: A Study Controlling for Age." *Journal of Public Health Medicine*, forthcoming.

Zung, W.W.K. 1965. "A Self-Rating Depression Scale." *Archives of General Psychiatry* 12:63-70.

10

Hindu Asian Indian Women, Multiculturalism and Reproductive Technologies

Vanaja Dhruvarajan

Introduction

In a recent paper I have argued that for racial minority women in Canada experiences of racism and sexism are equally salient (Dhruvarajan, 1990b). Even though there are some exceptions, most of these women live at the margins of several boundaries. Within their own ethnic group they occupy a position of marginality because of patriarchal bias of ethnic culture. As members of racially stigmatized groups they occupy a position of marginality in the larger society and because of sexism in this larger society, these women share a marginal position along with other women.

The objective of this research project is to examine the lived experiences of first generation Hindu Asian Indian women at this historical juncture. An example of one aspect of reproductive technologies was used to illustrate the experience of racism and sexism. These women were asked to speak to their own lived experiences and state their perceptions and evaluations regarding these issues.

Historically, Asian Indians as an ethnic group have suffered because of racist policies and practices. Studies have documented the prevalence of stereotyped attitudes and opinions regarding Asian Indians (Buchignani and Indra, 1985). Colonial domination of India and the subsequent stigmatization of its culture and people are the major factors leading to these stereotypes. Early immigrants suffered from social isolation, employment and educational discrimination. They were denied rights and privileges of many aspects of citizenship, such as the right to vote until 1947 when India became independent of colonial rule (Bolaria and Li, 1988). Recent studies indicate that Asian Indians experience social exclusion and inequality in employment and educational opportunities and income levels (Driedger and Mezoff, 1981; Buchignani and Indra, 1985; Bolaria and Li, 1988).

The policy of multiculturalism within a bilingual framework promoted by the federal government in recent years is creating conditions to facilitate some cross-cultural understanding. But these policies do not address the issue of racism. The report of the special parliamentary committee, Equality Now, does address these issues but it has not yet resulted in any significant institutional responses (Buchignani and Indra, 1985; Bolaria and Li, 1988).

In addition to these racist policies and practices, Asian Indian women have also suffered from sexist policies and practices. During the early part of this century as Asian men were not permitted to bring their wives and children, women even could not enter as dependent spouses (Bolaria and Li, 1988). In recent decades they have been allowed to immigrate mostly under family class rather than independent class (Boyd, 1986). This has had important consequences for women's lives since many of the privileges such as access to language training and various social services were denied to those who immigrate under family class.

Stereotypes abound regarding the nature and characteristics of Asian Indian women (Naidoo, 1980). These stereotypes are often used to justify the kind of treatment these women get in the larger society (Agnew, 1990). These women are generally thought of as being docile, subservient and reserved, to identify a few stereotypes. As Henry and Tator (1985) argue: economic relations are embedded in social relations thereby impacting on the opportunity structure for minority groups. Ralston (1988) in her study in Halifax documents the experience of discrimination on the part of South Asian women.

It is well documented by studies done within India that Hindu women's lives are circumscribed by patriarchal ideology provided by Hinduism (Dhruvarajan, 1989; Desai and Kirshnaraj, 1987). But it is also documented that there are regional variations in terms of degree of adherence to this ideology (Dhruvarajan, 1990) which has been changing historically (Sengupta, 1974). In addition, it has been shown that Hinduism is not exactly monolithic, and even though the dominant pattern is patriarchal, there are strands of Hinduism which emphasize gender equality (Liddle and Joshi, 1986). Besides, these issues are being actively debated in modern India at the present time (Everett, 1981; Kishwar and Vanita, 1984). Studies done in North America reveal that there is a patriarchal bias in this ethnic culture but the degree and likelihood of adherence to these tenets varies within the ethnic group population (Dhruvarajan, 1992; 1993). In view of these findings, one has to be very cautious about essentializing this ethnic culture in its patriarchal mode.

The example of reproductive technology provides a very good illustration to understand how this ethnic culture is understood and evaluated. More importantly, it provides insights into the way women of this ethnic group are treated. The hope that reproductive technologies provide avenues for all women to better control their role in reproductive activity and thereby have more autonomy in their lives has not been realized. Instead, in a very important sense, reproductive technologies are being used to further the erosion of women's status in society (Overall, 1989). This observation is particularly true for Asian Indian women.

The particular aspect of technology being focused on is the imaging technique of fetal sex determination. An American doctor, John Stephens, has opened a clinic in Washington State close to the British Columbia border and has targeted his services to the Asian Indian community in Vancouver. He justifies his actions by claiming that his services are in demand in this ethnic group because of "cultural attitudes." This action has elicited some controversy from some members of the Asian Indian community. The fear expressed is that knowledge of the fetal sex in the early stages of pregnancy can lead to abortion of female fetuses. There is evidence to suggest that such a fear is justified. Within India, according to some studies, close to 98 percent of the fetuses aborted are female fetuses, indicating a preference for male offspring among Hindu parents (Desai and Krishnaraj, 1987; Manushi, 1990). This practice is justified on religious and economic grounds. The origin of these practices is shrouded in history leading to many speculations. Whatever the source of these preferences may be, the fact remains that at the present time this misogynist practice is prevalent.

While the actions of the doctor in this instance are motivated by personal gains, they are mostly justified on the bases of a woman's freedom to choose and the ethnic group's right to practice its culture under the multicultural framework. But close scrutiny reveals that belief in the woman's freedom to choose is spurious because the prevalent stereotype of Asian Indian woman is that of a docile victim rather than an autonomous agent. The notion of multicultural right deteriorates into a worst form of cultural relativism. It is not motivated by respect for this ethnic culture but rather contempt. This notion is dramatically revealed in a *Globe and Mail* article justifying the doctor's action (December, 1990). The writer of the article maintains "social distance" from the ethnic group and pictures it as the cultural "other." Such a stance helps him to escape from the moral dilemma posed by the doctor's actions. He states dramatically that "their god is not your god" and "they have a right to practice their culture." He further states that the doctor deserves a medal for his actions because it would promote national integration. He states that such an integration would be achieved by the marginalized Asian Indian ethnic group through assimilation into the mainstream as the men from this ethnic group seek brides from the larger society. He maintains that this is bound to happen as supply of females goes down in the Asian Indian ethnic group as more and more female fetuses are aborted. The *Globe and Mail* also published a critical response from the feminist community to the Matheson article (December, 1990). Mainstream feminists, both from the Asian Indian community and from outside this community, jointly wrote the critique.

Except for reports in the news media, there is no systematic data available on the responses of the community to this issue. This study attempts to document the reactions of Hindu Asian Indian women to this situation. Such an effort provides insight into the interaction between the factors of gender, race and ethnicity.

Methodology

Using an interview technique, data for this study were collected from 30 Hindu Asian Indian women living in Winnipeg. These women were chosen from a larger sample of 98 women who were part of survey research conducted earlier. All of them in the sample are married and can be classified as belonging to families from middle or upper middle class. Of the 30, nine women are in professional/managerial type of jobs, 17 clerical/sales and four are homemakers. All of them have at least a high school diploma, the majority of them have at least a Bachelor's degree.

The questions asked pertain to the respondents' attitudes and opinions regarding the issue of targeting Asian Indian women by the American doctor. Questions were also asked to get information about their immigrant experience and experience of racism in the larger society and sexism within their own ethnic group as well as in the larger society.

Findings

Most of these women immigrated to Canada under family class. Many women have had difficulties in adjusting to the new society. Most of them used their ethnic group as support to get themselves established. In the work world, the general position is that one has to make adjustments. Since almost all of them have voluntarily immigrated to Canada, they feel that it is incumbent on them to make the necessary adjustments. The first few years have generally been difficult for most of them but gradually they have learned to cope. In general they do not want to make a big issue of racism in the workplace, neighbourhood or anywhere else.[1] But they do admit to racial incidents in the neighbourhood in relation to their children, to problems with the accreditation of work qualifications from their home country and a feeling of being treated as outsiders in social relationships. Most of their friends are from their ethnic group and they have continued their ethnic lifestyle. They perceive themselves as different from the mainstream culture and choose to keep their style of life private. Relationships with mainstream society are predominantly on a formal level.

Most of them expressed disapproval towards the practice of targetting Asian Indian women to the imaging technique of fetal sex determination. The reaction varied from anger and sadness to general discomfort. They felt singled out and treated like outsiders. Many argued that such a treatment is unfair because preference for male offspring is universal[2] and this preference is as intense among many other ethnic groups such as Chinese and Portuguese.

All of them stated that they themselves do not take advantage of this procedure. Many of them admitted that there is a general cultural bias in favour of male offspring, but stated that there is a variation in the ethnic group regarding the intensity of feeling regarding this matter. Those who are relatively more religious, come from North India, subjected to pressure from older generation, and from rural background, are likely to express such desire more intensely.

Almost all of them were quick to point out that such a preference is more prevalent in India than it is here. It is because the socio-cultural environment in Canada is different from that of India. In India, male children are preferred because in the absence of old age security benefits from the government, sons are the social security for parents in their old age. The family system and system of property inheritance historically has been patriarchal and the system of residence patrilocal. In addition, religious influence in India is stronger and according to orthodox religious tenets, only male children have the right and duty to give oblations to dead parents thereby insuring their safe spiritual journey. The ideal of an extended family system provides conducive conditions for the influence of the conservative older generation. Sons carry the family name forward as the daughters become part of their husband's family after marriage. Under these conditions female children in general are devalued. The dowry system makes the daughters an economic burden for the parents. The expectation of female virginity until marriage adds to the burden of the parents since they are in charge of protecting their daughter's virginity.

In Canada, the family system in general is nuclear and the influence of the older generation is minimal. Canada has old age pension and social security systems available. Here, both daughters and sons can keep their family name. Opportunities for girls are more readily available to become economically self-reliant thereby de-emphasizing the need for a dowry. Besides, the family size is generally small thereby making the family resources available to both sons and daughters. Also, the influence of religion generally is not as strong as it is in India. Under these circumstances the degree of devaluation of female children in Canada is much lower than it is in India.

The best way of getting rid of this misogynist practice, according to the respondents, is to give these families enough time to adjust to the new cultural/social surroundings. The old cultural values take time to change, but given enough time people will adopt new values. Most families do not want to have more than two children - boys or girls. In fact, close to 25 percent of this sample have only one or two daughters. The family has become used to having daughters only and actually most of them consider their families as normal as any other. As one woman with two daughters pointed out, she is not sure whether she would have used the facility if it were available at the time. Because it was not available, they had their two daughters and now they do not think there is anything wrong with it. In other words, they have changed their outlook. But if the facilities were available to identify the sex of the child there would have been no need to re-evaluate their assumptions regarding the need for sons. Therefore the general opinion was that easy solutions to difficult problems should not be provided. People should be left alone to reflect on the old assumptions thereby making room for change. Otherwise the old way of life will continue unquestioned.

Many of them admit that the Asian Indian ethnic culture is patriarchal. They are self conscious about it and agree that it should be changed. In this context, one of the questions asked was whether feminists are of any help at all. There was no consensus among these women with regard to this issue. Homemakers completely rejected feminist interference in family affairs because they are believed to cause more harm than good. Those who are in clerical/sales argue that feminists can help them indirectly to build their self confidence and reduce the degree of guilt they experience when they think of their own personal welfare rather than thinking only of their families.

Those in professional/managerial positions argue that the feminist solutions to women's problems are applicable to white middle class women and they are not helpful to Asian Indian women because these solutions are culture-specific. They believe that Hindu culture is different. Even though Hindu practices have become corrupt, it has solid philosophical foundations for gender equality. The best strategy for Hindu women is to reclaim their lost heritage. They make these arguments on bases such as: (1) the divinity as conceptualized in Hinduism includes both male and female principles. This gives Hindu women an edge by providing symbolic leverage to argue for gender equality. It also gives women self confidence since it insures spiritual equality with men; (2) in the Hindu context, the women's ability to achieve in different fields of endeavour is not questioned. In fact, the men's need to dominate women in the Hindu context is motivated by fear and jealousy rather than contempt; (3) women as mothers are revered. Indeed the principle of motherhood is worshipped. This gives women a special status as mothers. Within the home they have an edge in controlling and directing the course of events. Some of these women actually go to the extent of arguing that it is the men that need reassurance and support which only women can provide.

Family for these women is of paramount importance. Their identity is tied to the role of mother and wife. This is true whether women are doing paid work or not. They consider it as their responsibility to maintain harmony within the home. The division of labour is sex-typed. Husband/father is considered as the head of the household. Caregiving is women's responsibility. They have profound respect for Hindu philosophy and culture. They consider the feminist position as being purely individualistic while they themselves favour familial value orientations. Competition with men is ruled out since they believe that men and women are basically different and should complement each other. The position they take is that men and women are different but equal. Decisions within the family, almost all of them report, are made jointly. Gender equality for Hindu women is not to de-emphasize difference between men and women but to respect the difference and consider both equally valid. Looking at feminists from this vantage point, these women feel very distant from them not only because of racism/ethnocentrism espoused by them but also the kind of feminism they promote.

In day to day life, adherence to ethnic culture varies among these people. In general, they most often practice their religion at least to moderate extent; speak their language at home in addition to English; eat a combination of their ethnic food along with other Canadian varieties; leisure time activities include getting together with friends from own ethnic group, participation in festivals, attending ethnic music concerts, watching ethnic movies; cultivate friendship mostly among members of their own ethnic group; make special efforts to encourage the younger generation to appreciate/respect their cultural heritage. These practices are more strongly adhered to by those who rank high on religiosity.[3]

Discussion

This study clearly reveals that scientific discoveries and inventions do not always promote human welfare. In a sexist and racist social context, it can actually do harm and impede human progress. One cannot put to use these discoveries without carefully evaluating their impact on the well-being of people. In this particular case, the reproductive technology has the effect of buttressing the sexist and racist domination. The assumption that this is a free market economy in a free country and everyone has a right to choose the kinds of services they need is incorrect. Free agency for Asian Indian women is elusive because of the historical legacy of patriarchy. In addition the women themselves may promote such traditions because of their vulnerability within the patriarchal family/culture.

The argument that Canada is a multicultural society and people should be free to practice their culture is, in this context, nothing but the worst form of cultural relativism. The effect of such a stance is not only strengthening patriarchal domination within the ethnic group but also can lead to the erosion of ethnic culture itself. The latter consequence is very probable if the utilization of this technology leads to a shortage of females in this ethnic group. Under such circumstances, the frequency of marrying out of the ethnic group can increase for men due to shortage of women in the ethnic group. This particular position, which at first glance appears to promote multiculturalism, in fact threatens the perpetuation of ethnic culture. As Brah (1992) points out, multicultural stance without addressing racism leads to devaluation of ethnic groups/cultures. This practice is motivated by both sexism and racism. Targetting of this ethnic group for this particular technology is a result of essentializing the culture in its patriarchal mode.

It is true that there are those who condone these practices because a woman's position in the patriarchal family is at risk if she does not bear sons and this service will help her to elevate her own status. Besides, some mothers are reluctant to bring into the world daughters who are not wanted because of the fear that the child may be unloved and uncared for.

It is also true that as first generation immigrants, these women's first loyalty is to their ethnic group/family. They are more concerned about projecting a positive image of their culture rather than addressing the issue of sexism which all of them admit is prevalent. In fact for many of them ethnic culture has become an ego extension.[4] In a society which they perceive as being hostile, their sole support is their own ethnic group, particularly their own family. The position they take is that whatever problems they have should be worked out among themselves. Public laundering of private troubles is considered taboo. But this does not mean that they are unaware of sexism within their culture.

The findings of this study clearly indicate that even though the dominant ethos of this culture is androcentric, the degree of adherence to these tenets varies on the basis of degree of religiosity. The stereotyped images prevalent in Canadian society about this culture is not valid in all cases. In fact, possibilities of transformation of this culture towards an egalitarian mode do exist. In this sample, close to 25 percent of the respondents do not have any sons. All of them consider their families normal even though some had reservations earlier. But if the facilities for sex selection were available, it is difficult to rule out the possibility of their having made use of them. Under the circumstances they have come to accept their situation as normal.

To transform the ethnic culture from patriarchal to egalitarian mode, support systems to strengthen women's claims/voices within their ethnic group must be provided. Such an objective can be achieved by making sure that gender equality rights are not compromised in favour of multicultural rights. This will mean that members of this ethnic group are treated just as everyone else. This will also mean that this ethnic culture is not essentialized in its patriarchal mode. This will strengthen women's claims/voices within the ethnic group because they can invoke the egalitarian traditions of their own culture and justify the position taken by the larger society.[5] Such a stance will mute the voices inspired by androcentrism thereby facilitating the transformation of ethnic culture to egalitarian mode.

Coalition building between mainstream feminists and women of this ethnic background is advantageous to both. Hindu women will get a support system to help them negotiate their way within their ethnic group. For the mainstream feminists to have clout to bring about systemic changes it is important to have a broad based support.

Under current circumstances, coalition building does not seem very promising. Even though there are common interests, these women do not feel a sense of affinity with mainstream feminism/feminists. They not only feel socially distant because of racial/ethnic factors, they also do not identify with the policies/practices espoused by mainstream feminists.

The joint feminist response to the *Globe and Mail* article is an important beginning. But, as Barret and McIntosh (1985) point out, feminist analysis has up to now focused attention on middle class women and that analysis is passed on as being relevant to all women. Racism and ethnocentrism are the most important issues of concern for racial/ethnic minority women. For women of this particular group accreditation of their qualifications, access to language training and welfare of their children in the school system and neighbourhood are some of the most important issues. They are also concerned about the stereotypes that prevail regarding Asian Indian women. As Trivedi (1984, quoted in Barrett and McIntosh, 1985:34) points out, such stereotypes are not in keeping with facts and cause tremendous hardship for these women. In addition, essentializing of this culture in its patriarchal mode tends to have the effect of foreclosing these women's options to negotiate their way within their ethnic group. If these issues are addressed, there is hope for the development of solidarity between Asian Indian women and mainstream feminists, which is in the best interest of both.

Conclusion

It is clear from the above discussion that multicultural policies/practices in a racist/sexist environment reinforce unequal relationships between dominant and minority groups. In this particular context, targetting of Asian Indian women for the reproductive technology of fetal sex determination has the potential of making these women an endangered species and the Asian Indian ethnic culture an endangered culture. Such an environment also precludes development of solidarity among women of dominant and minority groups. It is because ethnocentrism inspired by racism on the part of women in dominant groups maintains social distance from ethnic/racial minority women. For the latter, lack of cultural and economic security leads to defensive ethnic attitudes and exaggerated ingroup positive evaluations. The end result is that under such circumstances, gender inequality cannot be effectively addressed either within the ethnic group or in the larger society.

The findings of this study document the experience of

marginalization for Asian Indian women. They feel alienated and socially distant from the larger society. They have a feeling of being taken for granted within their ethnic group. The general experience of life is that of being isolated and dominated. Addressing racism/ethnocentrism leads to the reduction of social distance for these women with the dominant groups in society, which creates conditions for the development of multicultural attitudes and behaviors on the basis of equality and mutual respect. It also promotes development of solidarity among mainstream and Asian Indian women, thereby creating conditions favourable to addressing gender inequality in the larger society as well as within the ethnic group.

This research project was supported by SSHRCC Small University Grants.

Notes

1. Chan and Helley (1987) had similar findings in their research on Chinese immigrants.
2. Corea (1979) documents the preference for male offspring in North America.
3. Please refer to Dhruvarajan (1992; 1993) for more details regarding these issues.
4. Most of them agree with the dominant ideology which maintains that conjugal relationships are symbiotic. They adhere to the belief in the basic difference between men and women and their complementarity. They also maintain that feminine qualities such as patience, sacrifice, nurturance and tolerance are highly evaluated in Hindu context just as their spiritual equality is unquestioned. Under these circumstances, they can be quite confident about their worth as women. These opinions are echoed in the dominant cultural ethos of Hindu society (Gandhi, 1941). They justify their symbolic allegiance to male hegemony on the basis of women's physical vulnerability, because of their differential role in the reproduction of the species. They strongly believe that the best strategy is to strive to achieve chosen personal goals within this framework. In essence, the objective is to transform the outlook of men as well as women so that they can work together to discharge their relevant duties to society and to each other as well as achieving personal goals. Since familial values are considered as equally binding for both women and men these women think that achievement of equality is possible in this context. Further research is needed to find out whether these women have analyzed the inherent contradictions in the positions they take. At the present time, it appears that they consider this position is most realistic.
5. This process of reclaiming past egalitarian traditions is a complex one. They do not reclaim a particular past tradition but construct a version of the past. Such an effort is often mediated by current needs and circumstances.

References

Agnew, V. 1990. "South Asian Women in Ontario: The Experience of Race, Class and Gender." in *Women Changing Academe*. Edited by S. Kirby et al., Winnipeg: Sororal Publishing.

Arora, U. and A. Desai. 1990. "Sex Determination Tests in Surat." *Manushi*. No. 60.

Barrett, M. and M. McIntosh. 1985. "Ethnocentrism and Social-Feminist Theory." *Feminist Review*. No.20.

Bolaria, B.S. and P.S. Li. 1988. *Racial Oppression in Canada*. Toronto: Garamond Press.

Boyd, M. 1986. "Immigrant Women in Canada." In *International Immigration* by R.J. Simon and C.B. Brettell. New Jersey: Rowman and Allanheld.

Brah, A. 1992. "Difference, Diversity, Differentiation." In *Race, Culture and Identity*. Edited by J. Donald and A. Rattansi. London: Sage.

Buchignani, N. and D.M. Indra. 1985. *Continuous Journey: Social History Of South Asians in Canada*. Toronto: McClelland and Stewart Ltd.

Chan, K.B. and D. Helley. 1987. "Coping with Racism: A Century of the Chinese Experience in Canada." *Canadian Ethnic Studies*. Vol. XIX.

Corea, G. 1979. *The Mother Machine*. New York: Harper and Row.

Desai, N. and M. Krishnaraj. *Women and Society in India*. Delhi: Ajanta Publications.

Dhruvarajan, V. 1989. *Hindu Women and the Power of Ideology*. Granby, Ma.: Bergin and Garvey.

Dhruvarajan, V. 1990a. Religious Ideology and Hindu Women's Roles in India's Modernization Process." *Journal of Social Issues* 46(3).

Dhruvarajan, V. 1990b. "Women of Colour in Canada: Diversity of Experiences." In *Women Changing Academe*. Edited by S. Kirby et al. Winnipeg: Sororal Publishing.

Dhruvarajan, V. 1992. "Conjugal Power Among First Generation Hindu Asian Indian Immigrants in Canada." *The International Journal of Sociology of the Family*. Vol. 22.

Dhruvarajan, V. 1993. "Ethnic Cultural Retention and Transmission Among First Generation Hindu Asian Indians in Canada." *The Journal of Comparative Family Studies*. Vol. XXIV.

Driedger, L. and R.A. Mezoff. 1981. "Ethnic Prejudice and Discrimination in Winnipeg High Schools." *Canadian Journal of Sociology* 6(1):1-19.

Everett, J. 1981. "Approaches to the Women's Question in India: From Materialism to Mobilization." *Women's Studies International Quarterly* No.4:169-78.

ICSSR. 1975. *Status of Women Report*. New Delhi: Allied Publishers.

Gandhi, M. 1941. *To the Women*. Karachi, India: A.T. Hingorani.

Globe and Mail. December 7, 10, 1990. By Graham Matheson and Feminist Response to Matheson respectively.

Henry, F. and C. Tator. 1985. "Racism in Canada: Social Myths and Strategies for Change." In *Ethnicity and Ethnic Relations in Canada*. Edited by R.M. Beinvenue and J.E. Goldstein. Toronto: Butterworths.

Kishwar, M. and R. Vanita. 1984. *In Search of Answers: Indian Women's Voices from Manushi*. London: Zed Books.

Liddle, J. and R. Joshi. 1986. *Daughters of Independence: Gender, Caste and Class in India*. London: Zed Books Ltd.

Liddle, J. and R. Joshi. 1987. "Women of South Asian Origins: Status of Research, Problems, Future Issues." In *The South Asian Diaspora in Canada: Six Essays*. Edited by M. Israel. Toronto: The Multicultural History Society of Ontario.

Overall, C. (ed.). 1989. *The Future of Human Reproduction*. Toronto: The Women's Press.

Ralston, H. 1988. "Ethnicity, Class and Gender among South Asian Women in Metro Halifax: An Exploratory Study." *Canadian Ethnic Studies* XX(3).

Sengupta, P. 1974. *Story of Women in India*. New Delhi: Indian Book Co.

11

Racial and Ethnic Dimensions of Aging: Implications for Health Care Services

K. Victor Ujimoto

Introduction

There are two important demographic characteristics to observe with reference to contemporary Canadian society. First, it is a rapidly aging society. Stone and Fletcher (1980:10) predict that the population over 65 years of age will continue to grow until the year 2016 and Statistics Canada (1990) data tend to support this prediction. Second, the aging population is an extremely heterogeneous one and thus ethnic cultural differences must be taken into account when developing health care services and related policies.

The heterogeneity of our aging population is illustrated in Figures 1a and 1b. A recent report by Samuel (1992) on the demographic projections for the year 2001 provides further support on the changing demographic composition for Canadian society. Samuel's population projections indicate that the Chinese population will constitute 23 percent of the visible minorities, 19 percent for both South Asian and Blacks, 13 percent for West Asians/Arabs, 6 percent for Latin Americans, and 7 percent for others. These projections mean a substantial increase in the so called "visible minority" population. One very obvious implication of all this is that greater consideration must be given to ethnic and cultural sensitivity in health care services as our population ages.

Ethnic and Cultural Factors in Health Care

The importance of examining the ethnic and cultural factors associated with health and health care has been recognized by both social gerontologists and health care professionals in recent years. Ujimoto (1988:220) argues that an understanding of what is meant by ethnicity is crucial to the understanding of ethnic minority attitudes and behaviour towards health and health care services. Ethnic and cultural differences in perceptions of personal health and illness, responses to illness, health status, utilization of services, and coping responses vary considerably, thus rendering a standard regimen inappropriate or ineffective.

Figure 1a. Ethnic Origins, Canada 1986.

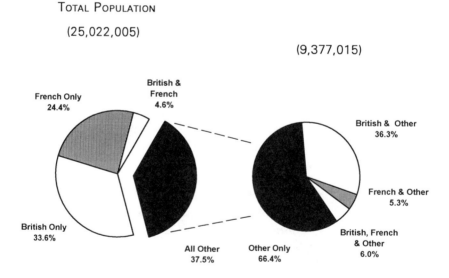

Source: Ledoux, Michel and Ravi Pendakur, *Multicultural Canada: A Graphic Overview*. Ottawa: Policy and Research Directorate, Multiculturalism Sector, Multiculturalism and Citizenship Canada, 1990, p.7.

Figure 1b. Visible Minority Groups, Canada, 1986.

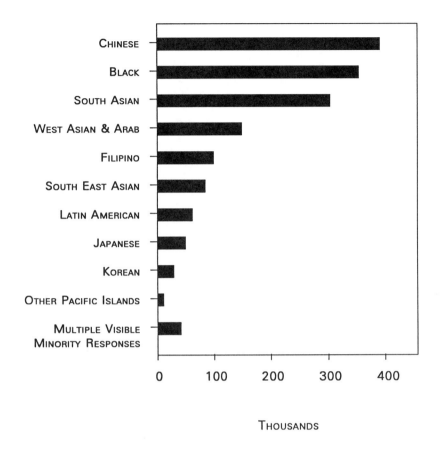

Source: Ledoux, Michel and Ravi Pendakur, *Multicultural Canada: A Graphic Overview*. Ottawa: Policy and Research Directorate, Multiculturalism Sector, Multiculturalism and Citizenship Canada, 1990, p.7.

The influences that ethnic and cultural factors may have on health and health care have been noted by Masi (1988:2173), Llorens (1988), Hikoyeda and Grudzen (1991), Gallagher, Grudzen and Wallace (1989) and more recently by Waxler-Morrison, Anderson and Richardson (1990:4). Masi (1988:2173) argues that "culturally sensitive health care is not a matter of simple formulas or prescriptions that provide a single definitive answer, rather, it requires understanding of the principles on which health care is based and the manner in which culture may influence those principles. That influence may affect or bias physicians, patients, and institutions serving the community." By culture, Masi means the patterns or standards of behaviour that one acquires as a member of a particular group. The standards of behaviour are influenced or modified through one's language use and the values and beliefs held by the individual. Let us briefly examine some of the health beliefs and values held by some ethnic groups to illustrate this diversity.

As Masi (1988:2430) has observed, many of our health beliefs concerning health stems from its relationship to nature or the natural environment. Health and illness are often attributed to natural causes and subsequent treatment is based on "elements or forces of nature." An example that is provided by Masi of a cultural health belief that is often categorized under natural causation is the belief that health is related to weight. Masi notes that this belief probably stems from the fact that in the past, illness was associated with emaciation and malnutrition. Based on this belief, it is observed today that many Italians and Portuguese encourage their children to overeat.

Two sub-categories under the natural classification noted by Masi are what he describes as "harmony" and "wind." Both are based on beliefs which involve the role of nature in health and illness. According to Masi, "Harmony beliefs maintain that the forces of nature in a normal or healthy person are in a state of balance. Health is considered to be the presence of an established harmony and/or balance. Disease is the result of an imbalance of this state." Health beliefs based on the concept of harmony are widely held in some of our ethnic communities and are expressed in a variety of ways.

The health beliefs based on the concept of hot and cold elements are most common in the Hispanic and Chinese communities. The Chinese concepts of *yin* and *yang* reflect the cold and hot elements respectively. As Masi has noted, the terms "hot" and "cold" do not refer to temperature but "to naturally inherent properties of an almost symbolic nature." Table 1 provides examples of various foods and medications that have hot and cold elements.

The hot and cold classifications illustrated in Table 1 are based on common Hispanic beliefs. Those who subscribe to these beliefs consider certain illnesses to be hot and others cold. In Western medical practice, penicillin which is considered to be a hot medicine, is very often prescribed for some illnesses also considered to be hot. Masi notes that a physician may allay the fears of patients who are concerned with the use of a hot medicine for a hot illness by having the patient take the penicillin with a cold food. Masi further notes that patients on liquid diets may refuse cold fruit juices, but will accept hot bouillon.

Table 1. Hot and Cold Classifications*

	HOT	NEUTRAL	COLD
FOODS	ALCOHOL COFFEE PEAS PEPPERS EGGS	CHICKEN RICE POTATOES BEANS	COCONUT BANANA AVOCADO MOST DAIRY PRODUCTS MANY FRUITS & VEGETABLES
STATES	PREGNANCY		POST-PARTUM
MEDICINES	PENICILLIN ASA DIURETICS MOST WESTERN MEDICINES		SODIUM BICARBONATE MILK OF MAGNESIA MANY HERBAL MEDICINES
ILLNESS	CONSTIPATION DIARRHEA ULCERS EAR INFECTION RASHES		ARTHRITIS COLDS MENSTRUAL PERIODS

* BASED ON COMMON HISPANIC BELIEFS.

Source: Ralph Masi, "Multiculturalism, Medicine and Health. Part II: Health Related Beliefs," *Canadian Family Physician* 34(November) 1988:2430.

Another example of a hot/cold health belief held by some members of the Hispanic community and considered to be of clinical importance by Masi is pregnancy. Pregnancy is considered to be a hot experience and thus pregnant women are often advised not to eat foods deemed to be also hot such as pork, peas, pepper and eggs. Thus, prenatal dietary counselling takes on added significance in that the physician must be aware of the cultural health beliefs of the patient. Sensitivity to the health beliefs and needs of the patient can reduce the anxiety or stress level of the patient.

One final observation noted by Masi is that hot/cold health beliefs are not limited to food selections only, but must be recognized in certain patterns of patient behaviour. In order to maintain or restore the hot/cold balance, some patients may be reluctant to wash their hair or to bathe. Again, the physician or nurse must be able to understand why the patient is reluctant to do so.

Similarities in the hot/cold beliefs are manifested in some Eastern cultures as well. The Chinese concepts of *yin* and *yang* correlate with the cold and hot beliefs respectively. In Taoism, the concepts of *yin* and *yang* are gender specific. *Yang* or male positive energy is associated with light, warmth, and fullness. In contrast, *yin* or female negative energy is associated with darkness, cold, and emptiness. It is believed that illness occurs when the *yin* and *yang* forces are not in balance. The *yin* and *yang* classifications are illustrated in Table 2.

Table 2. Yin and Yang Classifications*

	YANG (HOT)	NEUTRAL	YIN (COLD)
ORGANS	GALLBLADDER STOMACH LARGE & SMALL INTESTINES BLADDER		LIVER SPLEEN HEART LUNGS
FOODS	ALCOHOL COFFEE PEPPERS GINGER (&MANY SPICES)	RICE	BEER CHRYSANTHEMUM & MANY HERBAL TEAS WATER CHESTNUTS WATERCRESS TURNIPS CARROTS MELONS HERBAL MEDICINES
STATES	PREGNANCY YOUTH CONSTIPATION DIARRHEA EAR-ACHE FEVERS		POST-PARTUM OLD AGE COLDS ANAEMIA LEUKEMIA SHORTNESS OF BREATH

* Based on common Chinese beliefs.

Source: Ralph Masi, "Multiculturalism, Medicine and Health. Part II: Health Related Beliefs," *Canadian Family Physician* 34(November) 1988:2431.

Aspects of traditional Chinese medicine provides some insights into the health beliefs held by Asian elders. Lum (1988:5) argues that one of the basic beliefs is that there is no dichotomy in mind and body. In examining one's environment, Lum notes that the historical perspective is often used and that there is a need to examine "the internal and external, microcosm and macrocosm, *yin/yang*, positive which is external, and negative which is internal." To complicate matters, the Chinese elderly may associate or describe one's health problem or body condition with reference to one of the five body organs: the liver, heart, spleen, lungs and kidney. For example, "elevated liver fire" refers to a sense of tension or agitation. Reference to a feeling of an injured heart refers to sadness or melancholia. This practice or concretizing one's health problems makes it extremely difficult to provide the most appropriate treatment if the physician is not trained to be culturally sensitive.

Before we conclude our discussion on the harmony aspects of nature and health, it should be noted that the balance between mind and body is also recognized in Western society. Body fitness is often translated into improved mental outlook on life. In North America, the Chinese practice of *tai-chi* has been adopted and is quite popular in training both body and mind to maintain health. Similarly, *yoga* is practised widely as it encourages the development of mind and body in harmony.

In addition to "harmony" as a sub-category of the natural health model noted by Masi, "wind" is the second sub-category. Wind beliefs relate health and illness to air movements. One very common example of this belief is that drafts may cause an illness such as catching the common cold when sleeping near an open window. Masi (1988:2433) observes that many health related beliefs that belong to the wind sub-classification have incorporated the concepts of bacteria or viruses. He provides the following example which relates health or illness to some other external forces other than wind or air movements:

> In Chinese philosophy, the external force was called *ch'i* and was considered to be the basic "energy" of the universe. *Ch'i* would be taken in via the breath and would flow through the body meridians, or channels, as described in acupuncture teachings. It was believed that disruptions of the *ch'i* could upset the harmonious balance of the *yin* and *yang* and lead to illness. Loss of blood results in loss of *ch'i* and can result in either illness or further deterioration of someone already ill.

From the above quotation, it becomes abundantly clear that physicians must understand the fear experienced by some patients when blood samples are required for testing. In such cases, the patient believes that the removal of blood and subsequent loss of *ch'i* can adversely affect one's health. As Masi observes, however, the patient who refuses to allow blood samples to be taken is not challenging the physician's expertise, but merely expressing a fear based on traditional beliefs.

Ethnicity and Aging

Until very recently, the study of ethnic variations in the aging experience has received very little attention in Canadian gerontological literature. Earlier studies that attempted to examine the relationship between ethnicity and aging failed to differentiate between the various meanings usually associated with the term. One of the first attempts to give a conceptual clarification of what was usually meant by ethnicity is provided by Rosenthal (1986:19). From an extensive review of the literature, she derived the following three conceptions of ethnicity: ethnicity as culture, especially immigrant culture; ethnicity as a determinant of social inequality; and ethnicity as synonymous with "traditional" ways of thinking and behaving. As indicated by Rosenthal, each of the above conceptions of ethnicity will lead to a different model of aging of ethnic families because of the differential emphasis placed on the concept. Therefore, she argues for an integrative approach in which connections or linkages between various conceptions of ethnicity can be drawn together in the study of ethnic families. This approach makes considerable sense especially in the study of some ethnic families in which generational cohorts can be identified and thus different conceptions of ethnicity may be applied to each generation.

The first conception of ethnicity as culture, particularly immigrant culture, takes on added significance if we reconsider the demographic changes noted earlier that are taking place in Canadian society. It will be a fairly safe assumption to make that there will always be an immigrant or first generation of various ethnic groups in Canada. Therefore, the conception of ethnicity as immigrant culture requires a clear understanding of the various elements or components that constitute a given ethnic culture. Most definitions of culture include shared meanings (Gordon, 1964; Fry, 1980; Marshall, 1980; Hagedorn, 1986). As described by Hagedorn (1986:36), meanings are usually shared through the various components of culture such as beliefs, norms, mores, values, and symbols.

An interesting point to be made in the definition of culture has been noted by Rosenthal (1986:20), and that is while some definitions of culture include both shared meanings and patterns of behaviour, others do not. For our purposes, however, it will be argued that the various components of culture such as beliefs held, norms, mores, values, and symbols that constitute the shared meanings are only important in influencing behavioural outcomes. The extent to which each component of culture will influence behaviour will depend on the degree of institutional completeness, a term developed by Breton

(1964:193) to describe the extent to which various social organizations were developed in an ethnic community. For example, depending on one's age at the time of emigration, beliefs held by the immigrant were most likely influenced by the earlier socialization processes. The traditional norms or the rules of behaviour ingrained in the immigrant's mind may or may not be reinforced further depending on the size, density, ethnic composition, and the degree of institutional completeness of one's own ethnic community. Similarly, the enforcement of traditional mores and social interaction patterns based on a system of mutual obligations are also most likely to be influenced by the degree of institutional completeness.

Another important argument that is advanced by Rosenthal (1986:20) is that further distinction must be made between ethnic culture and immigrant culture. She argues that "if the conception of culture is limited to immigrant culture, then ethnic variability in family life should decrease over successive, new immigrant generations." While we have implied previously that immigrant culture is a "transplanted phenomenon," to use Rosenthal's term, and that its influence on behaviour will depend on the degree of institutional completeness, it must be underscored that ethnic cultural characteristics continue to exist although in slightly modified forms. Some of these characteristics that impinge on the general health status and well-being of the elderly will be discussed later in further detail.

The second conceptualization of ethnicity as a determinant of inequality by Rosenthal (1986:20) draws attention to the ways in which previous research has tended to equate ethnic group with minority group. While the main focus of current debate has been on the lack of distinction between social class and ethnicity (Holzberg, 1982) as key independent variables to account for variations in aging, there are nevertheless several key factors that are relevant to our present discussion on ethnicity and inequality. Since there are several different forms of inequality in Canadian society, we must be extremely careful in selecting the particular form of inequality that we wish to address, not so much in terms of ethnicity, but with reference to our dependent variable, for example, health status and well-being of our elderly.

The most common form of inequality is economic inequality or the variations in one's income and other material resources. A key to understanding economic inequality with reference to ethnic groups is to understand the long history of exploitation, especially of the immigrant or first generation ethnic group, and in many instances, that of institutional racism (Bolaria and Li, 1988). The adverse effects of institutional racism prevented equal access to many institutions and further increased economic inequality.

Another aspect of continued economic inequality which was deeply rooted in institutional racism was the eventual relegation of some ethnic groups to ethnic minority status. The concomitant effects of economic inequality, deprivation, lack of political power, minority status, and hence social inequality, all contributed to a lack of the individual's sense of who he or she is, that is, of one's identity. The sense of who we are and how we relate to others depends on the position occupied in the Canadian social structure. Another way of looking at this situation is to see which group or groups occupy a dominant position or a subordinate position in terms of influence and decision making. The numerical size of the group, where they are located in territory, their role in the economy, their level of education, and the occupational position held, all tend to influence not only the identity of the ethnic group members, but also the attitudes of the dominant groups towards the minority group. Attitudes in turn govern social relationships and the degree to which meaningful social interaction can take place. The development of one's ethnic identity and the strengths of this identity in relation to the extent of external or societal constraints is a complex issue that requires further investigation.

The third conception of ethnicity advanced by Rosenthal (1986:20) as being synonymous with "traditional" as opposed to the "modern" ways of thinking and behaving is based on several assumptions and misconceptions. As in the first conceptualization of ethnicity as culture, particularly immigrant culture, there is the implicit assumption that the traditional forms of family life and social discourse are retained and that ethnic culture does not change. Thus, there is a very strong tendency for researchers to over-idealize the ethnic family. Cultural change and generational differences in cultural retention have been subordinated or neglected all together. This tendency to both generalize and idealize the ethnic family in traditional family typology stems partly from the inclination to equate ethnic group with minority group and this latter labelling implied that the ethnic group was a relative newcomer to Canadian society. This implication was often based on the lack of appreciation of the history of the ethnic group concerned, which in many instances goes back several generations. By conveniently disregarding the history and social experiences of the ethnic groups in Canadian society, and also by failing to differentiate between various ethnic groups, it was possible to dichotomize ethnicity in terms of the traditional and modern orientations.

While the limitations of conceptualizing ethnicity in terms of the traditional and modern typology may be fairly obvious, it should be observed that the influence of traditional roles and values are still extremely important to our understanding of the variations in aging, health care, and mental health. Furthermore, it will be equally clear that a simple definition of ethnicity will no longer suffice and that we must draw upon several different conceptions of ethnicity in order to capture the dynamics of the aging process as it relates to the health status and general well-being of the elderly. However, before we proceed to examine the relationship between the various components of ethnicity and the social aspects of aging as they relate to health, a brief overview of what is meant by health, health care, and mental health will be provided.

Aging and Health

The well-being of the individual becomes a primary concern especially when one approaches retirement age. A crucial variable in assessing the individual's well-being regardless of one's age is health. What is meant by health? Shanas and Maddox (1985:701) note that the health in the aged is usually defined in terms of the presence or absence of disease, or in terms of how well the aged are able to function. The determination of one's health in terms of the presence or absence of disease is usually considered to be an objective assessment of health because it is based on medical examinations and laboratory tests to confirm the medical diagnosis. However, Shanas and Maddox (1985:701) note that a truly objective measure of health is difficult to achieve, and that the administration of the laboratory test to measure health varies from time to time. They provide, as an example, physiological measures such as blood pressure readings and glucose levels.

An alternative way to define health among the elderly suggested by Shanas and Maddox (1985:701) is based on how well the elderly is able to function in terms of day to day activities. They argue that the various things that the elderly can do, or think that they can do, are useful indicators of not only their health, but of the kinds of health services that they may require. This functional approach to the assessment of one's health is of particular importance especially with respect to ethnic minorities because it assumes that "both the individual and the physicians may have relevant and possibly conflicting information about health status" (Shanas and Maddox, 1985:701). Such conflicting information may easily occur as a result of different perspectives or different cultural perceptions of a given health condition. For example, symptoms such as a headache may be attributed to a particular disease by an ethnic elderly, however, this same symptom may be completely disregarded by the doctor as a sign of old age. Such a problem in the interpretation of the symptom may be doubly troublesome because various ethnic groups have different levels of pain threshold (Hayashida, 1984).

An excellent overview of the literature on recent trends in viewing the health status of the elderly from several different perspectives, as well as from several different levels of function, is provided by Shanas and Maddox (1985:703). They draw our attention to the growing acceptance and merging of the medical and functional models of health assessment especially by those in geriatrics. To underscore this latter observation, they quote the following from the World Health Organization:

> It is now accepted by the medical profession that morbidity should be measured not only in terms of the extent of the pathological process but also in terms of the impairment of the function in the person affected by a pathological condition . . . . Functional diagnosis is one of the most important elements that has been introduced in geriatrics. In this approach a distinction is made between an impairment and a disability caused by a pathological condition.

The utility in employing both models of health assessment becomes evident when we consider the distinction that is made between an impairment and a disability. From the World Health Organization report, Shanas and Maddox (1985:703) note that impairment is "a physiological or psychological abnormality that does not interfere with the normal life activities of the individual." They further note that disability is "a condition that results in partial or total limitation of the normal activities of the individual." It is important to keep these distinctions in mind when considering the health status of aged ethnic minorities. Some types of impairment may eventually result in disability.

While the physiological or physical aspects of aging are important considerations in terms of the functional capabilities of the elderly, it is also important to examine the effects of aging on one's mental health. In order to study the psychological aspects of aging, it is necessary to have an understanding of exactly what is meant by mental health. D'Arcy (1987:425) defines mental health as

> a state in which a person demonstrates his competence to think, feel and (inter)act in ways that demonstrate his ability to deal effectively with the challenges of life. The mentally healthy person is accepting of himself, able to give as well as receive in relationships and, having realistically evaluated his assets and liabilities, has an appropriate level of self confidence, making decisions based on sound judgement and accepting responsibility for his actions.

There are several key components in the above definition that merit our attention particularly with reference to ethnicity and aging. One such component concerns the individual's ability to think. As noted earlier in our discussion on ethnicity and its synonymity with traditional ways of thinking, it is quite conceivable that misunderstandings can occur if the traditional cultural backgrounds of the ethnic groups are not understood. Social behaviour as outward manifestations of the thinking process may often be interpreted as "bizarre" when it may be considered "normal" in one's own cultural group. Another important component which is noted in D'Arcy's definition of mental health is the ability to deal effectively with various day to day situations in life. As noted elsewhere by Ujimoto (1987a:131), there is accumulating evidence that coping plays a central role in reducing stress-related illnesses and in promoting good health. The coping strategies utilized by the elderly who have different socio-demographic characteristics are particularly relevant to the study of aging and health because constant psycho-social adjustments must be made throughout one's lifespan. Therefore, an understanding of the cultural context in which these adjustments occur is very important.

The final component of D'Arcy's definition of mental health that will be briefly discussed here concerns the types of social relationships that can realistically occur given the limited assets and resources of the elderly. The study of social relationships in terms of the cultural context in which they occur requires an understanding of the social exchange mechanisms of the particular group. For example, in the case of the elderly *Issei* (immigrant or first generation Japanese Canadian) and *Nisei* (second generation or Canadian born), it has been observed by Kobata (1979:100), Nishio and Sugiman (1983:19) and Ujimoto (1987a:116) that traditional Japanese values influence generational relationships. Intergenerational relationships based on a system of mutual and moral obligations as well as on social customs may be applicable only to certain groups, and at the same time, there may be less importance placed on them by subsequent generations. Social relationships based on concepts such as filial piety and familial dependency in old age are other factors that may intervene in social relationships depending on the ethnic group.

From our brief discussion of the three key components crucial to the definition of mental health provided by D'Arcy, it can be hypothesized that the negative effects of daily life situations will impact more severely on the mental health of recent immigrants to Canadian society than on subsequent generations. The recent arrivals to Canada are the ones who will experience the greatest changes in mental health because of value conflicts and other adjustment difficulties to their new environment. Support for this observation is provided by Kuo and Tsai (1986:133) who have documented that "an excessive amount of social stress among immigrants - resulting from social isolation, cultural conflicts, poor social integration and assimilation, role changes and identity crises, low socioeconomic status, and racial discrimination - has led to a high prevalence of ill health and psychological impairment among them." The plethora of factors that impinge on one's mental health are extremely difficult to disentangle. As Chappell, Strain and Blandford (1986:37) have noted, "Changes in mental health as we age are less straightforward. Mental health encompasses numerous aspects, including cognitive, psychological and emotional functioning. It is known to be related to both physiological conditions and social environments." At present, the social environment of aged ethnic minority groups is a relatively unexplored area of study.

Aging, Ethnicity and Health

While there are several recent Canadian publications on aging and health, for example, Simmons-Tropea and Osborn (1987:399), D'Arcy (1987:424), Connidis (1987:451), Marshall (1987:473), Chappell (1987:489), Schwenger (1987:505), and Shapiro and Roos (1987:520), the cultural variations in Canadian society and its implications for the future health care provisions of aging ethnic minorities are not considered. Since this is an important area of study, it is just beginning to receive more attention. As noted by Chappell, Strain and Blandford (1986:30), "the relevance of subculture (ethnic, minority and racial) for the elderly population and, in particular, for the provision of health care is an under-researched area in gerontology. Even though conceptually and theoretically it has been argued that subcultural cohesiveness is likely to result in more social support for its elderly members, this has not been established empirically."

One recent study that examined the relationship between aging and health as interpreted through culture is the study by Rempel and Havens (1986). In this study, they identified the differential perceptions of health of older persons based on twelve different ethnic groups in Manitoba. The Rempel and Havens (1986:18) data analysis indicates that ethnicity and education affect health perception. They note that the Asians and northern Europeans have the highest positive rating of their own health and the middle eastern and eastern Europeans the poorest health. Because of the small sample size for each of the ethnic groups represented in the sample, caution must be exercised in interpreting the data. The study is nevertheless useful as it suggests several new avenues for future research.

An area of study in health behaviour that is rapidly gaining attention concerns stress and coping behaviour. One study that examines the relevance of ethnicity in relation to stress and coping, particularly with reference to the minority elderly, is the study by Wong and Reker (1985:29). In their comparative study of elderly Chinese and Anglos, Wong and Reker were interested in determining how the Chinese and Anglos differed in their coping behaviour. The three categories of coping strategies that they examined were as follows:

1. Internal strategies are one's own instrumental efforts.
2. External strategies include various forms of dependence on others to reduce stress.
3. Palliative strategies are ways of coping that make one feel better without solving the problem.

Analysis of the Wong and Reker (1985:33) data revealed the presence of several stress producing health problems. In addition to arthritis or rheumatism, eye problems, and other health disorders, other stressful factors that influenced the well-being of the elderly included in-law problems, loss of a spouse, worries about the family, and economic problems. On the basis of their data analysis, Wong and Reker conclude that the "Chinese did not report having more problems, but they perceived their problems, especially the general problem of aging, as more serious than Anglos." The authors note that in addition to the normal biological constraints of aging, there are other compounding factors associated with the minority status of the Chinese aged such as "a language barrier, lack of information, and fear of racial discrimination."

In terms of coping strategies, Wong and Reker (1985:33) found that the Chinese relied more on external and palliative strategies than the Anglos. Although the Chinese relied more on external help, it is noted that the source of the outside help came primarily from family members and relatives. The Chinese also tended to reminisce and seek refuge in the past rather than attempting to solve a given stress situation except in coping with health related problems. Wong and Reker suggest that "Chinese elderly not only experience more stress, but possess less adequate coping resources." Since the aged Chinese were all first generation or immigrant Chinese while the Anglos were either born in Canada or were long time residents, the results are perhaps not too surprising. However, they do point out the concerns and health care needs of the first generation ethnic minority, and therefore, future health care policies should not be based on the common assumption that the aged are homogeneous.

A recently completed research project on the well-being of the aged Asian-Canadians included the coping inventory developed by Wong and Reker (1983, 1984) noted above. This project by Ujimoto, Nishio, Wong and Lam entitled, "Comparative Aspects of Aging Asian-Canadians: Social Networks and Time Budgets," examined the cultural aspects of ethnicity in relation to the allocation of time to various daily activities. By utilizing time-budget data, those activities most predictive of well-being were determined. A description of this research is provided elsewhere by Ujimoto (1987a:130 and 1990a: 381). Both time-budget and social network data enable us to differentiate between those individuals who rely upon external resources in order to cope with a stress situation rather than on internal strategies.

The Ujimoto, Nishio, Wong and Lam (1993) national survey also obtained self-reported data on health satisfaction by Chinese, Japanese, and Korean Canadian elderly. In their data, it was shown that a high proportion of respondents were satisfied with their health. The Chinese respondents appeared to be the most satisfied, followed by the Japanese, but the Japanese elderly tended to have the highest mixed feelings about their health compared to the Chinese and Korean elderly. Of those respondents who were dissatisfied with their present status, the Koreans were the most dissatisfied.

The relatively high percentage of Korean elderly who were dissatisfied with their own self-assessment of health appears to be in contrast to earlier studies which indicated that Koreans were well-adjusted. In a study by Kim and Berry (1986) that assessed the mental health of Korean immigrants who resided in Toronto, they found that the Koreans scored low on the Cawte Stress Scale and also on the Mann Marginality Scale when compared to other groups undergoing acculturation in Canada. Kim (1987) argues that these findings are consistent with several other studies. He notes that several factors may account for the successful adaptation of Korean immigrants. First, Kim states that since Koreans were voluntary migrants, their mental health status would be better than for others such as refugees. Second, Kim notes that the Koreans have developed better coping skills to deal with stressful life events. A third factor is that the Canadian government selection criteria are such that only the highly educated and those with occupation skills are chosen to immigrate. Finally, the relatively high degree of established Korean community institutions and the policy of multiculturalism both encourage Korean immigrants to retain their cultural identity. How can we account for the relatively high degree of dissatisfaction reported by the Korean elderly?

In terms of the possible contradiction between our data and the previously reported findings, caution must be exercised in interpreting and comparing data. By utilizing the standard stress and marginality instruments, it is conceivable that fairly consistent results can be obtained. However, if we attempt to seek health information from the Korean health professionals themselves, a much different picture emerges. Kim's (1987) intensive interviews with medical and social support staff revealed that the Koreans tended to internalize their problems, thus making it difficult for health care personnel to assess the real problems.

Kim (1987) reports that the Koreans do not want to admit that they are sick, or to show any signs of weakness and that they tend to somatize their illnesses because of the stigma attached to psychological illnesses. Korean doctors have reported to Kim that much of the Korean illnesses are psychological and stem from loneliness, depression, and anxiety. These, in turn, further aggravated the existing somatic problems. These illness characteristics and behaviour are not limited to the Korean elderly, but are very often manifested by other Asian Canadian elderly, particularly the first generation. Indeed, Liu (1986) notes that "somatization is culturally sanctioned in Chinese society, it is an adaptive coping response that allows the person to escape stigmatization." Our data from the Ujimoto, Nishio, Wong and Lam study indicates that the highest degree of self-reported health dissatisfaction is by the first generation and the most satisfied are the second generation and *kika-nisei.*

The dissatisfaction expressed by the elderly Korean and Chinese women may stem from the fact that both Chinese and Korean women immigrated to Canada as "captive immigrants," a term used by Kim to describe Korean parents or grandparents who came to Canada because of their sense of responsibility towards their family. In a Korean household that operates a small business or has dual income earners, the baby-sitting role is most often provided by the parents or grandparents. This appears to be the only role given to the elderly Koreans, thus compounding their sense of anxiety and depression. Such a limited role does not provide the elderly with the opportunity to become fully integrated into Canadian society. Kim (1987) notes that the Korean elderly are totally dependent on their children or grandchildren and that "they do not have the cognitive and social skills to participate in the larger society and their adjustment is limited to the ethnic pockets."

Cultural Factors and Aging

One of the key cultural variables that requires examination is the degree of obligations as perceived by the children towards their parents. The concept of filial piety has its roots in Confucianism and involves several types of obligations. According to Osako and Liu (1986:130), the child must obey his or her parents, support them in old age, and must succeed in one's career to bring honour to parents and ancestors. What happens then, when children do not fulfil the filial roles as expected by their parents? As a partial response to this question, it is suggested that intergenerational conflict is one possible outcome, and in those situations where conflict appears to be minimized, it is the parents who internalize their feelings and suffer the consequences in silence. This tends to be the case for elderly immigrants who arrived more recently than for those immigrants who have become acculturated to Canadian societal norms.

The data from the study by Ujimoto and colleagues (1993) revealed variations in responses to the question "What aspects of your cultural heritage do you feel have enabled you to grow old successfully?" Twenty-five percent of the Korean elderly indicated filial piety as the key cultural variable for successful aging. This contrasts with the Chinese and Japanese elderly respondents of whom 12.2 percent and 7.1 percent respectively had indicated filial piety. The Korean elderly also indicated that pride in their cultural heritage was important. It should be observed here, however, that the Koreans are the most recent immigrants to Canada among the Asian elderly studied here. This means that most of the socialization had taken place in Korea and thus it can be argued that there is a relatively strong attachment to traditional Korean values. For the Chinese, they tend to fall between the Korean and Japanese responses.

An extremely high percentage of Japanese elderly indicated that discipline and perseverance were important cultural factors that contributed to their successful aging. The Japanese term *gaman* was most frequently cited. According to Kobata (1979), *gaman* is literally translated as "self-control." The outward manifestation of this is the tendency to suppress emotions, whether they be positive or negative. In traditional Japanese society, *gaman* was seen as virtuous and Kobata argues that "the tendency to suffer in silence with a great deal of forbearance provides some insights into the nature of the family as the source for dealing with problems rather than the outside service providers." It is not surprising, therefore, to find that the Japanese elderly have the highest percentage of mixed feelings regarding their own evaluation of health. Both dissatisfaction and satisfaction appear to be suppressed in comparison to the Korean and Chinese elderly.

Associated with the concept of *gaman* of self control is *enryo*. According to Kobata, "the norm of *enryo* includes, but is not limited to, reserve, reticence, self-effacement, deference, humility, hesitation, and denigration of one's self possessions." Because of the plethora of terms that can be associated with *enryo*, it is extremely difficult to assess the well-being of the Japanese elderly. As Kobata notes, "the concept had its origins in the cultural norm of knowing one's position in relation to another when interacting with the others perceived as 'inferior' or 'superior' to oneself." Thus, in interactions with authority figures, for example doctors, the Japanese elderly very often do not volunteer their true feelings on how they feel. How can researchers differentiate empirically whether it is *gaman* or *enryo* or both that are operating in order to account for the lack of interaction? This is an extremely crucial aspect to understand if health care providers are to provide effective care. Our data revealed that 15.7 percent of the Japanese elderly respondents and 6.2 percent of the Korean respondents indicated that *enryo* or reserve was a negative aspect of their culture that impacted on their well-being. This is particularly true in health care settings in which those who are able to complain the loudest very often receive the most care.

More and more research on various aspects of aging and health are being reported in the literature. However, future studies will have to examine the influence of ethnicity on aging and health in greater detail. As reported by Ujimoto (1987a:117), difficulties with language and the inability to express one's innermost feelings by aged immigrants erect formidable barriers that prevent easy access to the available social, economic, and health support services. Whether it is the lack of health services available in one's own language or the cultural and psychological barriers that prevent ethnic minorities from utilizing various services, the net result is under-utilization of existing health services and facilities by ethnic minorities. Chan (1983:43) found that although the Chinese elderly women in his study were generally aware of medical and dental services in the Chinese community, they were unaware of other services and resources for the elderly available at other institutions and agencies outside of their own Chinese community.

While the under-utilization of health care services by various ethnic groups have been noted by Wong and Reker (1985:33), Rempel and Havens (1986:9), and Ujimoto (1987a:117), this is an aspect of aging, ethnicity, and health research that requires a controlled study to determine the reasons why this may be so.

Summary and Conclusion: Implications for Health Care Services

In this chapter, two important characteristics of contemporary Canadian society were observed. First, it was noted that the population of Canada is aging rapidly, and second, that it was a demographically heterogeneous population. Recent immigration trends tend to indicate that new immigrants from non-traditional source countries will continue and thus contribute even further to the heterogeneity of Canadian society. The most important implication of all these changes concerns the ethnic and cultural factors related to health beliefs and health care.

It was argued that health care providers must recognize and understand the variations in health beliefs, attitudes, and behaviour of our multicultural society, most particularly, the aging ethnic minorities. For the well-being of those who experience a combination of adjustment and health problems, a culturally sensitive health care system will provide some relief to the mental stress experienced in daily life.

An important aspect of coming to terms with a culturally sensitive health care system requires a knowledge of the diverse health beliefs held by many people. In particular, recent immigrants to Canada who were educated and socialized in Africa or in Asia are most often faced with language difficulties as well as differences in customs when communicating with persons in authority such as nurses and doctors. One way in which cultural misunderstandings can be reduced is to enable health care professionals to recognize the non-verbal aspects of communication in health care. This requires a greater sensitivity to the cultural dimensions of how illnesses are viewed in different ethnic groups. Barriers to communications must be reduced and this implies a continuing course of action for both patients and health care providers to learn what some of the cultural barriers to communication might be.

In addition to having a firm understanding of cultural barriers to communications, it is essential to know some of the traditional concepts associated with health beliefs such as *yin* and *yang*. In prescribing medication or food to combat illness, an understanding of the hot/cold classifications of health beliefs may prove to be positive in improving the health status of Hispanic and East Asian patients who may still cling to traditional beliefs.

The different meanings associated with ethnicity were also discussed in this chapter. Conceptions of ethnicity as traditional ways of thinking and behaving are most often associated with first generation immigrants and thus can not be generalized to all members of a given ethnic group. Intergenerational variations within an ethnic group may provide just as much diversity as between ethnic groups depending on the degree of assimilation and acculturation to Canadian society.

In terms of future research directions, it is necessary to secure adequate empirical data which differentiate health care needs for various ethnic groups. With the increasing heterogeneity of Canadian society, it is no longer appropriate to classify our research sample in the most convenient categories such as "Anglophones," "Francophones" and "Others." Precise differentiation of our research sample based on appropriate sample size will most likely provide much more valuable data upon which future studies can be based, either for baseline studies or for comparative longitudinal studies. Unless valid data are secured at the outset, effective methods of health care to address ethnocultural health needs will not be attainable. Furthermore, health care as well as health policies based on limited data will most likely result in a very wasteful use of limited resources. Alternative methods of less expensive health care may be possible if we examine how some ethnocultural groups deal with non-prescription and OTC (over the counter) drugs for certain illnesses.

The imposition of more ethnocultural health care information alone on the already over-burdened health care providers will not provide an easy solution to all of our health related problems. It is absolutely crucial that future health care services take advantage of the available health science and social science information and information technologies. Information technologies will facilitate the storage and retrieval of cross-cultural research information on illness and health. Perhaps the time has arrived to seriously consider establishing a central ethnocultural information resource centre to facilitate the sharing of ethnocultural health information.

Although the ethnic variable was emphasized in this chapter in order to illustrate the cultural diversity of Canadian society, it must be underscored that our aging population reflects the diversity of Canadian society as a whole. This diversity stems not only from ethnic and language differences, but also from socioeconomic status, religion, and Canadian regional differences. It does not take a visionary to foresee the implications of this diversity for social policy and programs. The urgent need for various social institutions in Canada to respond to the ever increasing diversity indeed provides an extremely interesting and worthwhile challenge.

References

Bass, S.A., E.A. Kutza, and F.M. Torres-Gil (Eds.). 1990. *Diversity in Aging: Challenges Facing Planners & Policymakers in the 1990s.* Glenview, Illinois: Scott, Foresman and Company.

Bolaria, B.S. and P. Li. 1988. *Racial Oppression in Canada.* (2nd edition) Toronto: Garamond Press.

Breton, R. 1964. "Institutional Completeness of Ethnic Communities and the Personal Relations of Immigrants." *American Journal of Sociology* 70: 193-205.

Chappell, N., L.A. Strain and A.A. Blandford. 1986. *Aging and Health Care.* Toronto: Holt, Rinehart and Winston.

Chappell, N. 1987. "Canadian Income and Health Care Policy: Implications for the Elderly." In V.W. Marshall (Ed.), *Aging in Canada.* Toronto: Fitzhenry and Whiteside.

Chan, K.B. 1983. "Coping with Aging and Managing Self-Identity: The Social World of the Elderly Chinese Woman." *Canadian Ethnic Studies* Xv(3): 36-50.

Connidis, I. 1987. "Life in Older Age: The View from the Top." In V.W. Marshall (Ed.). *Aging in Canada.* Toronto: Fitzhenry and Whiteside.

D'Arcy, C. 1987. "Aging and mental health." in V.W. Marshal (Ed.). *Aging in Canada.* Toronto: Fitzhenry and Whiteside.

Fry, C.L. 1980. *Aging in Culture and Society.* Brooklyn, New York: J.F. Bergin.

Gallagher, D., M.R. Grudzen and M. Wallace (Eds.). 1989. *Creative Coping with Caregiving: Clinical and Policy Making Areas.* Stanford: Stanford Geriatric Education Center.

Gordon, M.M. 1964. *Assimilation in American Life.* New York: Oxford University Press.

Hagedorn, R. 1986. *Sociology.* Toronto: Holt, Rinehart and Winston.

Hayashida, C. 1984. "Extending the Medical Center to a Multi-Ethnic Aging Population with Long-Term Care Needs." Paper presented at the 37th Annual Scientific Meeting, The Gerontological Society of America, Texas.

Hikoyeda, N. and M. Grudzen (Eds.). 1990. *Traditional and Non-Traditional Medication Use Amons Ethnic Elders.* Stanford: Stanford Geriatric Education Center.

Holzberg, C.S. 1982. "Ethnicity and Aging: Anthropological Perspectives on More Than Just the Minority Elderly." *The Gerontologist* 22: 249-257.

Kim, U. and J. Berry. 1986. "Predictors of Acculturative Stress: Korean Immigrants in Toronto, Canada." In *Ethnic Minorities and Immigrants in Cross Cultural Perspectives.* edited by L.H. Ekstrand. Lisse: Swets and Zeitlinger.

Kim, Uichol. 1987. "Illness Behaviour Patterns of Korean Immigrants in Toronto: What are the Hidden Costs?" In K. Victor Ujimoto and Josephine Naidoo (Eds.). *Asian Canadians: Contemporary Issues.* University of Guelph.

Kobata, F. 1979. "The Influence of Culture on Family Relations: The Asian American Experience." In P. Ragen (Ed.). *Aging Parents.* Los Angeles: University of Southern California.

Kuo, W.H. and Y. Tsai. 1986 "Social Networking, Hardiness and Immigrant's Mental Health." *Journal of Health and Social Behavior* 27, June: 133-149.

Lam, L. 1982. "The Chinese-Canadian Families of Toronto in the 1970's." *International Journal of Sociology of the Family* 12: 11-32.

Ledous, Michel and Ravi Pendakur. 1990. *Multicultural Canada: A Graphic Overview.* Ottawa: Policy and Research Directorate, Multiculturalism Sector, Multiculturalism and Citizenship Canada.

Liu, W.T. 1986. "Culture and Social Support." *Research on Aging* 8, 1: 57-83.

Liu, W.T. 1986. "Health Services for Asian Elderly." *Research on Aging* 8, 1: 156-175.

Llorens, L.A. (Ed.). 1988. *Health Care for Ethnic Elders: The Cultural Context.* Stanford: Stanford Geriatric Education Center.

Lum, O. 1988. "The Clinician's View of Ethnogeriatrics." In L.A. Llorens (Ed.). *Health Care for Ethnic Elders: The Cultural Context.* Stanford: Stanford Geriatric Education Center, 4-7.

Marshall, V.W. 1980. *Last Chapters: A Sociology of Aging and Dying.* Monterey, California: Brooks/Cole.

Marshall, V.W. 1987. "The Health of Very Old People as a Concern of Their Children." In V.W. Marshall (Ed.). *Aging in Canada.* Toronto: Fitzhenry and Whiteside.

Masi, R. 1988. "Multiculturalism, Medicine and Health. Parts I-III: Multicultural Health Cate." *Canadian Family Physician* 34: 2173-8; 2429-34; 2649-53.

Masi, R. 1989. "Multiculturalism, Medicine and Health. Parts IV-VI: Individual Considerations." *Canadian Family Physician* 35: 69-73; 251-4; 537-9.

Moon, S.G. 1982. "Adjustment Patterns Among Koreans in Canada." In Chang, Yunshik, Tai-Hwon Kwon and Peter J. Donaldson (Eds.). *Society in Transition with Special Reference to Korea.* Seoul: Seoul National University Press.

Nishio, H. and P. Sugiman. 1983. "Socialization and Cultural Duality Among Aging Japanese Canadians." *Canadian Ethnic Studies* 15(3): 17-35.

Ory, M.B. and K. Bond (Eds.). 1989. *Aging and Health Care: Social Science and Policy Perspectives.* London: Routledge.

Osako, M.M. and W.T. Liu. 1986. "Intergenerational Relations and the Aged Among Japanese Americans." *Research on Aging* 8(1): 128-155.

Rempel, J.D. and B. Havens. 1986. "Aged Health Experiences as Interpreted Through Culture." Paper presented at the Canadian Sociology and Anthropology Association Annual Meeting, Winnipeg, Manitoba.

Rosenthal, C. 1986. "Family Support in Later Life: Does Ethnicity Make a Difference?" *The Gerontologist* 26(1): 19-24.

Rothwell, T. and D. Phillips (Eds.). 1986. *Health, Race & Ethnicity.* London: Croom Helm.

Samuel, John T. 1992. *Visible Minorities in Canada: A Projection.* Toronto: Canadian Advertising Foundation.

Schwenger, C.W. 1987. "Formal Health Care for the Elderly in Canada." In V.W. Marshall (Ed.). *Aging in Canada.* Toronto: Fitzhenry and Whiteside.

Shanas, E. and G.L. Maddox. 1985. "Health, Health Resources, and the Utilization of Care." In R. Binstock and E. Shanas (Eds.). *Handbook of Aging and the Social Sciences.* New York: Van Nostrand Reinhold.

Shapiro, E. and N.P. Roos. 1987. "Predictors, Patterns and Consequences of Nursing-Home Use in One Canadian Province." In V.W. Marshall (Ed.). *Aging in Canada.* Toronto: Fitzhenry and Whiteside.

Simmons-Tropea, D. and R. Osborn. 1987. "Disease, Survival and Death: The Health Status of Canada's Elderly." In V.W. Marshall (Ed.). *Aging in Canada.* Toronto: Fitzhenry and Whiteside.

Statistics Canada. 1984. *The Elderly in Canada.* Ottawa: Minister of Supply and Services Canada.

Statistics Canada and Department of the Secretary of State of Canada. 1986. *Report of the Canadian Health and Disability Survey 1983-1984.* Ottawa: Minister of Supply and Services Canada.

Statistics Canada, Housing, Family and Social Statistics Division. 1990. *A Portrait of Seniors in Canada.* Ottawa: Minister of Supply and Services.

Stone, L. and S. Fletcher. 1980. *Canada's Older Population.* Montreal: The Institute for Research on Public Policy.

Toumishey, H. 1991. *Cultural and Racial Sensitivity: Implications for Health Curricula.* Toronto: Canadian Council on Multicultural Health.

Ujimoto, K. Victor. 1987a. "The Ethnic Dimension of Aging in Canada." In V.W. Marshall (Ed.). *Aging in Canada*.

Ujimoto, K. Victor. 1987b. "Organizational Activities, Cultural Factors, and Well-Being of Aged Japanese Canadians." In D.E. Gelfand and C. Barresi (Eds.). *Ethnicity and Aging: New Perspectives*. New York: Springer Pukblishing Company.

Ujimoto, K. Victor. 1987c. "Variations in the Allocation of Time Among Aged Japanese Canadians." In Karen Altergott (Ed.). *Daily Life in Later Life: A Comparative Perspective*. Beverly Hills: Sage Publication.

Ujimoto, K. Victor. 1988. "Aging, Ethnicity and Health." In B.S. Bolaria and H.D. Dickenson (Eds.). *Sociology of Health Care in Canada*. Toronto: Harcourt Brace Jovanovich.

Ujimoto, K. Victor. 1990a. "Time-Budget Methodology for Research on Aging." *Social Indicators* 23: 381-393.

Ujimoto, K. Victor. 1990b. "Health Care Issues For an Aging Multicultural Society: A Role for Information Technology." Paper presented to the House of Commons Standing Committee on Health and Welfare, Social Affairs, Seniors and the Status of Women. In *Minutes of Proceedings and Evidence of the Standing Committee on Health and Welfare, Social Affairs, Seniors and the Status of Women*, Issue No. 18, March 8.

Ujimoto, K. Victor, Harry Nishio, Paul T.P. Wong, and Lawrence Lam. 1993. "Cultural Factors Affecting Self-Assessment of Health Satisfaction of Asian Canadian Elderly." In R. Masi, L. Mensah and K.A. McLeod (Eds.). *Health and Cultures: Exploring Relationships*. Oakville, Ont.: Mosaic Press.

Verma, Ravi, Kwok B. Chan, and Larry Lam. 1980. "The Chinese-Canadian Family: A Socio-Economic Profile." In K. Ishwaran (Ed.). *Canadian Families; Ethnic Variations*. Toronto: McGraw Hill, 138-156.

Waxler-Morrison, N., J.M. Anderson and E. Richardson (Eds.). 1990. *Cross-Cultural Caring: A Handbook for Health Professionals in Canada*. Vancouver: University of British Columbia Press.

Wong, P.T.P. and G.T. Reker. 1983. "Face Validity of the Coping Inventory." Paper presented at the 12th Annual Meeting of the Canadian Association on Gerontology, Moncton, N.B.

Wong, P.T.P. and G.T. Reker. 1984. "Coping Behaviours of Successful Agers." Paper presented at the 30th Western Gerontological Society Annual Meeting, Anaheim, California.

Wong, P.T.P. and G.T. Reker. 1985. "Stress, Coping, and Well-Being in Anglo and Chinese Elderly." *Canadian Journal on Aging* 4: 29-37.

Yu, Elena S.H. 1986. "Health of the Chinese Elderly in America." *Research on Aging* 8, 1: 84-109.

12

Service Providers' Perceptions of Immigrant Well-Being and Implications for Health Promotion and Delivery

Alexander M. Ervin

Introduction

My goal here is to discuss some of the factors related to the health or well-being of immigrants in a much more holistic framework than it is normally conceived. This wider "casting of the net" has implications for health promotion and delivery in the contexts of communities and non-government organizations (NGOs), rather than leaving them as the primary or exclusive domains of medical professionals and agencies. Also, the chapter makes policy suggestions and considers health promotion within the complex framework of programming devoted to the resettlement of government-sponsored immigrants or refugees. For more perspectives on that more general process, readers might want to consult works by Bai (1992) Buchignani (1988), Chan and Indra (1987), Dorais (1987), Ervin (1991) Gilad (1990) and Taylor (1991).

In order to develop these health promotion themes, I will report on some preliminary, but relevant, findings from an ongoing research project that is being done on behalf of the Saskatchewan Association of Immigrant Settlement and Integration Agencies (SAISIA).[1] The research examines what people consider the significant "indicators" of immigrant "adaptation" and "integration." These concepts are central to the federal government's policies and programming directed to immigrant resettlement. Integration implies the capacity to freely participate in the Canadian society and economy, and adaptation suggests factors of personal adjustment to conditions of the host environment and the immigrant experience — ranging from climate, diet and values, to social relations and many other things. To date, indicators — social, medical, and economic — have been primarily quantitative and have been the subject of some general criticisms for their sometime superficiality or misrepresentation (see also, McKillip, 1987; Van Dusen and Parke, 1976), while at the same time being considered valuable potential tools for policy formulation, when they are made more sophisticated and accurate reflections of well-being.

In this regard, "front-line" workers, at immigrant settlement agencies (an NGO sector), have felt that policy makers and program evaluators at departments like the Canada Employment and Immigration Commission have been placing too much emphasis on economic indicators (e.g., how many weeks it takes for government sponsored immigrants to enter the work force) as measurements of both integration and adaptation. So, the research project was commissioned to gain a wider perspective on the whole gamut of important resettlement factors, taking into account what could be considered qualitative or more "subjective," yet highly germane "indicators."

Besides presenting some of these "indicators," I will also discuss them in the context of a literature that is informative of health delivery and promotion issues for ethnic minority populations in Canada. Overall, the implications relate mainly to psycho-social and mental health factors, but aspects of health delivery and promotion relevant to biomedical concerns can be derived from this discussion. And as Beiser (1991:7) points out, physical and psychological distinctions are more likely "in the minds of service providers than their clients." Finally, as emerging from the literature and my own experiences of practice and research (see also Ervin, 1991; Welin and Ervin, 1991), I will suggest some policy and research directions.

The total project itself is too multifaceted, regarding research questions and methodologies, to discuss here. Suffice it to say that it involves over 120 people (primarily immigrants from over thirty nationalities and ethnic groups, but also some service providers) and it utilizes four methodologies — key-informant interviews, focus groups, a likert-scaled questionnaire, and a Delphi panel.

For this discussion I will present the findings from the Delphi questionnaire, not only because that component is complete, but because its findings, derived from experienced immigrant service providers, are self-contained and rich in understanding of the processes and contexts of immigrant resettlement and well-being.

The Delphi Questionnaire: Its Purpose, Methodology and Participants

Our Delphi posed a single question: "What do you feel are the most important indicators of successful adaptation and integration for immigrants and refugees in Saskatchewan?" The participants were chosen on the advice of the three member agencies of SAISIA (the Regina, Saskatoon and Yorkton Open Door Societies). They were asked not to represent policy aspirations of their own agencies, but to reflect upon their own perceptions as service deliverers and, when relevant, as immigrants themselves.

The panel members were first asked to provide a list of the most important indicators. The researchers then standardized the phrasing of overlapping or identical indicators. Participants were then asked to choose the top fifteen in rank order from the composite list (numbering over 80) and provide supporting comments. The results were sent back to them and they were asked if they wished to change any of their responses, add any further comments, or indicate their satisfactions. Altogether, the process took three months. (For more details on the methodology of Delphi questionnaires or conferences, see Delbecq et al., 1975 and McKillip, 1987.)

Twenty-two service providers from Yorkton, Saskatoon and Regina were contacted and nineteen cooperated with full participation. Twelve were female and seven were male, ages ranging from twenty-nine to fifty-nine. Twelve were Canadian born (usually of European descent), while seven were immigrants. The nationalities of the immigrants included: 1 Indian; 1 Swiss; 1 Cambodian; 2 Vietnamese; 1 Latino; 1 Eritrean. Most were well-educated, with post-secondary and professional certification predominating.

All of the participants work directly with immigrants, most as paid workers, but several as knowledgable board members with settlement agencies. Those working outside of settlement agencies included an employee of the Canada Employment and Immigration Commission, a doctor, a medical secretary, an accounting clerk, a race relations program coordinator, a clergyman, coordinators of English as a Second Language (ESL) programming at a community college and at a university.

The Results

The scores were determined by giving those indicators in the first position 15 points, those in the second position 14 points, and so on, so that indicators ranked in the last position (i.e., 15th) would receive a single point. The total points allotted to each indicator produced a raw score. Those indicators having higher *raw scores* represent the indicators perceived by the respondents as having higher priorities. The *range of scores*, as well as the actual number of votes each indicator received, demonstrates how the perception of such indicators fluctuates among the participants involved. These data are summarized in Table 1. (For a detailed list of the range of scores for each indicator, and a composite of verbatim responses given by the respondents in support of these indicators, see Note 2). To preserve space and allow for the amplification of a discussion of health implications, I have included only the first 15, rather than all 56. It should be noted that consensus and patterning starts to break down at this point anyway.

It must also be conceded that if the Delphi questionnaire had been administered to a different panel we would not have achieved precisely the same rankings and weightings. However, it is quite likely, given its potential members' parallel and expert familiarity with immigrant resettlement, that the first ten to fifteen issues would have arisen. The overall patterns of ranking and identifications probably would have been similar.

Although 40 percent of the respondents are immigrants themselves, it must be remembered overall, that the opinions expressed are those of service providers rather than immigrant clients *per se*. We are currently testing these indicators, along with another six derived from a set of focus groups, with a total of 50 immigrants. The immigrants themselves may, for instance, place more emphasis on jobs and other matters. Also, if we had involved more service providers employed at multicultural associations, we may have had more emphasis placed on cultural persistence and heritage languages.

Furthermore, those familiar with immigrant resettlement know that it is a very complicated process. Needs and indicators will vary with individuals and factors of age, sex, ethnicity, cohort or "vintage" of arrival, education and many other factors. Timing, and consideration of what needs or markers have already been accomplished (family reunification, acquiring jobs and second language competency, etc.) will all have different importances for individuals at different times in their developmental cycle as adapting and integrating individuals. Also, most of these indicators are inextricably linked in actual context, so they cannot be so easily detached as they are here.

Nonetheless, I am convinced that these indicators are very effective and useful perceptions. They are important for those wishing to gain knowledge of the resettlement process and they also have significant implications for health promotion and delivery for immigrants.

Table 1. Fifteen Most Important Indicators of Successful Adaptation and Integration of Immigrants and Refugees - by Rank Order.

Indicators	Raw Scores	Number of Votes	Range of Scores[1]
1. Ability to speak and listen in English and to be able to understand the subtleties of ordinary and slang English	181	13	(13, 15)
2. Maintaining or establishing a functional, harmonious family life	135	14	(2, 13)
3. A sense of well-being, optimism (good mental health as well as a general sense of physical well-being	129	11	(4, 15)
4. Settlement in a safe, permanent home or apartment and acquiring satisfactory household goods	121	10	(8, 15)
5. The willingness to accept available as well as suitable employment	104	11	(4, 14)
6. Capacity to make friends in the host as well as the ethnocultural community	93	11	(5, 14)
7. Being able to support oneself and/or one's family	91	13	(1, 13)
8. Being able to adjust to life and culture in Canada and to know what is acceptable and ordinary	86	14	(2, 14)
9. To have skills for finding and acquiring employment	86	8	(1, 15)
10. To have proficient and non-verbal communication skills relevent to the host culture	83	6	(12, 15)
11. The gaining of suitable employment and feeling comfortable at work, as well as showing the capacity to advance in career	81	7	(5, 15)
12. To maintain self-confidence, a positive self-image, and pride in oneself	76	9	(5, 12)
13. The capacity to show realistic expectations for oneself and others	73	9	(3, 12)
14. Has capacity to make use of community support services such as medical and legal facilities on his/her own	70	8	(4, 13)
15. A good knowledge of community, including awareness of community services and resources	57	9	(3, 10)

[1] For a detailed range of scores for each indicator and composite of verbatim responses in support of each indicator, see Note 2.

Implications of the Findings for Health Delivery and Promotion

There was no surprise in the first place ranking for "the ability to speak and listen in English and to be able to understand the subtleties of ordinary and slang English." That need can be considered in conjunction with the tenth indicator focusing on "proficient non-verbal skills relevant to the host culture." It is obvious and highlighted in practically every review of immigrant settlement (see also Dorais 1987; Ervin et al., 1991; Report of the Task Force on Mental Health Issues Affecting Immigrants, 1988), yet it is still highly important. Communication skills are enormously complicated; the lack of them can lead to various forms of isolation — physical, social, economic and emotional — that can have negative health consequences. Wood (1988: 13) draws our attention to a literature linking schizophrenia, depression, and "behavioural deviance" among children, with some immigrants not being able to speak the host language, thus highlighting language competency as one risk factor. Similarly, the lack of communication skills, involving both patients and medical practitioners, could create significant dissonance (including misdiagnosis, subsequent non- or inaccurate compliance, etc.) in the clinical encounter, even when interpreters are present (see also Beiser, 1988:207).

Beyond that, any set of programming directed towards health promotion will depend on effective communication to immigrants, as individuals, and through families, natural networks, and community-based ethnocultural associations. Among individuals and groups, language skills vary considerably with our more recent, primarily non-European immigrants. Accordingly, there has been a growing recognition of the need to extend language programming with the current redesign of federal ESL programming oriented toward including more types of eligible immigrants and increased instructional periods. But the ultimate need — that of individual, competency-based instruction — may never be achieved.

Another set of indicators relates to employment and the fulfillment of basic material needs, providing the security for any subsequent attention to more psycho-social needs and other important things like reunification with immediate and extended family members. The cluster incudes "housing" (number 4) and several directly associated with employment — "the willingness to accept available as well as suitable employment" (number 5); "achieving financial independence from security supplements (being able to support oneself or family)" (number 7); "having skills for getting employment" (number 9); and "the gaining of permanent jobs that suit the skills of the individual" (number 11).

The service providers suggested that housing needs related to health, security and safety, more or less tend to be satisfactorily met in the Saskatchewan context. On the other hand, considering health holistically and in multisectoral context, employment and financial security weigh very heavily upon immigrants, and have health seeking implications. Just as one dimension, consider the following:

> ... many immigrants working in low paid, menial jobs do not have the benefits other Canadians take for granted. Many work in non-unionized jobs and get paid for the hours they are actually on the job. These factors add to the stresses of illness. From their reports, economic factors are usually paramount in the lives of many immigrants, and influence illness management and help-seeking. For example, failure to keep clinical appointments or to buy medicines could be the result of economic rather than ethnocultural factors (Anderson et al., 1990: 248).

In her review, Wood (1988:15-19) points out that occupational status (especially the household head's) has been directly associated with sense of well-being after several years of resettlement. Overall, she reminds us that satisfactory employment in the country of resettlement correlated more with emotional well being than other important factors such as pre-migration stress and family separation. Effective employment readiness programming, recertification and retraining programs as well as coherent job development strategies, should remain very high on the resettlement policy agenda.

Another cluster relates to psycho-social senses of identity, empowerment and generally being in some degree of realistic control over their lives. These would include "a sense of well-being" (number 3) as related to health, as well as "overcoming cultural shock and becoming steadily familiar with Canadian culture ; self-confidence and a positive self-image" (number 12); and "realistic expectations" (number 13).

The relevance of these psycho-social factors to health and well-being should be obvious. But attention should be drawn (Wood, 1988:17) to the importance of realistic expectations of future lives in the host country as indications of who is going to adapt more successfully as compared to those who are overly optimistic at the beginning. Many settlement workers have told me of having to deal with the anger, depression, and disillusionment of immigrants who have thought that Canada would be immediately able to provide a new prosperous life for them.

Another set relates to social support and social skills including "a functional harmonious family life" (number 2); "a social network and support system that includes people from the host as well as the ethnocultural community" (number 6); and "capacities to independently and effectively operate within the community no longer relying on the settlement agencies" (numbers 14 and 15).

Again, there are many implications to this cluster. A massive literature reinforces the perception that effective social support tends to be positively associated with well-being and health (see also Fuchs, 1991:147). As Fuchs (1991:155-156) also points out, immigrants require support networks that include balanced portions among the family, ethnocultural networks and "communities" and the general host community, in order to draw upon the socio-emotional and instrumental resources needed for well-being.

The indicators that came in at the second and third rankings — "family harmony" (number 2) and "a sense of physical and mental well-being or health" (number 3) — have the most significance for health promotion.

Regarding family, and using Vietnamese-Chinese as an example, Chan (1984:259) suggests that concerns about it are central to the refugee experience. The truncation of the family with significant loved ones still in the home country, or their whereabouts unknown, is a source of vulnerability with regard to physical and mental illness. This relates to the loss of social support and important confidants since their presence serves as a "buffer" with regard to such vulnerabilities (Chan, 1984:265). In his view, finding ways to reinforce, or reconstruct, such natural support systems should be central to any resettlement process (Chan, 1984:267).

Family relations have very complicated implications as buffers against, or as conduits for, poor health. Men and women may go through different adjustment processes in resettlement. For example, changing gender roles in Canadian society are significant in this regard. Although highly controversial, numerous people have suggested to me that spousal and child abuses need to be carefully studied with regard to immigrant contexts, recognizing that they are very serious health problems for the general population as well. Resettlement and economic stress; cultural antecedents regarding gender roles; and many other complications need to be unravelled in their appropriate contexts.

Another set of family problems can come about with growing communicative distance and conflict among generations within families. One of our focus groups stimulated a very lengthy and poignant discussion among middle-aged immigrants from Latin America, Northeast Africa, the Middle-East and Southeast Asia. The core of their anxiety related to the fact that they had sadly accepted a view of reality that they may not ever have the qualifications for full-time, satisfactory and secure employment in Canada. But, they felt that their long periods on social assistance or unemployment insurance were detrimental to their being effective role models for their children. In our current, unfinished questionnaire, 31 out of 47 immigrants (representing 30 ethnicities) agreed, or strongly agreed with the statement, "immigrants need more counselling and programs related to family problems." Only one disagreed and fifteen were neutral.

Wood (1988:33) suggests that family therapy, rather than individually focused treatment seems quite logical for immigrants. On the positive side she reminds us that the family, extended and nuclear, is probably the "most common coping mechanism for immigrants, enabling them to deal with normal life-crises in familiar ways." Beyond these considerations, most health promotion strategies that are developed for immigrants, should be directed towards families as natural units. Even further, there may be some need to reconsider all of the settlement programming and counselling, somewhat away from age and gender separation, and, instead, plan them more in holistic and familial contexts.

Most directly relevant to the health promotion and delivery themes is indicator number three — "a sense of well-being, optimism (good mental health) as well as a general sense of physical well-being." The service providers recognize that, although immigrants and refugees are resilient people, accumulated stresses from the home country and countless adjustments to the host context, can bear heavily on the health of immigrants. They feel that in order to effectively reconstruct their lives in Canada and to integrate satisfactorily into the Canadian job market, immigrants need to achieve a sense of optimism well-being and health.

With regard to the service providers perceptions of health and family harmony needs ranking above employment training and jobs, an informal conversation I had with several of them, along with a few immigrants, suggests that there might be some minor debate here. Immigrants might consider that, instead, the first priority would be to relieve major stresses by getting satisfactory work and that would subsequently improve their health and outlook. Service providers might argue that one has to be in the right state of mind in order to get the right job. Of course, the resolution of this "chicken and egg" type of controversy need not be precisely defined by ranking and obviously both fronts can and should be tackled at the same time.

It does remind us, though, that we should always be vigilant about an exclusive reliance on expert or normative opinion. Furthermore, many medical anthropology texts (see also Foster and Anderson, 1978:41) remind us that there are countless variations of cultural definitions of health and that many peoples will not necessarily define varied symptoms or syndromes such as trachoma, congenital hip dislocations, lower back pain, and other symptoms of illness or health problems, because they are very prevalent and sometimes considered normal patterns of life experience in their biocultural and ecological contexts. All of these latter sorts of realities remain to be negotiated among immigrants and health promoters in the Canadian context. People will only respond to what they genuinely consider to be health problems.

Beyond the fifteen core indicators that I have chosen to discuss, many of the other forty-one also have non-specific health implications. Before concluding this section I would like to mention one that has significant and direct health implications — "a capacity to adapt to the food habits of the host country" (number 47). It is likely that many of the ethnic diets, imported with immigrants, are in fact, as much or more healthy than "Canadian" regimes (for instance, as related to cardiovascular risk factors). However, in some cases the ingredients, marketing arrangements (supermarkets, secondary processing and packaging, etc.), along with some culturally-based misunderstandings can lead to undesirable situations. A number of years ago the Saskatoon Open Door Society started a nutritional class, with day care facilities, directed towards a particular ethnic group. Some mothers in that group had been reported as feeding their infants and toddlers 4-10 tablespoons of sugar a day in the hopes of having them grow up to be as large as Canadians. Members of this particular group tend to be quite a bit smaller than Euro-Canadians, and the foods available and their packaging are radically different from rural-based traditional, peasant markets in the tropical home country. These and many other potential dissonances need to be examined in the context of viable health promotion programs.

Policy Implications and Suggestions for Further Research

My major suggestion, influenced by a decade of association with immigrant settlement agencies as well as various research projects, is that much of the efforts of health delivery and health promotion could be effectively implemented at the settlement agencies themselves or at the facilities of multicultural councils and ethnocultural associations. Settlement workers and counsellors, as a result of on-the-job experience, generally have developed a fair amount of valuable and irreplaceable cross-cultural sensitivity that is otherwise difficult to train for. Furthermore, there are usually well trained, intelligent and effective outreach workers at each of these agencies representing the major ethnicities being served. Generally speaking, these settlement and outreach workers, as well as all the people who conduct direct services could be more formally trained in the procedures for health referrals and in the identifications of primary symptoms especially as they are relevant to mental health. Clinics and health assessments could be held at the agencies, because in many cases the immigrant clients feel more comfortable at the settings where there are already attempts to assess the needs of the "whole person" and trust has already been established.

Overall, there is a need at such settings, as one-stop resource centres, to refine and constantly improve capacities in individual and family assessments relating to a multitude of factors related to needs of economic, social and medical natures (see also Anderson et al., 1990; Welin and Ervin, 1991).

Clinics, when established, could be of the "walk-in" variety and they would have physicians, nurses and counsellors who are well-trained in cross-cultural sensitivity as well as the practical aspects of ethnomedicine. Clinics could be attached to the settlement agencies and multicultural centres, as mentioned, or they could be adjuncts of existing community clinics. It is exceptionally hard to generalize and we have very little systematic empirical information about health care utilization among the various ethnic groups and nationalities. But it could very well be that, in many cases, immigrants are not used to making appointments with family physicians but would be more inclined to seek emergency or *ad hoc* treatment and advice at such facilities. Incidently, depending on immigrant population sizes and resources available, such clinics need not be full-time, but instead strategically scheduled at appropriate hours, such as shortly after school or work.

With regard to general health promotion, there is a desirability to extend existing outreach services. An augmentation and further professionalization of outreach workers at settlement agencies would be productive. Settlement agencies frequently employ a small number of outreach workers, usually on a temporary basis (due to constraints of short-term government funding programs) from the most numerous ethnicities being settled in the community. These people are essential in primary resettlement (see also Crossley, 1991) which usually takes about one month and is focused on such things as getting appropriate clothing, housing and household goods. But beyond this period many immigrants may never again be in contact with the agencies. That may mean adaptation and integration is taking effect satisfactorily. But we do know that in many cases there are many significant problems and needs that are not being attended to.

Besides more effective delivery of services in the generic domain of adaptation and integration an enhanced cadre of properly trained outreach workers would likely be very useful as brokers of health promotion at individual, family and ethnocultural association levels. Supplemental to this suggestion is the possibility of mobilizing the efforts of immigrants with valuable medical experience from their home countries but who have not been able to gain Canadian credentials.

Emerging from the Delphi, from focus groups and preliminary results from another questionnaire, is the perception of a somewhat urgent need for effective family programming and counselling designed for immigrants. These might be delivered at the settlement agencies themselves or more collaborative programming and counselling arrangements could be made with local family service bureaus. A number of years ago when I did a community needs assessment for our local United Way (Ervin et al., 1991), I was surprised to find out that our local family service bureaus had very few Native or immigrant referrals and that they had no special programs available for them. In one sense this was understandable given the heavy case loads and waiting lists for the beleaguered social workers and counsellors. But obviously, given its importance in this survey and comments made by the immigrants themselves, much has to be done to effectively develop services and understandings in this domain.

Beyond these dimensions of service delivery there are a vast number of basic research questions that have to be addressed for effective community-based, health promotions serving our very diverse immigrant populations. I can only mention a few here. What are the modalities of "health-seeking" behaviours that are typical as well as being variable within such populations? They should be placed within the context of factors like explanations of illness; definitions and formulations of health (which have largely been elusive); ways of legitimizing sick roles and the ranges of illness behaviours and other topics appropriate to the study of ethnomedicine. Of particular interest here might be a detailed consideration of immigrant cultural views of prevention obviously for the design of promotion and prevention strategies that are more isomorphic with such views.

Fundamental to any consideration of health promotion, especially as it pertains to ethnically diverse peoples, is a consideration of the usual ways of communicating within immigrant social networks and communities. Clearly, the specifics of public health strategies and directives will be more effectively delivered through natural lines of communication and when couched in "discourses" or styles more familiar and acceptable to those being reached. We have barely begun this task. (Overall, for more discussion of similar dimensions see Allodi, 1984; Beiser, 1988, 1991; Chan, 1984; Ervin, 1991; Report of the

Canadian Task Force on Mental Health Issues, 1988; Wood, 1988; Waxler-Morrison et al., 1990). It should be noted that Waxler-Morrison and colleagues (1990) provide useful elaborations on the specifics of potential cultural clashes in clinical contexts.

Conclusions

It is difficult to conclude this paper because there have been so many complex but relevant issues that have not even been raised (e.g., racism, the appropriateness of immigration and multicultural policies), let alone the further implications and cautions regarding the findings that I have presented here.

Let me just point out three very broad concerns relevant to the underdeveloped domain of health promotion for immigrants in Canada. The first is that the well-being, or physical, psychological, spiritual and social health of immigrants, along with their capacities to freely integrate and adapt, will very much depend upon effective, holistic, comprehensive and multi-sectorial strategies of partnership. These would involve the host communities in terms of individuals agencies, services and programs, and the immigrants themselves as individuals, networks and associations. The indicators, as presented in this paper, and policies and programs emerging from their recognition will be significant in efforts to promote immigrant well-being and health. But even though they are already very broad and sometimes non-specific in scope, they cannot be separated from yet even larger political economic considerations of the structure and directions of Canadian society. Power, economic planning, regional disparities, demographics, racism and class variables must be included in discussions of this domain.

Second, health promotion, in terms of more directed strategies (such as dealing with nutrition, stress-reduction, transmittable diseases, etc.), will also have to be constructed with a much fuller understanding of the needs, factors and variables associated with immigrant well-being. For instance, immigrants may sacrifice personal long-term health and well-being by staying at health threatening or stressful jobs in order to accumulate sufficient savings to be able to sponsor the immigration of relatives from the home country. At the very least, on one level, that can be considered as a very rational health-seeking behaviour. Beyond situational, cultural and socio-economic factors relevant to each immigrants' background and point in time, more basic knowledge is required regarding expectations and the flows of communication in order to design effective but flexible health promotion strategies relevant to particular communities and the immigrants living there.

Third, as related to flexibility, the details of strategies of health promotion for immigrants must be formulated at the community level, rather than being "top-down" standardized formulations from federal and provincial departments of health. What works in Toronto or Ottawa may not work in Saskatoon. Realities, resources, special needs and strengths can be so variable in different communities, even with the same ethnic groups. Yet at the same time, the documentation of case studies, focused on health promotion emerging from these diverse settings will be essential in our constant need to improve health promotion for our multicultural populations. Our work has just barely begun.

Notes

1. I would like to acknowledge the valuable logistic advice of Michael Hanna (executive director) and Louise Welin (community programs coordinator), both of the Saskatoon Open Door Society. The research was funded through a small grant from Multiculturalism and Citizenship, Canada, and administered through the Saskatchewan Association of Immigrant Settlement and Integration Agencies. Randy Belon, a graduate researcher, effectively assisted the author with the Delphi questionnaire in the Spring and Summer of 1992.

2. **Indicator 1. RANGE OF SCORE** - 13, 13, 14, 15, 15, 15, 13, 14, 14, 13, 15, 13, 14. COMMENTS: Communication (including non-verbal communication) is the most important skill needed in all areas of adaptation and integration. People who can communicate in the mainstream language are better equipped to handle all the other areas of their lives in a new culture. An important factor in learning a language is the ability to listen. Listening will teach the learner many aspects/nuances of the new language - regardless of the personal ability to learn languages. To be able to communicate by listening and speaking, to be able to understand the ordinary person in an ordinary situation is imperative. To be at ease with the common person and interact socially creates a bonding and acceptance in human relationships. This does not happen over night, especially for someone with no English whatsoever. Nevertheless, this need must be met with priority. Failure to give quality language training to new residents promotes isolation and, eventually, friction. In Saskatchewan, this must come before other adaptation and integration processes can be met. Once this barrier is surpassed, life in general becomes easier and employment is then viewed as a more hopeful possibility.

   Indicator 2. RANGE OF SCORE - 11, 3, 12, 12, 2, 12, 12, 7, 10, 9, 6, 13, 12, 14. COMMENTS: This is an inclusive or general statement which may include such things as finding suitable daycare, harmonious roles, good communication within the home (and with schools, etc.). Maintaining or establishing a functional family life is probably the best support system for anyone. For the majority of people, their family is the first and, at times, only supportive feature and centre point of their lives. This provides a base of security and well-being which permits a person to go forward in other areas outside the family (education, vocation, social). A functional harmonious home is an indication of adjustment and general happiness of all family members.

However, the stresses of the process of migration itself often causes such strain and discord that the family may even break apart. If there is no happiness or harmony in one's family, then the purpose of coming to a new country will fail. There is a general need for counselling, support, and stress management skills for families and singles who have been dislocated from their families as a result of the migration process. This does not mean, however, that we should be assisting singles in pursuits to form families.

Indicator 3.   RANGE OF SCORE - 12, 4, 13, 11, 15, 13, 15, 11, 13, 12, 10.
COMMENTS: Mental and physical health are often measures or indicators of stress involved with adaptation. Physical and mental problems may accompany immigrants to the host country, but are apt to be exaggerated when coupled with the new culture, new climate, new language, new mores, and different educational, financial and legal systems. A sense of general physical and mental health is necessary to cope with adjustments and pressures that confront the immigrant during the integration process. This is an area that affects all aspects of one's life. A sense of well-being is the ultimate achievement because it indicates an absence of negative stress and possibly a satisfaction with general, current situations. Not everyone is able to manage to have this kind of mental attitude, though. Ensuring that good support systems exist would be very helpful to settlement in Canada.

Indicator 4.   RANGE OF SCORE - 11, 14, 10, 13, 8, 11, 15, 10, 15, 14.
COMMENTS: This is a very stabilizing factor. The privacy and security of having one's own home (or apartment) plays an important role in settlement. A lot of people have not had a permanent, safe home and have only a few possessions. Basic needs (i.e food, shelter, etc.) must be met before moving forward to adaptation and a home can provide a safe, nurturing environment in which to foster individual and familial social needs. The emphasis on 'satisfactory goods' is somewhat less important than housing. As well, this indicator is linked with health and financial indicators. Some feel it is important to have settlement near one's own ethnic area. However, cautions arise regarding turning hotels and reception houses into 'mini refugee camps' prior to satisfactory settlement. Both satisfactory housing and household goods are available in Saskatchewan.

Indicator 5.   RANGE OF SCORE - 14, 12, 11, 13, 12, 14, 14, 14. COMMENTS: This is key. We cannot even guarantee every current resident of Canada a job in the field that most interests them. Immigrants must not be led to expect an employment opportunity that is not really available. It is important for the newcomer to realize and understand that their skills, education or occupation may not necessarily be absorbed immediately into the work force. The ability to accept available as well as suitable employment will encourage or help the newcomer to adapt to the new country, to meet and socialize with Canadians when the opportunity presents itself and finally, to hear about other possible and better employment - using improved or new skills learned on-the-job. That is, realistic expectations and a plan of action will enable the immigrant to integrate into the Canadian fabric in a timely process. Unrealistic goals and inflexibility can increase the stress levels of the newcomers. This may in turn have a spiral effect on the mental health of the immigrant as well as the family unit.

Indicator 6.   RANGE OF SCORE - 10, 7, 11, 14, 3, 9, 5, 6, 13, 4, 11. COMMENTS: This is an extremely important indicator which helps to avoid ghettoization and promotes equal opportunity and participation in all aspects of life. To feel part of a society one needs to feel comfortable enough to interact with the peoples of that society/community. This indicates a healthy acceptance of both the past and current cultural experiences, and is important to help a person understand the mentality of the community. This makes one feel at home in the country and not like an 'alien'.

Indicator 7. RANGE OF SCORE - 9, 12, 6, 6, 10, 5, 1, 11, 13, 1, 7, 7, 3. COMMENTS: This indicator goes beyond simply using banking services, etc. to include one's total ability to handle money - i.e., the economics of the individual and the household. The meeting of basic material needs is necessary before the individual(s) can identify and fulfil other psycho-social needs ultimately leading to self-worth/dignity, independence and pride in accomplishments. This could only help the newcomer to feel assured about the future in Canada - a definite asset to successful settlement in their new home-country. This is not, however, an easy indicator to meet given the scarcity of jobs. It was indicated that this is not an essential indicator given the numerous social assistance services which are available. However, in most countries in the world it is still shameful to accept money from the government and a person who cannot support himself/herself and the family is a failure and a burden on society. Accepting financial assistance is a serious blow to the self-esteem and puts a person into the category of "those who milk the system."

Indicator 8. RANGE OF SCORE - 2, 14, 4, 9, 14, 8, 4, 2, 2, 3, 9, 2, 10, 3. COMMENTS: Knowing what is acceptable and ordinary in Canada is always very confusing. It takes time but this type of orientation is viewed as very important to newcomers, as it aids the next generation in adjustment. Simply coming to a new country as a tourist can be traumatic, but when one is coming to live, there must be a psychological acceptance of that fact - this acceptance can be crucial in the initial settlement phases for the newcomer. Further, in order to integrate, an individual would have to be cognizant of Canada's acceptable life and culture - knowledge of the 'acceptable' behaviours eliminates many obstacles and misunderstandings. Successful integration is nearly complete as the immigrant has accepted adjustments to life and culture, recognizes what is acceptable, ordinary, and can react appropriately to various situations.

Indicator 9. RANGE OF SCORE - 1, 12, 10, 14, 10, 13, 11, 15. COMMENTS: The Canadian way of finding and acquiring employment may vary from the immigrant's previous experience. For many immigrants the competitive job search is very difficult. To be able to reach the goal of employment one must have job search skills. Job skills are further desirable as they may lead to a sense of economic and personal achievement through financial independence and an improved self-image. Any employment preparation or job-finding program should always be seeking to equip the participants for independence, rather than continuous dependence upon an agency.

Indicator 10. RANGE OF SCORE - 13, 14, 14, 15, 15, 12. COMMENTS: Non-verbal language is just as important as words. Studies show that more communication is non-verbal. Movements of face and body do not universally mean the same - not even a friendly smile. Knowledge of non-verbal communication shows that a person is learning about the mainstream culture and the people. This also aids them in integration. Without proficient language skills, individuals can become ghettoized at home and in various job situations. Language skills are required to access the labour market, to access community support services and enable one to understand the host's laws. Without language, many of the other factors are not accessible or achievable. Language is the key to open other doors.

Indicator 11. RANGE OF SCORE - 15, 13, 10, 9, 14, 5, 15. COMMENTS: This indicator is, obviously, only appropriate for those immigrants who are work-destined. For example, this may exclude the elderly, youth, mothers or fathers of pre-schoolers and/or severely disabled persons. This area significantly affects one's 'sense of self.' The gaining of employment, especially in a field that the person was working in their own country, greatly supports a person's well-being. As well, a job means stability and a means of supporting the family. Often the biggest challenge is 'gaining' employment. A major barrier for newcomers is "Canadian experience" in any field of work. Obtaining suitable employment can indicate contentment as well as initiative.

Conversely, some who have not found suitable employment and have no chance of advancing in their non-careers can become depressed and bitter. Most immigrants come for a better life. Employment that can help them 'fulfil their dreams' will also help them to 'settle down.'

Indicator 12. RANGE OF SCORE - 12, 7, 8, 11, 5, 9, 12, 5, 7. COMMENTS: This area determines how a person reacts and interacts with everyone and everything in their life. One's feelings about oneself can open or shut doors for a person. Maintaining self-confidence, a positive self-image and pride is extremely important in developing a positive attitude that is necessary to reach one's goals. To feel good about oneself is to be able to keep the situation in perspective, to see experiences as learning experiences, and see negative situations as challenges - not a strike against you. Once self-confidence and positive self-image can be maintained, culture shock is not quite so severe. This is, of course, assuming these qualities were present in the individual prior to immigration. These elements are indicators of one's mental health and poor mental health may inhibit the process of integration.

Indicator 13. RANGE OF SCORE - 9, 7, 3, 6, 11, 9, 7, 12, 9. COMMENTS: 'Realistic' is the key word, especially considering the current economic climate; yet this realism must cover all facets of life in a new country. A sense of well-being and understanding of the culture is needed to have a balanced outlook on one's life in a different culture than that of birth. This demonstrates that the person is fairly grounded within the society. Should the newcomer not be able to accept the reality of a situation, the risks are that the adjustment period for the newcomer will take longer and this may adversely affect mental and physical well-being. That is, unrealistic expectations foster frustration and disappointment which, in turn, prolong the integration process. Once newcomers come to terms with realistic expectations, understanding all phases of settlement is easier.

Indicator 14. RANGE OF SCORE - 4, 13, 11, 10, 5, 7, 12, 8. COMMENTS: The effective use of community support services indicates a sense of self-empowerment, self-reliance, and independence from settlement agencies, thereby encouraging more independence and facilitating integration. Being able to locate and use formal support systems such as health, educational and legal agencies with no assistance indicates the immigrant had developed problem solving and coping skills. This enables one to be independent and live with all the comforts and services available and can be accomplished even before full language proficiency.

Indicator 15. RANGE OF SCORE - 10, 3, 5, 4, 8, 9, 7, 3, 8. COMMENTS: To be an independent member of Canadian society an immigrant must be able to access community resources and services and recognize what is available to them. They must also know how to obtain information about what is available - an information base is essential in order to take advantage of the resources. This is both an individual and family indicator.

References

Allodi, F. 1984. "Cultural Psychiatry and the Dynamics of Primary Prevention." In *Community Mental Health Action*. Edited by D.P. Lumsden, pp. 289-299. Ottawa: Canadian Public Health Association.

Anderson, J., N. Waxler-Morrison, E. Richardson, C. Herbert and M. Murphy. 1990. "Conclusion: Delivering Culturally Sensitive Health Care." In *Cross-Cultural Caring: A Handbook for Health Professionals in Western Canada*. Edited by N. Waxler-Morrison, J. Anderson and E. Richardson, pp. 245-269. Vancouver: University of British Columbia.

Bai, D. 1992. "Canadian Immigration and the Voluntary Sector: The Case of the Edmonton Immigrant Services Association." *Human Organization* 51:23-35.

Beiser, M. 1988. "The Mental Health of Immigrants and Refugees in Canada." *Santé/Culture/Health* V:197-215.

Beiser, M. 1991. *Research Priorities in Multiculturalism and Mental Health: Report of a National Workshop*. Ottawa: Health and Welfare Canada.

Buchignani, N. 1988. "Toward a Sociology of Indochinese Social Organisation: A Preliminary Statement." In *Ten Years Later: Indochinese Communities in Canada*. Edited by L.-J. Dorais, K.W. Chan and D. Indra, pp. 13-37. Montreal: Canadian Asian Studies Association.

Chan, K.W. 1984. " Health Needs of Indochinese Refugees: Toward a National Refugee Resettlement Policy and Strategy in Canada." In *Community Mental Health Action*. Edited by D.P. Lumsden, pp. 259-270. Ottawa: Canadian Public Health Association.

Chan, K.W. and D. Indra (eds.) 1987. *Uprooting Loss and Adaptation: The Resettlement of Indochinese Refugees in Canada*. Ottawa: Canadian Public Health Association.

Crossley, B.T. 1991. "Fundamentals of Government Sponsored Refugee Resettlement." In *Immigrants and Refugees in Canada: A National Perspective on Ethnicity, Multiculturalism and Cross-Cultural Adjustment*, edited by S.P. Sharma, A.M. Ervin, and D. Meintel, pp. 159-166. Saskatoon: University of Saskatchewan and Université de Montréal.

Delbecq, A., A.H. van de Ven, and D.H. Gustafson. 1975. *Group Techniques for Program Planning*. Glenview Ill.: Scott, Foresman.

Dorais, L.-J. 1987. "Language Use and Adaptation." In *Uprooting Loss and Adaptation: The Resettlement of Indochinese Refugees in Canada*. In K.W. Chan and D. Indra, pp. 52-65. Ottawa: Canadian Public Health Association.

Ervin, A.M. 1991. "Roles for Applied and Practising Anthropologists Working with Immigrant and Refugee Resettlement Agencies." In *Immigrants and Refugees in Canada: A National Perspective on Ethnicity, Multiculturalism and Cross-Cultural Adjustment*. Edited by S.P. Sharma, A.M. Ervin and D. Meintel, pp.196-206. Saskatoon: University of Saskatchewan and Université de Montréal.

Ervin, A.M., A. Kaye, G. Marcotte and R. Belon. 1991. *Community Needs, Saskatoon - The 1990's: The Saskatoon Needs Assessment Project*. Presented to the United Way of Saskatoon. Saskatoon: University of Saskatchewan.

Foster, G. and B. Anderson. 1978. *Medical Anthropology*. New York: John Wiley and Sons.

Fuchs, L. 1991. "Factors Affecting Happiness Among Southeast Asian Women in Saskatoon." In *Immigrants and Refugees in Canada: A National Perspective on Ethnicity, Multiculturalism and Cross-Cultural Adjustment*. Edited by S.P. Sharma, A.M. Ervin and D. Meintel, pp. 147-159. Saskatoon: University of Saskatchewan and Université de Montréal.

Gilad, L. 1990. *The Northern Route: An Ethnography of Refugee Experiences*. The Institute for Social and Economic Research, St John's: Memorial University of Newfoundland.

McKillip, J. 1987. *Need Analysis: Tools for the Human Services and Education.* Newbury Park CA: Sage.

Report of the Canadian Task Force on Mental Health Issue Affecting Immigrants and Refugees. 1988. *After the Door Has Opened: Mental Health Issues Affecting Immigrants and Refugees in Canada.* Ottawa: Health and Welfare Canada.

Taylor, D. 1991. "Vietnamese Refugees in Three Contexts: A Life History Approach." In *Immigrants and Refugees in Canada: A National Perspective on Ethnicity, Multiculturalism and Cross-Cultural Adjustment.* Edited by S.P. Sharma, A.M. Ervin and D. Meintel, pp. 139-147. Saskatoon: University of Saskatchewan and Université de Montréal.

Van Dusen, R.A. and R. Parke. 1976. "Social Indicators: A Focus for the Social Sciences." In *Anthropology and the Public Interest: Fieldwork and Theory.* Edited by P.R. Sanday, pp. 333-345. London: Academic Press.

Waxler-Morrison, N., J. Anderson and E. Richardson (eds.). 1990. *Cross-Cultural Caring: A Handbook for Health Professionals in Western Canada.* Vancouver: University of British Columbia.

Welin, L. and A.M. Ervin. 1991. "Refugee Clients and Social Service Agencies: Some Aspects of Cross-Cultural Misunderstandings." In *Immigrants and Refugees in Canada: A National Perspective on Ethnicity, Multiculturalism and Cross-Cultural Adjustment.* Edited by S.P. Sharma, A.M. Ervin and D. Meintel, pp. 178-185. Saskatoon: University of Saskatchewan and Université de Montréal.

Wood, M. 1988. Review of the Literature on Migrant Mental Health. *Santé/Culture/Health* V: 1-93.

PART 3:

Health Status and Health Care of Aboriginal Peoples

13

Colonization, Self-Determination, and The Health of Canada's First Nations Peoples

Terry Wotherspoon

Introduction

The struggle for adequate health care, although not as prominent in headlines as land claims and economic development issues, is a crucial prerequisite for the self-determination of Canada's First Nations peoples. Because health status is strongly interrelated with both the socioeconomic status and general vitality of a population, strategies to improve health standards and health care delivery are crucial components of Native self-government initiatives. The first part of this chapter provides an overview of health indicators, demonstrating the serious need for improved health care for much of the Native population in Canada. The remainder of the chapter examines issues related to jurisdictional reorganization and trends towards the devolution of health care for Canadian Native peoples. It is argued that, unless self-determination addresses significant socioeconomic inequalities and political problems, it is likely that disparities in health care among First Nations peoples will be perpetuated.

Indicators of Health Status Among Native Peoples in Canada

An overview of various indicators shows that the health status of Canada's Native peoples, in general, tends to be substantially poorer than that of the general population, although there have been improvements in several important respects in recent years. Unfortunately, analysis of detailed comparisons between First Nations and the general population, and within particular subgroups of each population, is often difficult given limited sources of comprehensive data (Muir, 1991:7). Nonetheless, those data that are available reveal several significant trends.

Canada's Native population is relatively young in comparison with the population as a whole. Data from the 1991 census reveal that 54 percent of persons of aboriginal origin are aged 25 or less, compared to 34.9 percent of the general population (calculated from Statistics Canada, 1992:6; Statistics Canada,1993:128-134). There are also important regional and provincial variations in the size and growth rate of Native populations, with the highest concentrations of registered Indians in Ontario and the Prairie provinces, and the fastest growth rates in the Prairies and the North (Department of Indian Affairs and Northern Development, 1992:6).

These demographic and regional patterns have important implications for health care, influencing the kinds of health care problems experienced by Native peoples as well as the organization and dissemination of health care services. Specific subgroups, such as children, the elderly, men and women, and persons in particular socieconomic circumstances, for instance, are likely to have differential health status and health care needs.

Table 1 contains data for registered Indians and the Canadian population as a whole on three indicators commonly used to make comparisons of general health status among populations. The trends indicate marked improvements in the crude death rates and infant mortality rates for registered Indians relative to the general population, while the birth rate for registered Indians remains about double the Canadian rate. However, the crude death rates are highly influenced by the different age structures of the two populations, recognizing that the chances of death tend to increase with age. When standardized for age, and within each age cohort, death rates are higher for Indians and Inuit than for the general population (Brady, 1983; Muir, 1991:13). While the average life expectancy at birth (not shown in the table) has improved for registered Indians, increasing from 59.2 years in 1975 to 66.9 years in 1990 for males and from 65.9 years to 74.0 years over the same period for females (Department of Indian Affairs and Northern Development, 1992:23), Indians can expect to live on average about eight to nine years less than other Canadians (Muir, 1991:22).

Table 1. Birth Rates, Crude Death Rates, and Infant Mortality Rates, Selected Years, 1960-1990, Registered Indian and Canadian Populations

YEAR	BIRTH RATE (LIVE BIRTHS/1000 POP.)		CRUDE DEATH RATE (DEATHS/1000 POP.)		INFANT MORTALITY RATE (DEATHS OF CHILDREN ONE YEAR OR UNDER/ 1000 POP.)	
	CANADA	REGISTERED INDIANS	CANADA	REGISTERED INDIANS	CANADA	REGISTERED INDIANS
1960	26.8	46.7	7.8	8.8	27.3	82.0
1967	18.2	39.9	7.4	8.4	20.8^A	48.6^A
1976	15.7	29.0	7.3	7.3	13.5	32.1
1978	15.3	28.0	7.2	7.4	12.0	26.5
1979	15.5	27.3	7.1	7.1	10.9	28.3
1980	15.5	27.5	7.2	6.8	10.4	24.4
1981	15.3	27.2	7.0	6.3	9.6	21.8
1982	15.1	28.7	7.1	6.2	9.1	17.0
1983	15.0	27.1	7.0	5.6	8.5	18.2
1984	15.0	26.3	7.0	5.7	8.1	19.0^B
1985	14.8	30.3^C	7.3	6.0	7.9	17.9^C
1986	14.7	26.1	7.2	5.6	7.9	22.2^C
1987	14.4	27.6	7.2	5.4	7.3	13.7
1988	14.5	29.3^C	7.3	5.4	7.2	12.8^C
1989	15.0	N.A.	7.3	4.8^D	7.1	9.9^D
1990	15.3	N.A.	7.2	3.8^D	6.8	10.2^D

A   Figures are for 1968.
B   Data not available for Yukon.
C   Data not available for Pacific Region.
D   Data do not include Northwest Territories Indians because of the transfer of health services to the government of the Northwest Territories.

Sources: Department of Indian Affairs and Northern Development, *Basic Departmental Data 1992*. Ottawa: Minister of Supply and Services Canada, 1993:25, 27; Statistics Canada, *Deaths, 1991*. Ottawa: Minister of Industry, Science and Technology, 1994:22; Bernice L. Muir, *Health Status of Canadian Indians and Inuit 1990*. Ottawa: Minister of Supply and Service Canada, 1991:10-14.

Infant mortality remains a persistent problem for many Native people and communities. While the infant mortality rate, calculated as the number of deaths of children of one year of age and under expressed as a proportion of every one thousand live births in a given year, declined dramatically among registered Indians from 82.0 in 1960 to 10.2 in 1990, these rates remain considerably higher than those for the general Canadian population. While data from the 1980s indicate that the highest rates of mortality existed at the perinatal stage (from 28 weeks after conception to seven days after birth), mortality rates for Native infants between four weeks and a year were nearly four times those for infants of the same age range in the general population (Muir, 1991:14-15). Additional evidence that pregnancy and early childhood problems exist among portions of the Native population is provided by trends that reveal increases in fetal death rates between 1982 and 1985 (Assembly of First Nations, 1987:10).

It is possible to conclude, as some commentators have, that genetic factors account for the observed differences between Natives and the general population. Careful examination of the data, however, indicate that health problems among First Nations peoples are more likely a consequence of poverty and other socioeconomic conditions. Leading causes of death among Indian infants include respiratory ailments, infectious and parasitic diseases, and accidents, all of which are indicators of inadequate housing, sanitary conditions, and access to medical facilities (Department of Indian Affairs and Northern Development, 1980:16; Muir, 1991:16). Poverty contributes to infant mortality and other health problems among mothers and young children. Wilkins, Sherman and Best (1991:28) conclude from their analysis of health conditions for children in urban Canada that, "infants from poorer neighbourhoods were 30-50% more likely to be born too small, too soon, or with growth retardation, they were two-thirds more likely to die before their first birthday, and more than twice as likely to die in the post-neonatal period (28-364 days)." Similarly, Muir (1991, 14) observes that the probability of infant mortality and other health risks is increased by low birth weight, which in turn is associated with poverty through the interaction of poor nutrition, high stress, obstetric complications, smoking, alcohol and drug use by the mother during pregnancy, and other problems in the mother's health status.

The impact of socioeconomic factors is also evident in other indicators of health status among Native people. Death rates from diseases of the circulatory system and neoplasms (cancer), characteristic of urban, industrial lifestyles, are lower for Native people than for non-Natives, but Natives have much higher than average rates of death from injury and poisoning at about four times the national average (Assembly of First Nations, 1987:12; Department of Indian Affairs and Northern Development, 1992:28-29). Native people have experienced declining death rates from diseases of the respiratory and circulatory systems, but such rates remain between two and three times the national average. Death rates from infectious and parasitic diseases, which for Native people remain consistently above national levels, began to increase in the mid-1980s after several years of steady decline. These trends, as with infant mortality rates, reflect pronounced differences in lifestyle and living conditions among population groups.

Causes of death and illness patterns for Native people are commonly associated with risk factors that accompany poverty or inadequate standards of living, although it is important to recognize at the same time that there are significant differences within as well as between populations. A recent study of housing conditions on Indian reserves, for example, revealed that poor health was linked to such problems as lack of central heating and poor ventilation systems, inadequate water sources and sanitation facilities, fire hazards from wood stoves and improper air circulation, and mental and physical stress from overcrowding (Young et al., 1991). Oberle (1993) reports that nearly half of registered Indian families living on reserves in Canada have incomes below poverty lines, compared with an overall Canadian rate of 14.4 percent, but notes, as well, that there are many Indian families, especially those outside of the Prairie and Atlantic regions, that have incomes substantially above poverty lines.

Certain diseases are more prevalent among Native people than among the general population. As with death rates, Indians have high rates of hospitalization associated with injuries and accidents, pregnancy and childbirth, diseases of the digestive and circulatory systems, and infectious and parasitic diseases. In addition, Indians have high rates of diseases like tuberculosis and diabetes that are directly attributable to lifestyle and nutrition patterns (Assembly of First Nations, 1987:19). These trends are amplified when age and geographic distribution are taken into consideration. In Saskatchewan, for example, rates of diabetes and essential hypertension (linked to increased risk of heart disease) were higher for registered Indians living on reserves in the southern regions than in the north, reflecting differences in diet, lifestyle, and level of health care and monitoring services (Health and Welfare Canada, 1988:31-32, 50). A survey conducted in the early 1970s by the federal government on the nutrition status of Canadians revealed that Indian and Inuit populations, amplified by factors such as age, regional distribution and gender, had serious deficiencies in terms of calcium, iron and vitamins A and D intake, indicating improper diet, often because of inadequate supplies of fresh fruit, produce and dairy products in isolated and northern regions (Nutrition Canada, 1975). Moreover, Indian populations had considerable variations in body weight and caloric input. Pregnant women frequently had inadequate levels of caloric intake while, among children and other adults, there was such widespread excessive caloric intake that the survey concluded "that overweight, obesity and elevated cholesterol levels are health hazards of major proportions" (Nutrition Canada, 1975:37). Overall, comparisons among age cohorts within the Native and non-Native populations reveal that Native children and youth face much greater and more varied diseases, disabilities and health risks while among the elderly, given the general pattern in which health problems tend to increase with age, the health indicators in the two populations are relatively similar.

As noted above, one of the most striking aspects of Indian health status is the high rate of death from accidents, injuries and poisoning. Throughout the 1980s, injury and poisoning remained the leading cause of death among Canada's on-reserve registered Indian population, although death rates from these causes declined from 205.3 per hundred thousand (about one-third of all cases of death among registered Indians) in, 1982 to 107.2 per hundred thousand (28.2 percent of all deaths among registered Indians) in 1990 (calculated from Department of Indian Affairs and Northern Development, 1992:29).

These trends have been relatively consistent across age groups and regions. Within the registered Indian population, data from the mid-1980s reveal that injury and poisoning constituted the leading cause of death for all age cohorts below 65, accounting for 87 percent of all deaths among those aged 15 to 24, and just under two-thirds of deaths among persons under 15 and among those between 25 and 44 (Muir, 1991:21). Injury and poisoning were also the leading cause of death among registered Indians in the North and in every province west of Ontario, and the second leading cause of death in Ontario, Quebec and the Atlantic (Muir, 1991:18). Siggner and Locatelli (1981:23) report that in British Columbia, based on data from the mid-1970s, "deaths due to accidents, poisonings and violence account for over 38 per cent of all Indian deaths in comparison with less than 11 per cent of all such deaths in the provincial population." In Saskatchewan, deaths from accidents, suicides, homicides, and poisoning accounted for six of the top ten causes of death in 1987 (Health and Welfare Canada, 1989:23). Motor vehicle accidents constituted the single leading cause of death among Saskatchewan's registered Indians for all age groups between 5 and 44 years, while the potential years of life lost due to injuries and poisoning were calculated as 5,901, or 60 percent of the total potential years of life lost from all causes of death (Health and Welfare Canada, 1989:25-27). On a national basis, the rate of deaths among First Nations peoples by motor vehicle accident was about three times the Canadian average, the rate of deaths by drowning was double the national average, and the rate of deaths by firearms was about nine times the Canadian average for the period from 1980 to 1983 (Assembly of First Nations 1987:13). High rates of death by other forms of injury and poisoning are also common, especially among Indians between the ages of 10 and 20.

Although rates are declining and are not included in most of the statistics cited above, suicide constitutes the largest single cause of injury- and poisoning-related deaths among the Native population. Data from 1982, for instance, reveal that suicides accounted for 36.1 percent of violent deaths among status Indians compared to a rate of 14.3 percent among the general population (Health and Welfare Canada, 1987:33). Among the registered Indian population, suicide rates for the 1984-88 period were 57.8 per 100,000 for males and 14.5 for females, compared to rates (from 1986 data) of 22.8 for males and 6.4 for females among the total Canadian population (Muir, 1991:40). The highest rates, and the highest disparities between the two population groups, were for males aged 15 to 29, while a disturbing trend in the 1980s was an increase in rates of suicide among Indian children below the age of 15 (Muir, 1991:40).

The high rates of suicide, poisoning, accidental injury, and other health risks identified for large segments of the Native population are often associated with above-average incidences of alcohol and drug abuse. Though comprehensive data are not available, virtually all reports on First Nations health status and social conditions emphasize the serious nature of alcohol and drug-related problems. A federal government survey in 1980, for instance, indicated that, "Officials working in health services for Indians estimate that between 50 and 60 percent of Indian illnesses and deaths are alcohol-related" (Department of Indian Affairs and Northern Development, 1980:21). Health and Welfare Canada estimates indicate that, for Natives, 75 percent of deaths by accident, poisoning and violence, and 90 percent of deaths by fire, are linked to alcohol abuse (Health and Welfare Canada, 1985:5). About one third, or 42 out of a total of 130 Indian deaths in Saskatchewan in 1987 were attributed to alcohol and drugs (Health and Welfare Canada, 1989:29). Data from Alberta show that 14.1 percent of all deaths among registered Indians in the province in 1987 were alcohol-related while Manitoba reported that, for 1988, 11.4 percent of deaths among registered Indians were alcohol-related and an additional 4.1 percent were drug-related (Muir, 1991:41). Jarvis and Boldt (1982), by utilizing data derived from key informants in Indian communities throughout Alberta, suggest that heavy use of alcohol contributes to more deaths and related health problems than are officially reported. Moreover, alcohol and drug abuse are associated with other chronic conditions such as cirrhosis, heart disease, and birth defects. The combination of drug abuse, alcoholism, and inadequate or overcrowded living conditions is further linked to other problems such as the rapid spread of AIDS and other sexually-transmitted diseases among Native communities. Fritz and Darcy (1983) report also that Indians have much higher rates of institutionalization and treatment than do non-Indians for psychiatric disorders related to alcoholism and drug addiction.

Consistent with these observed patterns of illness, death and other health disorders, available data (which, unfortunately are not comprehensive) reveal that Native people tend to have higher than average rates of utilization of health care services. Data from the late 1980s show that hospitalization rates for registered Indians in Manitoba, Saskatchewan, and British Columbia, for instance, were between 1.4 to 2.2 times higher than those for the general population (Health and Welfare Canada, 1988:22; Muir, 1991:23-24). Similarly, Fritz and Darcy (1983:73-76) observe with respect to Saskatchewan data that the Indian population had a higher rate of hospitalization than the non-Indian population for treatment of psychiatric disorders, although Indians had a lower rate of treatment on an outpatient basis than did the general population.

Rates of hospitalization and medical treatment by particular reasons or disorders are similar to patterns revealed in causes of death. Registered Indians and Inuit populations have much higher than average recorded rates within several disease categories, notably injury and poisoning, pregnancy and childbirth-related complications, diseases of the respiratory, digestive and nervous systems, diseases related to the skin and nutritional factors, immunity disorders, infectious and parasitic diseases, and mental disorders. Several highly infectious diseases, such as tuberculosis and hepatitis B, that are relatively rare or contained within the general population are often prevalent among pockets of the Native population. By contrast, rates of cancer (neoplasms) and diseases of the circulatory system, that are common within the general population, tend to be lower within Native populations, although there tend to be higher rates of cancer among the Inuit than the other groups (Muir, 1991:23-38). As with other health indicators, population differences in incidences of disease and disorders can be traced directly and indirectly to people's life circumstances.

High degrees of interaction among socioeconomic conditions, physical and mental health, and the availability of health care services and resources, contribute to the general image of two distinct realities of living and dying for Native people and non-Natives. As the data have shown, in terms of disease and illness, injury, causes of death, and forms of treatment, First Nations peoples in Canada tend to experience conditions which, though improving, continue to be unsatisfactory in the context of an industrially and medically advanced society. This does not mean that Native people are inherently more illness- or injury-prone, but reflects instead the highly disadvantaged position occupied by large segments of the Native population. However, on indicators such as birth and death rates, life expectancy, rates of cancer and heart disease, and other disorders, there are signs of a gradual convergence between the general Native and non-Native populations. Moreover, the trends show that several factors other than race, including gender, class, age, and area of residence, where comparable data are available, contribute to the explanation of differential health status. The remainder of this chapter examines further prospects for change in health care among First Nations peoples in relation to diverse socioeconomic circumstances and inequalities in the arrangement and delivery of health care services.

Socioeconomic Determinants of First Nations Health Status

For First Nations, as for other social groups, changing dimensions of health status can be understood as a product of peoples' lived experiences. All societies require at least minimal standards of health care in order to ensure that necessary social tasks are fulfilled and the population is able to maintain itself. The degree to which these conditions are adequate will vary in accordance with a society's resources and needs. As Marx (1970:72) observed, so long as living standards and skill requirements are low, "A quick succession of unhealthy and short-lived generations will keep the labour market as well supplied as a series of vigorous and long-lived generations." Under real historical conditions, however, it is necessary to maintain a supply of workers and other individuals with particular types of needs, skills, know-how, and physical attributes. The higher than average and often severe health care risks and problems outlined above are telling indicators of Native peoples' historically marginalized position in Canadian society. It is important, however, not to ignore significant variations in these conditions both within First Nations populations and in the changing relations between First Nations and the Canadian state.

European contact and colonization of the First Nations, while not the sole cause of declining health standards, clearly posed health risks and lifestyle changes that were often destructive to Native populations. Although, like many pre-industrial societies, Native populations were frequently depleted by natural and social forces, available evidence suggests that traditional Native populations were relatively healthy and free of major infectious diseases and other disorders (Young, 1988:32-33). With contact, however, exposure to new social practices and epidemiological factors posed both direct and indirect health risks. Europeans sometimes carried with them viruses to which Natives had not previously been exposed, for example. Cultivation of land, the domestication of animal herds, and settlement in communities and, later, reserves, contributed to the spread of diseases, infections and parasites. Alcohol was often associated as cause and consequence with the destruction of family and community life. Overfishing and depletion of game led to widespread starvation, which was sometimes exacerbated by the withholding of food, supplies, and medicine by government or fur trade officials. The impact of epidemics and other health problems was intensified by the breakdown of cultural support systems and the frequent absence of alternative forms of medical assistance (Dobyns, 1983:16). Although many Natives were incorporated successfully into non-traditional pursuits through the fur trade and eventually into agricultural and industrial activities, the gradual process of displacement of Indians from traditional lands and migration patterns posed major risks to the Native population. The substitution of a cash economy for traditional subsistence patterns resulted in a notable decline in Natives' health status. The authors of a medical survey of nutrition among Indians in northern Manitoba observed in 1946 that,

> It can be stated that without exception in those areas where the dietary habits of the Indian have changed from the consumption of foods from the country itself to "store food," which is largely white flour, lard and sugar, the physical condition of the Indian has markedly deteriorated in recent years (Moore et al., 1946:228).

Moreover, until relatively recently, the state has been slow to respond to serious health problems that exist for much of the Native population in Canada. In 1933-34, for instance, just under $10 per capita were paid out of public and band trust funds for Indian health services, well below comparable expenditures of at least $30 per capita for the national population, and at least one-third below levels considered by the Director of Medical Services to be sufficient to provide highly effective service delivery to Indians (Department of Indian Affairs:1934). The evidence suggests that health care problems are magnified for those segments of the population that are dispensable, through either neglect, lack of adequate resources, or some combination of related factors.

Jurisdictional Reorganization and Devolution of First Nations Health Care

In the latter half of the twentieth century, the combination of political struggle by First Nations peoples with the desire by employers and state officials to maintain access to a stable workforce and capital resources has stimulated a drive to improve Native health care. Interrelated processes like northern development and off-reserve migration signified changing social and economic relationships within Native communities and between those communities and Canadian society in general. Both in negative and positive ways, Natives were increasingly identified as a "problem" population.

Initially, the political and economic crises which surrounded the depression in the 1930s provided an impetus to re-examine funding and service delivery arrangements that prevailed among different levels of government in Canada. Status Indians, officially under the care and protection of the federal government until such time as they could be assimilated, were placed in an increasingly ambiguous position as federal and provincial governments began to contest jurisdictional and funding arrangements in areas like health care and social services. Serious concerns were also raised over the provision of services to non-status and off-reserve Indians and Metis peoples.

One of the first measures to recognize these changing relationships was the transfer of Indian health care services from the Indian Affairs Branch within the Department of Mines and Resources to the newly constituted Department of National Health and Welfare in 1945. The move helped to consolidate administrative responsiveness to Indians' health problems, resulting in the expansion of public health services, hospitals, and other medical resources. Definite improvements were made over earlier efforts to deal with Native health care through the systematic collection of data, the monitoring of particular disease trends, and the employment of personnel committed to finding solutions to pressing health care problems. The identification of tuberculosis as a major health problem among Indian people, for example, stimulated the expansion of treatment centres and testing and inoculation programs which contributed to declines in the official rate of death among Indians from the disease from levels of 579 per hundred thousand in 1946 to 48 in 1955 (Graham-Cumming, 1967:141-142).

Nonetheless, general health care services for Native peoples tended to remain severely inadequate. The removal of health care from the Indian Affairs Branch caused sufficient interdepartmental bitterness that concern for administrative procedures often took priority over actual service delivery (Graham-Cumming, 1967:128). Such problems were compounded by the isolated locale of most Indian bands which necessitated costly transfers, usually by air transport, of medical personnel into Native communities and reserves, or of Native people who required hospitalization out to larger centres. In the meantime, major reviews of Canada's health care system, notably the Royal Commission on Health Services which reported in 1964 and the 1970 Task Force on the Cost of Health Services, failed to acknowledge or investigate fully the needs and problems associated with Indian health care (Badgley, 1973:158; Young,1984:262).

As Canada and the provinces moved towards a national health insurance program in the late 1960s that included the establishment of federal standards and cost-sharing for health programs delivered by the provinces, the status of health care services for First Nations peoples became even more indefinite and confusing. While Indians, like other Canadians, received coverage under the national health insurance program, there were no clearcut guidelines for the actual entitlement and delivery of service, and Native peoples often received irregular or inadequate health care services. Final determination of eligibility for insurance coverage was often left to health care professionals at the point of service delivery (Badgley, 1973:153).

First Nations' organizations recognized and began to press the government to address three main areas of concern in relation to the delivery of health care services. First, levels of service and financial arrangements for health care on and near reserves were inconsistent and usually inadequate. Indians expressed their dissatisfaction with several aspects of the health care system, including variations in the range of services covered under medical insurance and treaty rights, irregular billing patterns, delays in federal reimbursement to medical practitioners for services rendered, and lack of monitoring to ensure that funds earmarked by the federal government for Indian health services were actually spent for that purpose by provincial governments. Severe inequities in health care delivery existed between northern and southern regions of the country. Second, increasing patterns of migration from reserves to urban areas meant that many Indians lost their health care entitlements either formally through loss of status or, more importantly, through the process of becoming uprooted from a community environment in which informal support networks could provide direct care or service referrals. The National Indian Brotherhood (1976:2), for instance, pointed to the existence of about one hundred registered Indians whom they termed "medical foster children" in medical care away from home, whose parents were given no visitation rights or information concerning the children's condition and discharge dates. Third, Indian organizations became increasingly sensitive to the connection between socioeconomic conditions and health status, recognizing that political and administrative ambiguity over Indian affairs were prolonging what was clearly an intolerable situation. In 1976, the National Indian Brotherhood (1976:7), drawing upon position papers from its member organizations, recommended "a policy of free and complete medical care to Indian people" that included a comprehensive health plan and free dental care, eye care and drugs, funded completely by the federal government. In a submission to the federal government's special commissioner on national health services in 1979, the Federation of Saskatchewan Indians expressed the prevailing view of First Nations peoples that, for Indian people, demographic, health and socioeconomic indicators all "clearly portray a situation that is getting worse rather than better" (Health and Welfare Canada, 1980:89).

By the 1980s, Indian organizations and federal and provincial government representatives agreed that some recognition should be given to aboriginal self-determination over many areas of life, including health care. The federal government approved an agreement to transfer control over local health services to Indian bands in 1981, and in 1986, a federal Indian Health Transfer Program specified the conditions under which devolution to Native control could proceed (Frideres, 1994:206-297; Muir, 1991:8). In addition to these general agreements, there emerged in the 1980s a growing array of health-related programs offered through private and community agencies in response to specific health care needs.

Growing formal attentiveness to the organization of health care services for, and the health status of, First Nations peoples, is a consequence of both political and economic factors. Native leaders and organizations, building upon the anger produced by the immediate experience of widespread ill health and suffering, have made health issues a major focus within their demands for official recognition of Native rights and self-government. At the same time, significantly, growing reliance upon Native peoples' labour power on and off reserves by both Native and non-Native employers has made it imperative that increasingly greater proportions of First Nations populations be relatively healthy and ready to work. Moreover, there is a high degree of affinity between, on the one hand, the emergent prominence on national agendas of the apparent contribution of rising health care costs to government deficits and public debt and, on the other hand, the political attractiveness of community health services and traditional healing practices that potentially can be provided in an environmentally sensitive way at relatively low cost.

It is important to a consideration of prospects for increased First Nations involvement in health care to recognize a distinction between Native people's control over a predominantly white, capitalist model of health care and development of an alternative model of health care based upon First Nations traditions. The National Indian Brotherhood (NIB) in 1978 issued a statement of principle that highlighted the contrast between these two health care models. The NIB argues that, on the one hand, as an Indian people,

> Our whole culture, our knowledge of thousands of years, has been devoted to developing ourselves as wise children, to changing ourselves rather than changing our environment, to humbling ourselves before the forces of nature, the forces and will of the Creator, to prevent our own egos from destroying us or our environment, to seeking balance and harmony within ourselves and to extend that balance and harmony to all our daily acts, to our very way of life (National Indian Brotherhood, 1978:1).

By contrast, the destructive forces of a dominant society are seen to have devastated a harmonious and integrated approach to life:

> So today we are living with our fellow man who is in conflict with himself, whose attitude, values and culture are adverse to nature and the creation, a people who develop and inflate their egos and force all things in their sphere of influence to humble themselves to the will of those few whose way of life is that of adversity, conflict and imbalance. A people who freely manipulate the environment and yes, even the lives of their fellow men. A society whose culture and every act is one of manipulation, control and adversity to every living organism, even their very own (National Indian Brotherhood, 1978:2).

The vivid representation of these two world views presents a compelling case for First Nations control over health care and other aspects of Native life. From the perspective of many Native peoples who are seeking to regain control over their lives, the loss of traditional healing practices under the onslaught of a manipulative dominant medical model has drastic consequences that go beyond health care. O'Neil (1988:30) observes that traditional Indian medicine "is a broad constellation of values that underpins the respectful relationships that Indian people insist characterize their relationships with each other, the physical environment and the spiritual world." Referring to attempts to revive sacred rituals, one Alberta healer says that "many people have gotten careless about the rituals or have forgotten how to do them properly.... Thus, a kind of double bind exists: it is dangerous to take part in ceremonies conducted by incompetent people, but it is even more dangerous not to do the ceremonies at all" (Young, 1989:34).

However, to understand these problems, it is also necessary to take into account the particular economic and political realities that affect health status and within which health care systems operate. While some sociocultural factors are unique to the health care concerns of Native peoples in general, Natives also enter into the health care system through their wider social relations compounded by distinctions of class, gender, age, and other characteristics. The high concentrations of Native people who are in the younger age cohorts, for example, mean that Natives are more likely overall to demonstrate greater susceptibility to afflictions like childhood diseases and accidental deaths and injuries. Similarly, Native women living in poverty are exposed to higher than average risks of problems such as malnutrition and pregnancy-related disorders. In short, health care conditions reflect both the socioeconomic circumstances experienced by First Nations peoples and the way in which these are managed politically (Culhane Speck, 1987).

First Nations control and delivery of Native health care services is potentially a preliminary step in the direction of recognizing that environmental factors rather than individual and cultural pathologies are the basis of health problems. This is a progressive step insofar as it represents a rejection of dominant models of medicine and health care that reinforce social inequalities under capitalism by emphasizing the medicalization of health problems, corporate and profit-driven services and decision-making structures, and responsiveness to system rather than consumer and community needs (Doyal and Pennell, 1979; Waitzkin, 1983).

Recent initiatives for band control of health services and recognition of traditional healing methods place health care in a context that takes into account peoples' life experiences. Several Native communities have followed the prominent example of British Columbia's Alkali Lake Band which in 1972 began a program of abstention from alcohol, personal development workshops, community cultural activities, and employment initiatives in order to counter serious alcohol-related problems. The Four Worlds Development Project (1985:59-60) in southern Alberta, for instance, integrates health care with a broad set of strategies for community development.

General policy orientations that favour a shift towards Native self-government have made health care a central component in band development. Landmark agreements such as those beginning in 1975 among the federal and provincial governments and the Cree, Naskapi and Inuit peoples of the James Bay and northern and northeastern Quebec regions provide a framework to enable the establishment both of special federal and provincial health programs to meet local needs, and of administrative and fiscal transfers to facilitate the involvement by district and band councils in health care assessment and delivery processes (Peters, 1989:196-198).

However, as a wide diversity of interests, historical considerations, and local needs enter into the health care field, there is no single path along which self-government initiatives are likely to be established. At most, all that can be concluded, as Boisvert (1985:57) emphasized in an analysis of self-government alternatives, is that, "A judicious sharing of responsibilities among governments including aboriginal governments seems the only approach to use in the social policy field" in general. Ongoing jurisdictional disputes over the organization, financing and delivery of First Nations health care services are further complicated by a general political sentiment to reduce health care expenditures and rationalize services. Under such conditions, the availability of sufficient resources to provide Native communities adequate health care remains in continual jeopardy.

First Nations health care concerns must also take into account the recognition that effective changes in health status require major transformations in the organization of social life that go beyond what Native peoples can accomplish on their own. There is an increasing need to acknowledge that health is a product of social circumstances. The politicization of environmental concerns, for example, provides an opportunity to link Native health care issues with broader reform strategies. But there are also deeper political and economic realities that must be confronted before any substantial progress can be made in the area of Natives' health.

In particular, health prospects for First Nations peoples tend to be disadvantaged at two levels. First, as persons who tend to occupy primarily subordinate class positions, Native peoples continue to face higher than average health risks. As observed earlier, there is a systematic association between poverty and illness, with persons of lower socioeconomic status much more likely than those of higher socioeconomic status to experience physical, medical and mental health problems (see, e.g., Health and Welfare Canada, 1981; Millar and Stephens, 1993; Oberle, 1993). Deficiencies or inadequacies in areas like housing, sewage, nutrition, and general living conditions, for instance, contribute directly and indirectly to increased health risks.

Second, Native peoples' health is subject to further jeopardy by many of the strategies that are being pursued by Natives and non-Natives alike for economic development. Exposure to environmental hazards and social displacement through massive mining, energy and hydroelectric projects both alter traditional patterns of life and produce new health and safety risks, such as those illustrated in Figure 1.

Figure 1. Selected Contaminants and their Impact on First Nations Health Conditions

Source & Contaminant	Areas of Major Concern (Number of Projects or Developments)
Impact: Destruction of wildlife; restrictions on hunting & fishing rights; contamination of food, air & water	
Flooding of First Nations lands through dams and hydroelectric developments	Atlantic (8) Northern Quebec (11) Ontario (17) Manitoba (4) Saskatchewan (2) British Columbia (9)
Acid rain and toxic chemicals from smelters, coal-fired electricity, transportation and industrial processes	Quebec & Ontario (43% of lakes contaminated) Ontario (Serpent River, Big Trout Lake, Weagamow, Wawa-Sudbury, 65% of headwaters in Muskoka-Haliburton area) Arctic & Northern Canada (lakes & coastal regions contaminated) Canada (40% of forest affected, a dozen rivers no longer support trout or salmon)
High water temperature from large-scale forest harvesting	British Columbia (Meares Island, Lyell Island, Moresby Islands, Stein watershed)
Aquaculture and fish farming in marine water	Bays traditionally harvested by First Nations in Maritime waters
Oil and gas exploration, drilling, pipelines, refineries, and potential for spills	West coast offshore High & eastern Arctic (Beaufort Sea, MacKenzie Delta) Northern Alberta
Noise from military	Northern Canada
Impact: Water Contamination and Destruction of Fisheries	
Mercury and other heavy metals from mining, smelters and acid rain	Northwest Territories (lakes and rivers) Ontario English-Wabigoon River system, St. Clair River, Sarnia
Toxic chemicals including PCBs, DDT, dioxin, and endusulfin	Great Lakes (1000 chemicals) Ontario (Niagara River) Quebec (St. Lawrence River system) Northern Canada
Impact: Social and Economic Disruption	
Dislocation of whole communities, disruption of industries, depletion of resources	All regions noted above

Source: Data from Assembly of First Nations, *Current Indian Health Conditions: A Statistical Perspective*. Ottawa: Assembly of First Nations, 1987:23; and Bernice L. Muir, *Health Status of Canadian Indians and Inuit 1990*. Ottawa: Minister of Supply and Services Canada, 1991:54-55.

Discharges of pollutants and hazardous waste materials such as mercury, PCBs, and other toxins pose direct health risks, but they also contribute to longer-term problems as they accumulate in fish, waterfowl, game, soil, and drinking water (Bolaria, 1991:230-232; Muir, 1991:54-55). Processes of northern and community development, whether accomplished through massive public projects, corporate ventures, band initiatives, or some combination of these, have in general tended to emphasize immediate economic priorities over social and cultural factors. Despite negotiated agreements to provide compensation as well as environmentally and socially responsible development practices through such initiatives as massive hydroelectric and energy projects, the drive to gain access to land and resources as quickly as possible has resulted in major social, economic and ecological upheavals that sometimes have had devastating consequences for whole communities or regions (Berger, 1977:148; Lysyk, 1977:94; Cree-Naskapi Commission, 1988:40-41; Waldram, 1988). Even economic development strategies based upon ventures like gambling and tourism that have no immediately apparent impact on health are potential contributors to problems such as alcohol and drug abuse, violence, and other health concerns that arise from poverty and social dislocation.

It is possible that projects under First Nations guidance may alleviate the most serious injustices by a concern for the general welfare of Native peoples. However, conflicting agendas mean that human justice and social service concerns are often subordinated to priorities for immediate economic gain or for projects whose benefits will not be equitably distributed throughout Native communities.

Conclusion

This chapter has examined historical and contemporary dimensions of First Nations health care and health status. It has been argued that the health status of Native peoples is a consequence of social and economic circumstances which, in turn, reflect the positions that Natives occupy within the wider social system. Current socioeconomic changes, including First Nations initiatives in economic development, self-determination, and increased control over areas like health care, contain prospects for a marked improvement in Native peoples' overall social opportunities and life conditions. There are likely to be benefits for health status and health care services insofar as health care issues are closely integrated into strategies to alleviate poverty and equalize life chances. There are also dangers, however, that development strategies that perpetuate socioeconomic inequalities and advance the deterioration of the environment and community life will pose continuing and new health risks to large segments of First Nations populations.

This chapter incorporates material revised and updated from chapter six of Vic Satzewich and Terry Wotherspoon, *First Nations: Race, Class, and Gender Relations* (Toronto: Nelson Canada, 1993).

References

Assembly of First Nations. 1987. "Current Indian Health Conditions: A Statistical Perspective." Assembly of First Nations research document. Ottawa: Assembly of First Nations.

Badgley, R.F. 1973. "Social Policy and Indian Health Services in Canada." *Anthropological Quarterly* 46(3): 150-159.

Berger, T. 1977. *Northern Frontier, Northern Homeland: The Report of the MacKenzie Valley Pipeline Inquiry*, Volume I. Ottawa: Minister of Supply and Services.

Boisvert, D.A. 1985. *Forms of Aboriginal Self-Government*. Kingston, Ont.: Institute of Intergovernmental Relations Background Paper Number 2.

Bolaria, B. Singh. 1991. "Environment, Work, and Illness." In B. Singh Bolaria (Ed.), *Social Issues and Contradictions in Canadian Society*. Toronto: Harcourt Brace Jovanovich, 222-246.

Brady, Paul D. 1983. "The Underdevelopment of the Health Status of Treaty Indians." In P.S. Li and B. Singh Bolaria (Eds.), *Racial Minorities in Multicultural Canada*. Toronto: Garamond, 39-55.

Culhane Speck, Dara. 1987. *An Error in Judgement: The Politics of Medical Care in an Indian/White Community*. Vancouver: Talonbooks.

Cree-Naskapi Commission. 1988. *Report of the Cree-Naskapi Commission*. Ottawa: Indian and Northern Affairs.

Department of Indian Affairs. 1934. *Annual Report of the Department of Indian Affairs, 1933-34*. Ottawa: King's Printer.

Department of Indian Affairs and Northern Development. 1980. *Indian Conditions: A Survey*. Ottawa: Minister of Supply and Services.

Department of Indian Affairs and Northern Development. 1992. *Basic Departmental Data 1992*. Ottawa: Department of Indian Affairs and Northern Development.

Dobyns, H.F. 1983. *Their Number Become Thinned: Native American Population Dynamics in Eastern North America*. Knoxville: The University of Tennessee Press.

Doyal, L. with I. Pennell. 1979. *The Political Economy of Health*. London: Pluto Press.

Four Worlds Development Project. 1985. *Developing Healthy Communities: Fundamental Strategies for Health Promotion*. Lethbridge: The Four Worlds Development Project.

Frideres, J.S. 1994. "Racism and Health: Case of the Native People." In B. Singh Bolaria and Harley D. Dickinson (Eds.), *Health, Illness, and Health Care in Canada*, second edition. Toronto: Harcourt Brace & Company Canada, 202-220.

Fritz, W. and C. D'Arcy. 1983. "Comparisons: Indian and Non-Indian Use of Psychiatric Services." In P.S. Li and B. Singh Bolaria (Eds.), *Racial Minorities in Multicultural Canada*. Toronto: Garamond, 68-85.

Graham-Cumming, G. 1967. "The Health of the Original Canadians, 1867-1967." *Medical Services Journal Canada* 23 (February): 115-166.

Health and Welfare Canada. 1980. *Canada's National-Provincial Health Program for the 1980's: A Commitment for Renewal*. Ottawa: Health and Welfare Canada.

Health and Welfare Canada. 1981. *The Health of Canadians: Report of the Canada Health Survey*. Ottawa: Minister of Supply and Services.

Health and Welfare Canada. 1985. *National Native Alcohol and Drug Abuse Program: A Progress Report*. Ottawa: Minister of Supply and Services.

Health and Welfare Canada. 1987. *Suicide in Canada*. Report of the National Task Force on Suicide in Canada. Ottawa: Minister of National Health and Welfare.

Health and Welfare Canada. 1988. *Health Status of Canadian Indians and Inuit, Update 1987*. Ottawa: Health and Welfare Canada.

Health and Welfare Canada. 1989. *1989 Vital Statistics for the Registered Indian Population of Canada*. Ottawa: Health and Welfare Canada.

Jarvis, George K. and Menno Boldt. 1982. "Death Styles among Canada's Indians." *Social Science and Medicine* 16:1345-1352.

Lysyk, K.M. 1977. *Alaska Highway Pipeline Inquiry*. Ottawa: Minister of Supply and Services.

Marx, Karl. 1970. *Wages, Price and Profit*. Peking: Foreign Languages Press.

Millar, W.J. and T. Stephens. 1993. "Social Status and Health Risks in Canadian Adults: 1985 and 1991." Statistics Canada, *Health Reports* 5(2): 143-156.

Moore, P.E., H.D. Kruse, F.F. Tisdall, and R.S.C. Corrigan. 1946. "Medical Survey of Nutrition among the Northern Manitoba Indians." *Canadian Medical Association Journal* 54 (March): 223-233.

Muir, Bernice L. 1991. *Health Status of Canadian Indians and Inuit 1990*. Ottawa: Minister of Supply and Services Canada.

National Indian Brotherhood. 1976. "Policy on Indian Health Services: Working Draft." Ottawa: National Indian Brotherhood.

National Indian Brotherhood. 1978. "National Indian Brotherhood Commission Inquiry on Indian Health: Statement of Principle," adopted November 9, Ottawa: National Indian Brotherhood.

Nutrition Canada. 1975. *The Indian Survey Report*. Ottawa: Department of National Health and Welfare.

Oberle, Peter R. 1993. *The Incidence of Family Poverty on Canadian Indian Reserves*. Ottawa: Minister of Supply and Services Canada.

O'Neil, J.D. 1988. "Referrals to Traditional Healers: The Role of Medical Interpreters." In D.E. Young (Ed.), *Health Care Issues in the Canadian North*. Edmonton: Boreal Institute for Northern Studies Occasional Publication Number 26.

Peters, E.J. 1989. "Federal and Provincial Responsibilities for the Cree, Naskapi and Inuit Under the James Bay and Northern Quebec, and Northeastern Quebec Agreements." In D.C. Hawkes (Ed.), *Aboriginal Peoples and Government Responsibility*. Ottawa: Carleton University Press, 173-242.

Siggner, A. and C. Locatelli. 1981. *An Overview of Demographic, Social and Economic Conditions among British Columbia's Registered Indian Population*. Ottawa: Minister of Indian Affairs and Northern Development.

Statistics Canada. 1992. *Age, Sex and Marital Status,* 1991 Census Catalogue Number 93-310. Ottawa: Minister of Industry, Science and Technology. 1993. Ethnic Origin. 1991 Census Catalogue Number 93-315. Ottawa: Minister of Industry, Science and Technology.

Waitzkin, H. 1983. *The Second Sickness.* New York: Free Press.

Waldram, James B. 1988. *As Long as the Rivers Run: Hydroelectric Development and Native Communities in Western Canada.* Winnipeg: University of Manitoba Press.

Wilkins, Russell, Gregory J. Sherman and P.A.F Best. 1991. "Birth Outcomes and Infant Mortality by Income in Urban Canada, 1986." Statistics Canada, *Health Reports* 3(1): 7-31.

Young, D.E., with G. Ingram and L. Swartz. 1989. *Cry of the Eagle: Encounters with a Cree Healer.* Toronto: University of Toronto Press.

Young, T. Kue. 1984. "Indian Health Services in Canada: A Sociohistorical Perspective." *Social Science and Medicine* 18(3): 257-264.

Young, T. Kue. 1988. *Health Care and Cultural Change: The Indian Experience in the Central Subarctic.* Toronto: University of Toronto Press.

Young, T. Kue, Linda Bruce, John Elias, John D. O'Neil, and Annalee Yassie. 1991. *The Health Effects of Housing and Community Infrastructure on Canadian Indian Reserves.* Ottawa: Ministry of Supply and Service Canada.

14

Health Promotion and Indian Communities: Social Support or Social Disorganization

James S. Frideres

Introduction

Health needs assessments carried out in Indian communities over the past decade reveal that health conditions are not comparable to that of non-Indians. The results of these needs assessments show individuals residing in Indian communities have health problems different from and more severe than in non-Indian communities. Waldram and O'Neil (1989) document that these needs assessments show that many Indian communities throughout Canada are dysfunctional, both reflecting and contributing to poor living conditions and high incidence of specific diseases.

The task of this chapter is first to identify the institutional structure in place which provides health care services to Indians in Canada. We will then provide a profile of Indian health in their communities, followed with tentative answers as to why Indians exhibit high levels of illness, mortality and a general low quality of life. Finally, we will present possible alternative strategies to deal with the situation regarding health conditions found on reserve communities.

The Canadian Health Care System

The provision of health care before 1945 was largely a private matter, although the federal government covered some of the costs for the establishment of hospitals and the training of medical doctors. However, after this time, the federal government took control of health services and implemented a universal health plan. The Hospital Insurance Diagnostic Services Act (1957) and the Medical Care Act (1966) are just two examples of major legislative measures introduced as the federal government began to exert its influence on the number of medical practitioners and facilities available to Canadians.

As health care costs began to escalate in the 1970s, the federal government unilaterally decided that it could no longer singularly support the system it had put in place. It began to withdraw funding and insisted that the provincial governments pick up part of the cost. By the late 1970s, policies had been put in place to ensure an orderly transfer to the province of both control and financing of health care for Canadians. When the provinces began to take on the additional costs for providing health care, some introduced financial strategies which threatened the universal access principles of medical care, e.g., double billing. After considerable negotiation between the federal and provincial governments, these procedures were stopped when the Canada Health Act was passed. The provisions of this Act reaffirmed the concept of universal access and the support of both levels of government would ensure its success.

Until the late 19th century, the provision of health services for Indian people was infrequent and minimal. Questions about whether or not Indians were human and then later questions about their lack of religion (pagans), prevented the creation of any systematic policy by which health care would come to be directed toward them. When health care was provided for Indians, it was through the Hudson Bay Company or by various religious groups which provided a limited range of health services. Later, when Treaties were established, the federal government took on additional responsibilities for the overall care of Indian people. In some cases, Treaties specifically outlined the government's responsibilities regarding health care, e.g., Treaty 6, but in most cases the responsibility was not clearly defined. Nevertheless, under the *Constitution Act, 1867*, the welfare of Indians was clearly placed within the jurisdiction of the federal government. As such, the federal government began slowly to implement policies and programs which would have an impact on the general health of Indians. These programs and policies increased in scope and covered an increasing number of activities defined under the broad rubric of health. By the end of W.W.II, the existing bureaucratic structure could no longer handle the complex structure and health care for Indians was transferred from the Department of Mines and Surveys (the federal government's department dealing with Indian issues) to the Department of Health and Welfare. In 1962 the Medical Services Branch took over the health care of Indians and has continued to do so.

The basis of health care for Native people does not reside in the Constitution nor, in most cases, in the Treaties signed with the Indians. Yet, the federal government has taken on the responsibility of providing this important (and today very costly) venture. The federal responsibility seems to have emerged out of the resistance of provincial officials to provide services because of their lack of jurisdiction over Indians in both financial and other activities, e.g., provinces cannot tax Indian land or income received from the reserve.

The health care services provided for Indians today is comprehensive and similar to that provided to other Canadians. The structure, however, runs parallel to the organization established for provision of health care for other Canadians. The Medical Services Branch has its headquarters in Ottawa with a number of regions covering Canada. Within each region, there are a series of zones which coordinate the medical activities for Indians. The primary level of health care is provided through Nursing stations. The second level of health care consists of small hospitals. Finally, the tertiary level of health care is provided through provincial medical centres. In some cases the Medical Services Branch may contract out services they feel they cannot provide. While the Medical Services Branch provides health care services for all Indians, they are limited in their ability to influence certain factors influencing health. For example, our data suggests that much of the basic health issues of Indians are related to socio-economic issues. For example, sanitation facilities are an important determinant of health, yet, the Medical Services Branch has no control over the introduction of sanitation programs in an Indian community. Upon closer inspection, there is little cooperation between the Medical Services Branch and the Department of Indian and Northern Affairs, the organization responsible for Indian Affairs. In addition, the Medical Services Branch does not provide services to off-reserve Indians (of which nearly one third reside off reserve). Over time, the federal government has argued that urban Indians must use alternative sources of health care. As such, Indians off reserve must go to private health provisioners and provincial hospitals which are in turn reimbursed through federal transfer payments (Kramer and Weller, 1989).

As a result of the health care system put in place, Canadians are living longer and with fewer years of disability.[1] The reduction of infectious diseases, e.g., tuberculosis and typhoid, has been particularly important in decreasing the mortality rates and enhancing the quality of life for Canadians. Knowledge that nutrition and sanitation are crucial factors in health and health related diseases has led to extensive programs to ensure that Canadians' health is looked after. We are now cognizant of the impact that environmental conditions have on health and quality of life. Nevertheless, while we all have access to enhanced social programs, to health care facilities and to increasingly sophisticated medical services, it would seem that not all Canadians are able to take advantage of these facilities or programs. As Nathanson and Lopez (1987) point out, one's placement in the social structure has far more impact on lifestyle than individual choices. As a result of the position Indian people find themselves, they face barriers to optimal health status.

Health Profiles

Since the comprehensive health care structure has been put in place, substantial benefits have accrued to Native people. Mortality rates have dramatically been reduced as well as a general increase in the "wellness" levels of people. However, the decrease in mortality rates has been selective, e.g., specific infectious diseases. We also find that the relative increases in the health of Native people have not approached the health status of non-Indian people. As Kramer and Weller (1989) point out, the availability of modern medicine does not guarantee health. As such, there are additional determinants of health indicators which must be investigated. Furthermore, we need to look at why Indian communities are unable to utilize existing health care facilities and programs as well as how Indian communities are able to survive under social and structural conditions which are not conducive to good health.

Early improvements in health and life expectancy for all Canadians (41 years in 1851 to 61 in 1930) were due largely to reduction in infectious diseases, e.g., tuberculosis, diphtheria, typhoid and smallpox. These reductions seem to be a result of increased standard of living and an enhanced medical knowledge of diseases. Subsequent increases in life expectancy (now approximately 80 years) are a result of other factors such as improved survival of low birth weight babies, improved treatment of heart disease and lower rates of accidents (Beaujot, 1991). For example, in 1986, nearly half of the deaths recorded were due to heart problems with another quarter due to cancer (Nagnur and Nagrodski, 1988). The following data provide us with some useful insights into the health issues of Indians.

Overall, we find that the Indian population in Canada is the most disadvantaged ethnic group with regard to life expectancy and mortality. As data in Figure 1 show, the Indian population continues to have a lower life expectancy than the non-Indian population. Data in Figure 2 show the age-standardized death rates for both Indians and the general

Canadian population for the past decade. While the rates for both groups have decreased, Indian death rates remain substantially higher than the general population over time. Figure 3 shows the death rates by age grouping and reveal that the younger Indian population reveals the highest death rates. Figure 4 compares the deaths from accidents and violence during the 1978-88 period. In the period of 1983-86, adult Indian males experienced an accidental death rate nearly four times that of the overall population. Mortality rates are presented in Figure 5. While the rates of both the Canadian population and the Indian population have decreased, the rate of decrease for Indians has been substantially greater.

Figure 1. Life Expectancy at Birth: Status Indians and All Canadians, 1981, 1991, 2001.

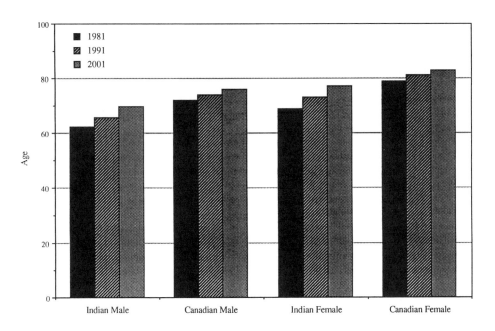

Source: Ellen Bobet, *Inequalities in Health: A Comparison of Indian and Canadian Mortality Trends*, Health and Welfare Canada, Ottawa.

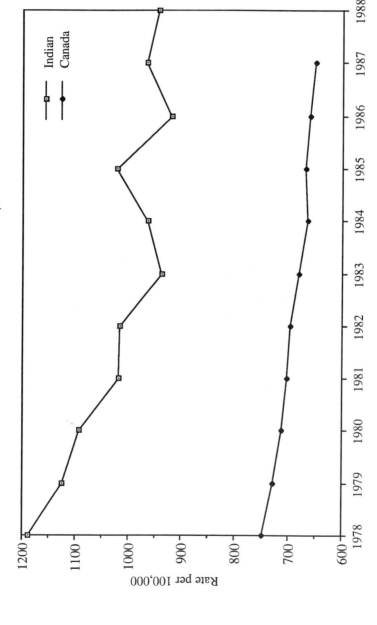

Figure 2. Death Rates, 1978 - 1988: Indian and Canadian Populations*

* Age-standardized

Source: Ellen Bobet, *Inequalities in Health: A Comparison of Indian and Canadian Mortality Trends*, Health and Welfare Canada, Ottawa.

Health Promotion and Indian Communities

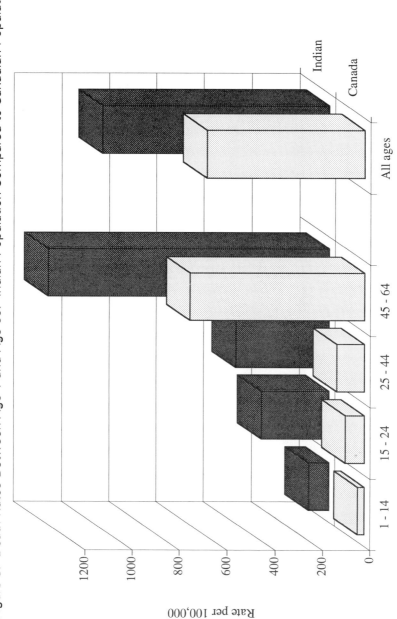

Figure 3. Death Rates Between Age 1 and Age 65: Indian Population Compared to Canadian Population

Source: Ellen Bobet, *Inequalities in Health: A Comparison of Indian and Canadian Mortality Trends*, Health and Welfare Canada, Ottawa.

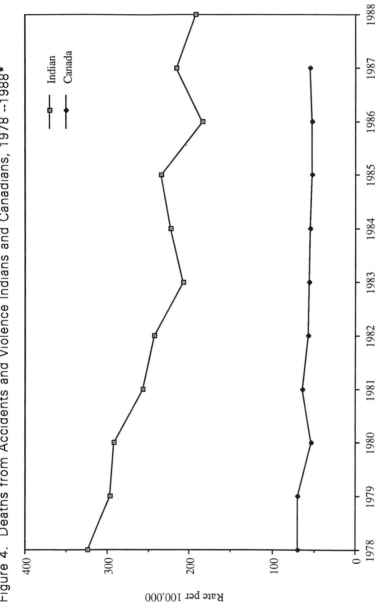

Figure 4. Deaths from Accidents and Violence Indians and Canadians, 1978–1988*

* Age-standardized

Source: Ellen Bobet, *Inequalities in Health: A Comparison of Indian and Canadian Mortality Trends*, Health and Welfare Canada, Ottawa.

Figure 5. Infant Mortality: Indian and Canada, 1960 – 1988*

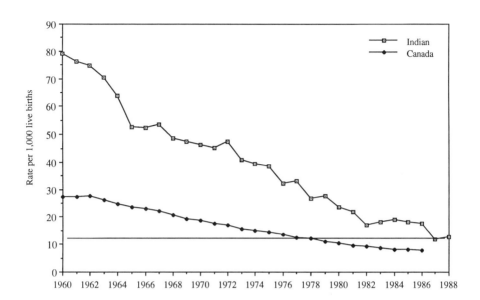

Source: Statistics Canada, cat. 84-206

However, in the end, the Indian rate still exceeds the national standard. A closer look at the source of infant mortality reveals that while the neonatal rates for Indians are similar to the general population, the perinatal rate is twice the Canadian norm and the post-neonatal rate is over three times as high. Figure 6 shows the specific cause of deaths in those involving accidents and violence for three time periods. In almost all cases (with the exception of exposure), there has been a decrease in the deaths. This is particularly true for deaths by firearms. On the other hand, suicides had increased to nearly three per 10,000 population, well over five times the national average.[2]

Figure 7 reveals the patterns of deaths by accident and violence for specific age groups over a ten year span. The data show that causes of death for 0-1 year olds has changed dramatically. On the other hand, for others (except the 55+ group), the pattern seems unchanged. Figure 8 identifies Indian deaths by type of disease. The data show that the impact of most diseases has been constant since 1979 withthe exception of injury/poisoning and circulatory system diseases, which have been reduced substantially. Compared to a rate of nearly 20 per 10,000 in 1960, these incidences have decreased to less than 12 in 1989.

278 Racial Minorities, Medicine & Health

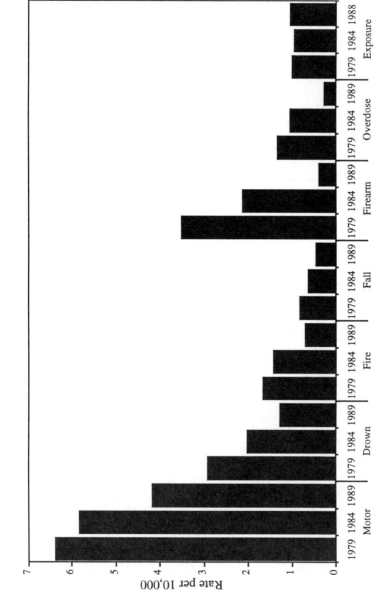

Figure 6. Native Deaths (Accidents and Violence) by Year 1979 – 1989*

* Other rates for cause of death in 1989 were: suffocation, 0.57; homocide, 1.14; suicide, 2.85

The data also show that while the rank order of diseases is similar by gender, males were much more likely to die of these two diseases than were females. Using age-standardized rates per 100,000, Bobet (1990) compared death rates from neoplasms of Indians to the general Canadian population. Her results showed that in 1978, the Indian rate was 129 while the Canadian population stood at 167. However, a decade later Indian rates had increased to 136 while the general population stood at 175. She also showed that death (using age-standardized rates) from diseases of circulatory system for both Indians and the general Canadian population were about the same although both had decreased from 1979 to 1989.

The results reveal that the Canadian population has benefited from the increased medical technology and quality of life generated from an enhanced knowledge of illness. Unfortunately, this cannot be said for Indians. While they have achieved some benefits, the effects have been mediated by socio-economic factors. As such, while mortality rates of young Indians have decreased, they still remain substantially higher than non-Indians. In addition, because of the low standard of life and cultural disorganization, Indians are not utilizing western medical knowledge nor the medical knowledge of their elders. As a result, many types of illness for Indians are at all-time highs, e.g., suicides.

We also find that over the past half century, the general Canadian population experienced a shift in the causes of death from infectious diseases to degenerative diseases. For example, in the 1930s, nearly half of the "years lost in life" were due to respiratory system diseases. An additional quarter were from "early infancy" diseases. Today, in the general population these causes account for eight and six percent respectively (Beaujot, 1991). However, for Indians, the infant mortality rate is twice as high as the national average and diseases of the respiratory system are almost double the national average — 91.1/50.4 (average for the 1984-88 period). As such, these causes contribute to "years lost" which are comparable to those of the general population in the 1930s. Today two major diseases in Indian communities — AIDS and diabetes — are rampant as they exceed the national rates by substantial amounts. The incidence of AIDS also reflects that communicable disease, so prevalent at the beginning of the 20th century, is now one of the leading causes of death of Indians as we move into the 21st century.

The above data suggest both a lower standard of living and an inability by Indians to access technological advances in health care services for Indians. Such factors as poorer housing and other environmental conditions on the reserves have contributed to these high death rates and other indicators of poor health. However, there

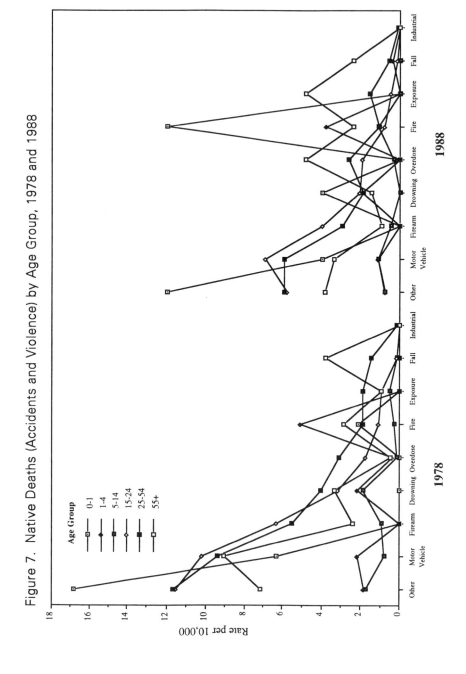

Figure 7. Native Deaths (Accidents and Violence) by Age Group, 1978 and 1988

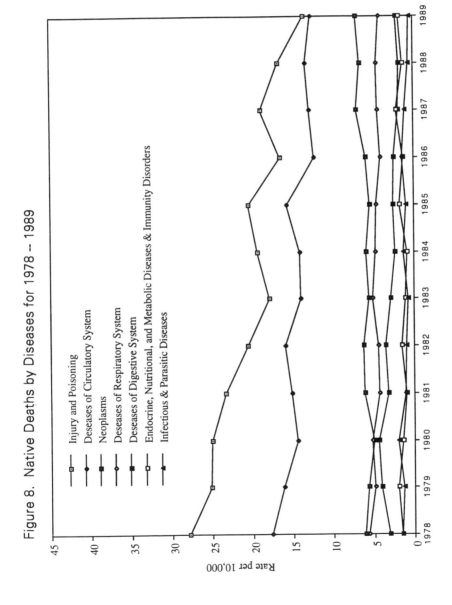

Figure 8. Native Deaths by Diseases for 1978 – 1989

are social and structural factors which have equally contributed to the poor health of Indian people. The lack of community organization, dependency upon urban centres and the federal government, and the history of colonization have all had substantial impacts upon Indian peoples access and use of medical services. These structural and historical factors also have prevented Indians from engaging in major educational programs on the issue of health.

Decolonization

The process of change is slow and the changes in health care services are no exception. The changing of institutional structures and linkages require massive modifications in organizational models as well as values of those working with the organizations. Furthermore, the definition of change and the perspectives therein are dependent upon the dominant group's explanation. As Indian people begin the process of taking over control of their lives, they find that they must first challenge the vocabulary used by the dominant group. For example, since the 1970s, government officials have talked about devolution, and the process by which they were turning over control to Native people.[3] From the perspective of Indian people, it was not the federal government acting in a manner to bring about decolonization; rather it was the actions of Indian people who were creating the process of decolonization.

The process of colonization of Indian people has been carefully recorded and causes and consequences have been identified. At the same time we have been oblivious to the process by which Indian people were striving toward and implementing the process of decolonization. This thrust by Indian people to regain control over their lives has not been the subject of research nor has it been part of the vocabulary of the dominant group. The push for self determination or in more specific forms, self government, has been the basis of decolonization. Whether the focus is upon politics, education, business or health, Indian people are attempting to take control of their lives and live within the institutional structure of the dominant society while maintaining some control over the structures which influence their behaviour and the organization of their community. Recently, negotiations have taken place among the federal, provincial and Indian leaders regarding this issue.

While the federal government has, for some time, embarked on a policy of implementing "devolutionary" policies focusing on business issues, there is an equal insistence on the part of Indian people that they want to maintain control over their land, their children's education and the health of their people, enacting the process of decolonization. There is no doubt that economic issues are important in the overall picture of Indian people, but it is equally important that Indians have the ability to influence their children through educational institutions, health care services, legal institutions and political structures. Indian people have also realized that economic issues pursued by the government reflect an assimilative and control function. Outside government agencies or private businesses are encouraged to stimulate economic activities on reserves or rural enclaves but always retain ultimate control and encapsulate the Indian population. These devolutionary decisions have tried to integrate Indians into the mainstream economic activities while at the same time making sure that executive powers remain in the dominant group. In short, devolution is not the same as decolonization.

The process of decolonization is rejecting the strategies that have been promoted by the federal and provincial governments and is moving toward an autonomous (self government) model of control. Although there is no existing structure for Indians which reflects this goal, it remains the objective of many Indians. Some examples of approaching the autonomous model are evident and have demonstrated dramatic impacts. The Montreal Lake Band in Saskatchewan is a good example. Within three years after primary health care was placed under Band control in 1988, health indicators showed marked improvement. Support for the process of decolonization has, in recent times, come from an unlikely source—the legal profession and the courts. The various "task forces" set up by the Nova Scotia, Manitoba, Saskatchewan and Alberta governments with regard to justice have set the stage. The Law Reform Commission of Canada also has supported the concept of self government and has recommended that autonomy and self determination become the manner in which decolonization is implemented. Each of these Task Forces has also noted the "progressive" steps taken by both the United States and Australia regarding self determination of Aboriginal peoples.

The process of decolonization is resisted on many fronts. Provincial governments, while objecting to taking over the provision of services to Indian people, have equally rejected Indian people becoming autonomous because of the implications such an arrangement would have in the entire area of provincial responsibilities; the first of many groups outside the influence and scope of provincial government legislation. At a more general level, many people will argue that Indians are not yet ready to take over control of their lives. Depending upon the evidence marshaled, there will always be some support for this claim. Selective examples will be brought forward to illustrate the validity of such a claim.

However, a more global perspective will need to be utilized with the view that change does not come overnight and corrections can be implemented as the community is undergoing change.

The decolonization process is also rejected by government agencies as well as non-government agencies. Many of these organizations have been created out of the mandate to "save" Indians. Their *raison d'être* is based upon the belief that they are able to help Indians. While the pathologies of Native communities have emerged because of colonization (Taylor-Henley and Hudson, 1992), various organizations refuse to allow Indians to invoke the process of decolonization and initiate their resolution to the many problems confronting Indian communities. Until these agencies and organizations are convinced that Indian programs will solve the problems, they are unwilling to give up their power or share it with Indian communities. This reaction by non-Indians is equally prevalent in Indian communities where local Indians supported by the colonization process are also unwilling to give up and share their power they obtained through the process. Still others claim that decolonization cannot proceed until the government ensures that resources be retained if problem solving is to occur.

Etiology of Illness

In addition to genetic based causes of illness (which we will not be dealing with), there are two general determinants: biological and social-psychological. The medical model adopted in Canada is based solely upon a biological theory of disease. Using this as the basis of our beliefs about illness, we have created a medical structure which directs its actions on the belief that illness is a result of various infections resulting from improper dietary intake, sanitation or resistance to infections. As a result, we have taken medical and organizational steps to deal with these abnormal conditions. Unfortunately, we have only looked at the symptoms of the these diseases and have not tried to address the causes. For example, many Indians live in communities which are not served by adequate water supplies, housing or transportation. Furthermore, many of these same communities have not been able to establish an economically viable economy, which has adverse impacts upon health. The lack of education of these same individuals has also reflected poorly on their health. However, our health care system does not deal with any of these socio-economic factors, which if remedied, might enhance the health of the population. While the inclusion of socio-economic factors in the medical model is certainly a step forward from just looking at the symptoms of the illness, it does not take into account the second cause of illness- social-psychological factors.

Selye (1956) was one of the first to propose the theory that diverse external stimuli could generate ill health — either mental or physical. His theory linked stressful life events with the onset of ill health. As Lin and Ensel (1989) point out, there is considerable research which shows a moderate relationship between ill health and various stress factors. Certainly Indian people, living in conditions of "underclass," have experienced and continue to experience stress. The high rates of illness and mortality seem to be related to these high stress levels. How these factors are interrelated with "disease" factors is yet to be determined but there are links which seem to be present. Some have argued that these relationships are direct and independent of life events while others suggest that the level of social support mediates the effects of life events on health. It is our contention that the social support factors ameliorate the impact of stress factors on Indian people which reduce the stress impact. However, data from a variety of sources show that some stress continues to impact upon these people with the result that rates of some illnesses are much higher than others.

Definition of and Response to Illness

The definition of health varies from one societal context to another. People defined as ill in one society may not be so defined in another. Furthermore, labels of illness will vary over time. For example, people defined as having a specific illness today may be rediagnosed tomorrow, particularly in the case of mental illness. Nevertheless, in each society, there is some form of a *sick role* — a pattern of behaviour expected of individuals who are ill. In most cases, sick people are defined as deviants and must take steps to move out of that role to become normal participants in the community. To refuse treatment can bring about negative sanctions from other individuals or in some cases, institutional reaction, e.g., courts impose action on the ill person. To deal with individuals who are placed within the *sick role*, our society is organized in such a manner which will allow universal access to health care and, hopefully, benefit from it.

How individuals are dealt with in regard to their illness will also vary. In our society, health care activities that were formally organized within a broader social context now come under the regime of a special institutional structure. This decomposition has become a central feature in our institutional structure (Albercht and Otto, 1991). Traditionally, as each member of society participated in the educational system, religious institutions, leisure activities and work organizations, the values and norms of each of the institutions were linked to and accepted by the other organizational structures. In short, health care was considered part of the overall social system, the work context and within other institutional arrangements, e.g., religion. Over time this structure became embedded in our social organization and this mutual reinforcement of the institutional structures has allowed us to approach health in a segmented fashion. As a result, we have established large bureaucratic structures focusing on one type of health program—reactive acute care.[4] Unfortunately, over time this institutional arrangement has presented problems. For example, as Kramer and Weller (1989) point out, the health bureaucracies are not organized to attack the root causes of the problems which seem to be related to illness. As noted above, only direct biological disease issues are dealt with by the Medical Services Branch while DIAND is solely responsible for the social, economic and educational factors impinging upon Indian people. In addition, while there are many other agencies and government departments which have control over various segments of Indian lives (e.g., Department of Justice and the Treasury Board) few engage in coordinated efforts.

Furthermore, being ill in an Indian community is quite different than being ill in a non-Indian community. First of all, conceptualizations of mental health are quite different from the general Canadian population. For examples, the idea of a "strong" woman are incomprehensible in a non-Indian community. Yet within an Indian community, the belief that some women have powers well beyond those of the average individual are not uncommon. Within the Indian community, these individuals also have power to bring about mental and physical ailments which are disabling to the individual. Visiting a doctor, hospital or taking prescribed medicines to cure such illnesses will usually not cure the illness being experienced. The use of certain substances are also not defined as contributing to illness within the community. Smoking, drinking and the use of certain other drugs are not normally considered causing certain illnesses. Furthermore, when certain actions are considered potentially harmful, Indian residents may not have any alternatives so an acceptance of fate is the preferred response. For example, if the fish in a nearby lake or river are contaminated but an alternative source of food is not available, the contaminated food will continue to be consumed. The resultant illness will be accepted or tolerated and thus the individual experiencing certain symptoms associated with an illness will not be defined as enacting a sick role. Hence, the structure and make-up of an Indian community provides a conceptualization of illness and health which is different than those identified in the general Canadian population.

Social Support

Social support is the process by which resources in the social structure are brought to bear on the needs of people (both functional and symbolic) in both routine and crisis situations (Lin and Ensel, 1989). For purposes of this paper, we make the assumption that the support system available to people is a function of the structural conditions they operate within as they exist in a stratified system where institutional arrangements have been in place over time. From a sociological perspective then, the social structure experienced by Indian people determines their social relationships, their health and the subsequent definitions of illness. Thus we find that structural organizations in which Indian people operate are not similar to other groups of Canadians and result in different health patterns, definitions of illness and eventually disease and mortality profiles. The general model underlying the following argument has been referred to as "structure seekers" by Pearlin (1992:2) where structure is defined as those arrangements among the parts of a system that are more or less stable through time, though not immutable. As noted above, the unique organization and structure of an Indian community suggests that the concept of illness must be reviewed carefully when assessing the social importance of health indicators explicated earlier in the paper.

Given our knowledge about Indian communities on reserves which show that they are rural, small and heavily kin-related, we should expect them to exhibit, in the Durkheim tradition, *mechanical solidarity*.[5] We would expect this *mechanical solidarity* to provide strong social support for all residents. This social support, it is expected, would reduce the impact of structural effects on illness for individuals. However, it is clear that we do not find this evident in Indian communities. Why not? The first explanation centres on the definition of the *sick role*. Individuals exhibiting behaviour which might, in the larger society, be defined as sick, are not so defined within the reserve, even though the outcome may lead to death. Secondly, many causes of death are not considered abnormal within an Indian community after decades of living with similar social and economic conditions. Therefore, in many cases, social support mechanisms are not put in place to deal with a "problem." A third reason is that certain structural conditions are not sufficient to produce illness, but when interacted with certain behaviours, e.g., substance abuse, impact upon the health of individuals in some cases is potentially lethal. For example, the use of motor vehicles and firearms are not sufficient causes of mortality. However, when mixed with substance abuse, they become the leading causes of death on the reserve.

A fourth explanation focuses on the degree of social support that the community members provide to their co-residents. In this context we need to focus on the extent of market exchanges, institutional distributions and coercive appropriations that take place in an Indian community (Wellman, and Wortley, 1990). Supportive ties in Indian communities vary by the strength of the relationship and the access that individuals have to each other. Furthermore, as the community intensifies its capacity to communicate and coordinate their activities, additional support to members should be evident. Other relationships such as access to resources and kinship will impact the support provided. Thus, it would seem that because Indians live in isolated enclaves, engaging in frequent contact with other community members; this would provide support through shared values, mutual awareness of needs, mitigating feelings of loneliness and facilitating the provision of resources. It is anticipated that various types of coping behaviours are taught to young people and carried out as Indians strive to live in dysfunctional communities. In short, we would expect the mechanical solidarity to mediate the impacts of structural factors causing illness.

However, this general hypothesis does not seem to be confirmed for Indian communities. Our assessment of Indian communities reveals that the nature and extent of social support on Indian communities is low. Our task is to explain this state of affairs. First, it is important to realize that reserve culture is a product of civil servants. Reserves were never intended to be integrated communities; they were simply tracts of land given to Indians to carry out subsistence agriculture with the hope they would fail within a few years after being established. Secondly, the organization of the Indian community is bureaucratically and arbitrarily constituted (Carstens, 1991). As a result of the intense and constant imposition of bureaucratic structures over the past half century, Indians have incorporated these rigid structures into their personalities and relationships with other people. Carstens (1991) points out that Indians living on reserves are subject to the process of *administrative determinism* which reflects the total impact of the *Indian Act* which influences the behaviour of individuals in almost every form and juncture. The resultant political conditioning has reduced the extent and form of social support networks.

Third, there are different categories of people living on or connected with the reserve community. As Carstens (1991) notes, members of the community may or may not reside on the reserve. The resultant complexities of a reserve consisting of permanent residents, off-reserve, sojourners, return migrants, Bill C-31 and out-migrants have led to considerable factionalization of the community. In addition, those people living on the reserve differ in their involvement and integration into the larger society. For example, as

Carstens points out, the family living on welfare is quite different than the one who is actively employed either on or off the reserve. This increasing heterogeneity has produced polarized social structures as evidenced in other communities (Menahan, 1992). Deep social divisions, each with differing amounts of power and resources have emerged, producing permanent social cleavages within the community.

Fourth, patterns of residence are a function of historical and contemporary factors, e.g., inheritance, subdivision of land and changing patterns of wealth. As such, Indians do not control their residential patterns nor can they always determine who will be their neighbour. Fifth, as DIAND has relinquished its day to day administrative control, a nucleus or core of Indians have moved into these positions. These positions represent power positions in the community and control large amounts of resources. Networks with 'powerful' individuals will be coloured by who occupies positions of control. Previous research has indicated, as noted above, a sixth source of potential disruption of social support; that family or kinship networks have an impact upon the degree of social support offered to individuals. Lithman (1978) and Carstens (1991) among others, have indicated that within an Indian community, there are two different layers of kinship networks. The general patronymic networks are the most complex and encompass the largest number of kin. At a lower level, we find family compacts (bunches) are small groups of consanguine kin and affines. These networks are vacillating and ever-changing as the political and economic structure of the community varies over time. A seventh issue leading to the lack of social support is the complexity of organizational structure of Indian communities. Government officials, assuming that small communities were not complex, introduced simplistic organizational structures to implement their decisions and allow residents to carry out their daily activities when reserves were created. Today it is clear that smallness does not easily translate to simple. We are now aware (Wolfe, 1989) that small rural communities are complicated, requiring intricate and precise organizational responses to their unique characteristics. Residents of small communities are frequently called upon to serve in important positions, respond to actions by agents both in and outside the community and take on activities dealing with a large range of problems for themselves and their communities. For example, "burn out" is a common phenomenon in Indian communities as individuals are expected to perform in a number of roles.

An additional problem for small communities is the lack of communications between government agencies/departments and the leadership of the community. Most residents of small communities are kept "in the dark" about policy changes, programs and other information which might serve the communities' purposes but not the government's.

As Wolfe (1989) points out, a clear dependency relationship between small communities and the government exists. As Wilkinson (1986) points out, a ninth factor is that small rural communities are always subject to a "dependency relation" with nearby larger urban centres — centres which supply the rural population with most of their daily needs and all of their specialized requirements. He goes on to show that rural dependency is associated with poverty, community instability and malintegration. However, rural communities have tried to overcome these aspects by using their isolation and shared experiences to create and sustain local community control. This then requires an active process of public participation in addition to social support.[6]

Finally, most reserve communities are factionalized. This does not mean that each of these factions is long standing (although it might be) or acts in a 'corporate' fashion. Nevertheless, these factions compete for scarce resources, power and influence. In addition, these factions are open categories and fluid, with changing membership over time. The result is that interpersonal relations on reserves are generally characterized by far greater levels of conflict than in non-Indian communities.

Indian Control

Indian people have consistently argued that local control of various institutional spheres needs to be within the jurisdiction of Indians. The reasoning is that institutions which accommodate and encourage community control tend to be more sensitive to Indian political cultures and such cultures can be a basis for effective governance (Conn, 1985). In short, local, self government will perform along the lines understood by the villagers (Cassidy, 1991). There is a belief that real community control will result if decolonization and self government are achieved. While we will not argue against such claims, we want to point out that self government is not a complete panacea for any community in terms of creating social support, reducing illness, enhancing health and/or facilitating socio-economic development. Nevertheless, many Indian leaders have accepted the concept of self government as the means of achieving all the desired goals of the community. The obvious goal is to achieve *final power* which will allow the community to make decisions in its best interest, not someone else's.

In order to achieve community control, the process of decolonization must be complete. This will require organizational shifts during which a power transfer will take place. How these will take place and the institutional arrangements of the new structure will be dependent upon a variety of factors. The success of the reorganized community in terms of maintaining authority and self government will also be dependent upon the actions of the various stakeholders in the community. Figure 9 identifies the overall model for achieving a state of balanced (spiritual, psychological, physiological, community) health for Indian communities. It clearly outlines the strategies and mechanisms necessary for reducing the inequities, increasing prevention and enhancing coping behaviour of Indian people.

Figure 9. A Framework for Health Promotion

A FRAMEWORK FOR HEALTH PROMOTION

AIM		ACHIEVING HEALTH FOR ALL	
HEALTH CHALLENGES	REDUCING INEQUITIES	INCREASING PREVENTION	ENHANCING COPING
HEALTH PROMOTION MECHANISMS	SELF-CARE	MUTUAL AID	HEALTHY ENVIRONMENTS
IMPLEMENTATION STRATEGIES	FOSTERING PUBLIC PARTICIPATION	STRENGTHENING COMMUNITY HEALTH SERVICES	COORDINATING HEALTHY PUBLIC POLICY

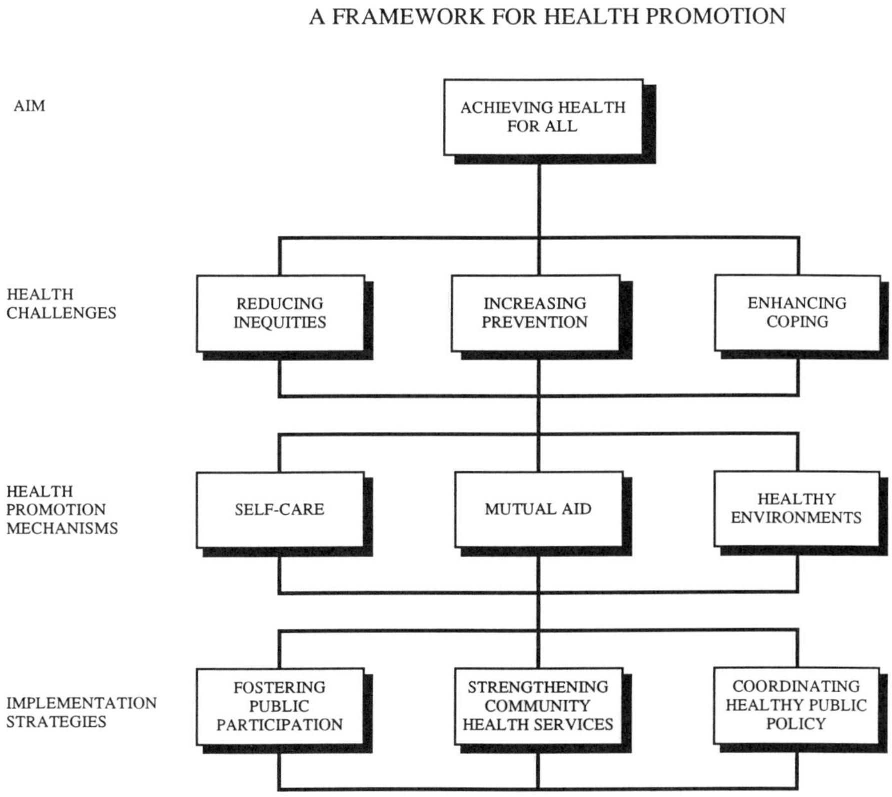

How will the process of decolonization be carried out, and for what goal? Once put in place, how will community control best serve the goals and objectives of the community? Previous research has indicated that success in goal achievement and maintenance of control was achieved when the organizations created are broadly based, nonpartisan, have an independent public identity, have a functional independence from any single sponsoring organization and are connected to existing networks of active volunteers and community leaders at the local level (Jennings, 1988). Crosby and colleagues (1986) also point to the need for organizations which provide clear, correct and current information to community residents. However, to ensure these attributes are in place, the community must be aware of how these structures operate and change over time. In addition, at what level does intergovernmental cooperation entee into the relationship? Residents must appreciate that participation changes in character over time. Wilkinson, (1986) has shown that communities act, but only under special circumstances. It is important that community leaders correctly time the issues facing the community with specific action on the part of the community residents. That is, community leaders must organize their activities around the issues at the appropriate time in order to ensure their ability to make decisions in their best interest.

Indians must also be aware that there will be substantial resistance to shift control to the community level. Montgomery (1979) notes that the "bureaupathology" which emerges out of bureaucratic organizations will lead to "patron-client" relationships with local leaders which will lead to a suppression of local issues in favor of issues decided upon by the bureaucrats. Yap (1990) cogently points out that people in power are reluctant to give up their power because they feel that it will never be satiated. Finally, there is a reluctance to give up power because of potential conflicts between community needs and professional standards. In the end, there may also be a financial conflict as limited resources mean that decisions will have to be made with regard to the placement of funding. In summary, a good organizational structure may be in place but if not funded properly, the goals and objectives of the community will not be achieved.

Conclusion

The current health system cannot deal with Indian health problems for many reasons. Our health system is based upon the belief that only large technologically sophisticated organizations housed within a hospital setting are appropriate for providing health care for the individual. Second, the health care system refuses to accept the importance or significance of group and community health. There is a consistent refusal of western health individuals to accept the notion that health can be provided communally; all diagnoses and treatment must take place at the individual level. Finally, there is an unwillingness of the government and health care officials to introduce alternative health care initiatives. The reluctance to accept the provision of health care by anyone other than a certified medical doctor is just one example.

There is, however, a willingness by the government to accept "self government" which might include the provision of health care for Indians by Indians. However, if this is to occur, there must be safeguards to ensure that the transfer of health care services is adequately funded, reflect true decolonization of government authority to Indian people and allow Natives to achieve the necessary training before the transfer takes place. Finally, there is the need for a modification of the types of services provided. In short, there needs to be a better integration of community health and social services. For example, there needs to be a stronger linkage with nondirect health services. Non-health factors such as unemployment, poor housing and lack of sanitation will need to be integrated into the health provision for Natives. In the end, it is important for Canadians to realize that medicine is not health.

Notes

1. Wilkins and Adams (1983) estimate that on average, 13 years of an individual's life will be spent in some state of disability. For Indian people, it is estimated that the length of time is nearly double that figure. In addition, for Indian people, states of disability occur continually throughout life, beginning in the early years while for non-Indians, disability is generally associated with old age.
2. When gender is controlled for, the pattern of accidental and violent deaths is very different. While motor vehicles is still the leading cause of death, males have a rate well over twice that of females. Firearms is the second leading cause of death for males while it is nearly the lowest cause for females. Similarly, drowning is the second leading cause of death for females while for males it is the lowest.
3. Devolution is the process by which the dominant group defines the process and outlines the procedures by which control is handed over to the subordinate group. Decolonization occurs when the subordinate group is able to determine the conditions of self determination.
4. While we also have engaged in a direct biological prevention program, e.g., inoculation, we have not expanded other proactive procedures.
5. Tonnies has also suggested that communities in the gemeinschaft tradition will exhibit characteristics which produce social support for community residents.
6. Public participation is the involvement of the community in planning and decision making rather than just contributing labour (Yap, 1990).

References

Albrecht, G. and H. Otto. 1991. *Social Prevention and the Social Sciences.* New York: Walter de Gruyter.

Beaujot, R. 1991. *Population Change in Canada.* Toronto: McClelland and Stewart Inc.

Bobet, E. 1990. *Inequalities in Health: A Comparison of Indian and Canadian Mortality Trends.* Ottawa: Health and Welfare Canada

Canada, Government of. 1957. *Hospital Insurance Diagnostic Services Act.*

Canada, Government of. 1966. *Medical Care Act.* Ottawa.

Carstens, P. 1991. *The Queen's People.* Toronto: University of Toronto Press.

Cassidy, F. 1991. "Organizing for Community Control." *The Northern Review* Summer, 7: 17-34.

Conn, S. 1985. "Inuit Village Councils in Alaska — An Historical Model for Effectuation of Aboriginal Rights?" *Etudes/Inuit/Studies* 9 (2): 43-59.

Crosby, N., J. Kelly and P. Schaefer. 1986. "Citizens Panel: A New Approach to Citizen Participation." *Public Administration Review* 46: 170-178.

Jennings, B. 1988. *A Grassroots Movement in Bioethics.* Community Health Decisions, Hastings Center Report, 18(3).

Kramer, J. and G. Weller. 1989. *North American Native Health: A Comparison Between Canada and the United States.* Lakehead Centre for Northern Studies, Research Report #5, Thunder Bay: Lakehead University.

Lin, N. and W. Ensel. 1989. "Life Stress and Health: Stressors and Resources." *American Sociological Review* 54, June: 382-399.

Lithman, Y. 1978. *The Community Apart: A Case Study of a Canadian Indian Reserve Community.* Stockholm: University of Stockholm.

Menaham, G. 1992. "Social Cleavage and Political Divisions in Community." *International Journal of Contemporary Sociology* 29(1): 97-114.

Montgomery, J. 1979. "The Populist Front in Rural Development: Or Shall We Eliminate Bureaucrats and Get On With the Job?" *Public Administration Review* 39(2): 58-65.

Nagnur, D. and M. Nagrodski. 1988. "Cardiovascular Disease, Cancer and Life Expectancy." *Canadian Social Trends* 11: 25-27.

Nathanson, C. and A. Lopez. 1987. "The Future of Sex Mortality Differentials in Industrialized Countries: A Structural Hypothesis." *Population Research and Policy Review* 6(2): 123-136.

Pearlin, L. 1992. "Structure and Meaning in Medical Sociology." *The Journal of Health and Social Behavior* 33(1), March: 1-9.

Selye, H. 1956. *The Stress of Life.* New York: McGraw-Hill.

Taylor-Henley, S. and P. Hudson. 1992. "Aboriginal Self-Government and Social Services: First Nations-Provincial Relations." *Canadian Public Policy* 18 (1), March: 13-26.

Tonnies, F. 1957. *Community and Society.* Lansing: Michigan State University Press.

Waldram, J. and J. O'Neil. 1989. "Native Health Research in Canada: Anthropological and Related Approaches." in Native Health Research in Canada (Special Issue), *Native Studies Review* 5(1): 1-17.

Wellman, B. and S. Wortley. 1990. "Different Strokes from Different Folks: Community Ties and Social Support." *American Journal of Sociology* 96(3): 558-588.

Wilkins, R. and O. Adams. 1983. *Healthfulness of Life.* Montreal: Institute for Research on Public Policy.

Wilkinson, K. 1986. "In Search of the Community in the Changing Countryside." *Rural Sociology* 51(1): 1-17.

Wolfe, J. 1989. "Approaches to Planning in Native Communities: A Review and Commentary on Settlement Problems and the Effectiveness of Planning Practice." *Plan Canada* 29(2): 63-79.

Yap, K. 1990. "Community Participation in Low Income Housing Projects: Problems and Prospects." *Community Development Journal* 25(1): 56-67.

15

Sick to Death: The Health of Aboriginal People in Australia and Canada

Carol Reid

Introduction

There are remarkable similarities in the contemporary health status of Aboriginal peoples in Australia and Canada.[1] To understand these similarities we need to recognize historical factors of colonization and settlement that have occurred in both countries. The continuance of a 'colonial mentality' (Morrow, n.d.) is reflected in the political and legal institutions that govern every aspect of Aboriginal peoples' lives in Australia and Canada. It is exhibited in the continuation of governments legislating on behalf of a group of people who have little or no say in those decisions. It is evident in the way institutions are ordered and structured to exclude and marginalize Aboriginal peoples.

Given that Aboriginal peoples in Australia and Canada have had somewhat different contact experiences it is interesting to note the striking similarities in rates of unemployment, recidivism, school attrition rates and health status. The reason for this is that the relationship between Aboriginal and non-Aboriginal peoples in both countries has, and continues to be, characterized by institutional racism. Institutional racism is "both a racist theory and a social practice embedded in institutions that systematically excludes subordinate members from equal participation and treatment in society" (Bolaria and Li, 1988:30). This chapter argues that the health of Aboriginal people in Australia and Canada must always be seen in the context of the political, economic and social conditions in which they live.

Interaction between Aboriginal peoples and the state is a central part of any analysis of how these conditions have emerged and how they can be improved. The argument advanced in this chapter is that structural change is required to reduce the pervading impact of institutional racism on the health of Aboriginal people in Australia and Canada. The focus is therefore on the role of structures in white society - rather than on the cultures of Aboriginal society - in generating sickness and premature death in Aboriginal society. Nevertheless, this change must be seen as resulting from "action within and upon" the limits set down by society (Fleras and Elliott, 1992:ix). The concept of agency must be central to understanding how change is shaped. Locally specific initiatives are important factors in that change because of the contemporary differences in which Aboriginal issues have been conceptualized in each country.

In the following pages I first outline the historical similarities and differences of the Australian and Canadian Aboriginal experience and discusses the most appropriate theoretical framework for an examination of the health of Aboriginal people in both countries. Data relating to indices of the disadvantaged socio-economic status of Australian and Canadian Aborigines - and relating to their inferior health status - are then introduced. Finally, the critical issue of the control and representation of Aboriginal people in health care and, more generally, social, economic and political institutions of Australian and Canadian societies is introduced. The chapter concludes by emphasizing the superiority of a political economy model of Aboriginal health over a culturalist model and suggests that Aboriginal health issues cannot be separated from the treatment of Aboriginal people in Australian and Canadian society as a whole.

Historical Overview and Theoretical Considerations

Historically, imported diseases, murder, rape, miscenegation and institutional neglect led governments in Australia and Canada to assume that their indigenous populations would gradually die out and disappear (Patterson, 1988; Reynolds, 1981). When Aboriginal people got in the way of expanding agricultural needs, their lands were further appropriated while they, the rightful owners, were moved to 'protected' reserves. In Canada, numerous treaties were signed to extricate the land from the Aboriginal population (Frideres, 1985). The very act of drawing up treaties meant that the land in question was actually acknowledged as being owned by Aboriginal people and that there could be a continuing legal basis for compensation. But the treaties did more than this; they effectively gave the government total control over Canadian Aboriginal lives. The Canadian state has continued to define and control the lives of Canadian Aboriginal people from the earliest days to the present.

In Australia, there were no such treaties, as the land at the time of settlement was presumed empty. 'Terra nullius' (Reynolds, 1981) was the legal term used to justify the separation of Aboriginal people from their Land. Since the British did not attempt to understand Aboriginal land tenure and social organization, they presumed none existed. In keeping with the ideology of social Darwinism they deemed themselves superior and therefore took their 'rightful' place in dominating and controlling every aspect of Aboriginal life. Their land was taken when needed - often violently because of resistance - with no treaties and no compensation.

It wasn't until 1960 in Canada, and 1967 in Australia, that Aboriginal people were granted citizenship rights. Furthermore, recognition of Aboriginal peoples as sharing a distinct cultural heritage in terms of specific economic, political and social histories didn't occur until 1972 in Australia and 1982 in Canada (Fleras and Elliott, 1992:13). The different historical and legal relationships of Aboriginal people to land in Australia and Canada have important repercussions in that these relationships continue to influence the way in which governments and Aboriginal people can and are responding in each country.

The results of this different basis for land acquisition is that in Canada there has been a policy of 'containment'of status Indians on reserves which persists today despite the drift of increasing numbers of status Indians to urban areas (Waldram, 1989; Frideres, 1988b). In Australia, this policy of containment of Aboriginal peoples on reserves was abandoned in the 1950s. In the 1960s and especially since 1972 when a policy of 'self-determination' began, there has been a rapid increase in the number of people moving to urban areas. The contemporary history of both countries diverges at this point although self-determination remains a common goal.

At the centre of this divergence are the ways in which Aboriginal peoples in both countries have resisted total domination and continued to argue for the rights of self-determination. This is a complex process because Aboriginal populations are spread over a vast area. This means that the delivery of services such as housing, health, education and legal representation is differential because of a sometimes rural, sometimes urban population. As O'Neil and Waldram (1989:13) argue,

... problems in Native communities, be they health problems or otherwise, must be understood in a wider historical and political context as reflections of colonial history. It also means that solutions to these problems must derive from processes set in motion at the community level which articulate with traditional values and local economic and political forces.

In Canada there is currently much more emphasis on control within the reserve system - that is, for band councils to be able to determine what is appropriate for their communities. There appears to be little consideration as yet for how self-government will affect all the status, non-status Natives and Metis who live in urban areas. Yet, according to a recent editorial, urban Aboriginals could be as large as two-thirds of the total Aboriginal population (*Globe and Mail*, June 3, 1992).

In Australia, Aboriginal communities are also spread across urban and rural areas in traditional and non-traditional living situations. But as prior ownership has never been recognized, the fight for Land Rights has united Aboriginal groups into national action. Groups that can satisfy the government about their relationship to Land may have rights granted while urban Aboriginal people, for example, argue for compensation and restricted Land Rights in terms of areas of historical significance. The diversity of contemporary Aboriginal living situations is at least nominally recognized if not understood by non-Aboriginal people. Until 1972 the definition of Aboriginality was based on racist biological definitions of 'blood.'[2] 'Real' Aboriginal people lived in the desert and were visibly different according to the social construction of Aboriginality and the resulting cultural stereotypes. This ideological approach denied the impact of historical factors such as miscegenation, rape, policies of assimilation and subsequent economic and political marginalisation and the resulting diversity of Aboriginal situations.

As a consequence, the use of the word 'traditional,' in terms of lifestyle and values, is problematic in the Australian context given the increasing number of Aboriginal people who today live in urban areas (approximately 65 percent, Australian Bureau of Statistics, 1991). The term 'traditional' evokes a static concept of culture and has inherent connotations of helplessness, stagnancy and inability to adapt to modern Australian life. It does not help us to understand the cultural renewal strategies of urban Aboriginals and it also creates an artificial division between the 'real' and 'true' Aborigines and others. This simplistic approach diverts attention away from the need to account for different historical junctures, responses and needs (see Langton, 1981). The term 'traditional' has come to encompass all that is 'good' or 'better' about Aboriginal culture juxtaposed with all that is 'bad.' The latter is typified by the social disorganization model that is used to define contemporary and specifically urban Aboriginal life (Reid, 1991). A more useful approach is to retain a distinctiveness regarding Aboriginal peoples that emerges from different specific historical, political, economic and cultural experiences that are constantly being adapted, transformed and reproduced. Waldram (1989) raises a similar concern regarding urban Aboriginals in Saskatoon and claims that many are in fact bicultural and bilingual, thus questioning the myth of Aboriginal people's inability to adapt and change.

In comparing the health status of Aboriginal peoples in Australia and Canada it is necessary to do so in relation to socio-economic and political factors. This is to avoid a culturalist model which uses an individualistic basis for explaining health issues. For example, the acceptance of 'germ theory' tends to "presuppose that health is the concern of the individual" (Frideres, 1988a) rather than dependent upon "socially determined ways of life" (Bolaria:cited in Frideres, 1988:135).

A World of Difference

Australia and Canada are demographically similar. A large part of the population clusters in the most hospitable parts of the country leaving vast and inhospitable tracts of land with settlements scattered few and far between. Not uncommonly, Aboriginal people live in these inhospitable lands that until recently were not prized for agricultural use but now offer riches to be gained by mineral extraction. The tenuous nature of land rights is poignantly obvious in these circumstances in Australia where mining companies have waged an expensive ideological war against Land Rights, particularly in the Northern Territory (Reid and Trompf, 1991). In Canada reserves have not meant self-sufficiency due to the limitations placed on land usage (Frideres, 1988b; York, 1990:5).

Canada and Australia share another distinction - that of having a Fourth World population living in a First World nation. The United Nations defines indigenous populations in this situation as people:

> . . . who live more in conformity with their particular social, economic and cultural customs and traditions than with the institutions of the country of which they now form part, under a state structure which incorporates mainly the national, social and cultural characteristics of other segments of the population which are dominant" (cited in Reid and Trompf, 1991:xiii).

This does not imply homogeneity since Aboriginal people live in many different environments, language groups and communities. What is common to Aboriginal and Torres Strait Islander people in Australia and status Natives, non-status Natives, Inuits and Metis in Canada, is a dramatically different life in terms of quality and 'quantity' compared to non-Aboriginal Australians and Canadians. This difference in life options and outcomes is directly related to their social, economic and political marginalization which can be directly related to their alienation from their land and traditional means of production (Brady, 1983:41). The removal of ancestral lands created 'a problem' for white administrators which they have historically grappled with, in paternalistic manner, from 'protectionism' through to blatant racist policies of assimilation which saw residential schools in Canada (Haig-Brown, 1988; York, 1990:22-53) and 'stolen generations' in Australia (Read and Edwards, 1988).

While historical atrocities are now widely recognized and documented, racist practices continue today. The Report of the National Inquiry into Racist Violence in Australia found in 1991 that "racism and racist violence permeates the day-to-day lives of Aboriginal and Islander people" (Muirhead, 1991:72). This, it was claimed, had a cumulative effect which expressed itself in feelings of hopelessness, powerlessness, anguish, distress and emotional disorders among Aboriginal people. It is important to stress that these psychological effects are not the result of cultural disintegration but of continuing legal, political and economic discrimination. For example, the imprisonment rate for Aboriginal people is fourteen times higher (Table 1) than for the total population and is largely for infringements such as drunkenness, violence and petty theft such as break and enters (Aboriginal Statistics, 1986). In the late 1980s there was concern at the large number of deaths in custody attributed to suicide. Justice Muirhead (1988) found that sentencing was often harsher for Aboriginal people and more likely to be handed out than alternative measures such as bonds or community service. Furthermore, medical assistance was often not procured when the prisoner appeared in distress.

Frideres points out that suicides among Aboriginal people in Canada account for over one quarter of accidental deaths and the rate is three times the national average (1988b:199). The containment of peoples on reserves with little prospect of continuous employment and therefore limited choices barely needs a mention. The Human Rights and Equal Opportunity Commission (1991)in Australia and York (1990) in Canada comment on the depressed conditions in which Aboriginal people live on and off reserves. Urban Aboriginal people are found in poor areas of cities in overcrowded and delapidated buildings. These areas are often targets for heavy-handed police activity in terms of surveillance and constitute a continual threat of physical violence. Racism in the police force, lack of employment, poor housing and shortages of water and sewerage systems are factors influencing health. On reserves in Canada, "fewer than 50 percent of Native homes have sewer or water connections; another 50 percent can be described as overcrowded" (cited in Fleras and Elliott, 1992:16).

Table 1. Selected Demographic Characteristics and Socio-Economic Status of Aboriginal People in Australia and Canada.

	RATES COMPARED TO TOTAL POPULATIONS	
	AUSTRALIA	CANADA
UNEMPLOYMENT	4x	3x
INPRISONMENT	14x	9x(APPROX.)
INFANT MORTALITY	2.7x	2x
LIFE EXPECTANCY	<20 YEARS	<10 YEARS
FERTILITY	3x	2x
INCOME (AS PORTION OF NATIONAL AVERAGE)	2/3	2/3

Sources: Australian Bureau of Statistics, Australia's Aboriginal and Torres Strait Islander People: Census of Population and Housing, June, 1986 (Commonwealth of Australia, 1991); James Frideres, "From the Bottom Up:Institutional Structures and the Indian People," in *Social Issues and Contradictions in Canadian Society*, edited by B.S. Bolaria (Toronto: Harcourt Brace Jovanovich, 1991); Mary Jane Norris, "The Demography of Aboriginal People in Canada," in *Ethnic Demography: Canadian Immigrant, Racial and Cultural Variations*, edited by S.S. Halli, F. Trovato and L. Driedger, (Ottawa: Carleton, 1990).

The data on age structure show that Aboriginal populations tend to be younger relative to the general population (Australian Bureau of Statistics, 1991; Norris, 1990). There are a couple of explanations for this relatively larger proportion of youth among the Australian and Canadian Aboriginal people. First, as Table 1 shows, fertility rates are higher for Aboriginal groups compared to the total population; second, higher mortality rates in the middle years contributes to this 'youthful' trend. While infant mortality rates in both countries have decreased significantly over time because of particular attention being given to this area (Norris, 1990; Reid and Trompf, 1991), these rates are still higher than the general population. However, little has been done to address the real basis for illness which is reflected in the health status of all ages.

It is the types of illnesses and causes of death that show a clear link between the wider issues in Aboriginal affairs and the differing health status of Aboriginal people. Gray, Trompf and Houston (1991:111) found that in Australia "the pattern of Aboriginal mortality resembled no model life table pattern. . . . what was found was a pattern of very high rates of mortality in middle adulthood." To understand this we need to assess the quality of life for most Aboriginal people. Because of recurring illnesses in childhood and chronic disease in adult years, most Aboriginal people are sick until their early deaths. As Table 1 shows, Aboriginal people in Australia have a life expectancy 20 years less that the national average, while Aboriginal Canadians live, on average, 10 years less than the national average. Continual sickness until early death is significant if we are to fully comprehend the extent of suffering caused by the policies of governments in Australia and Canada towards Aboriginal people. Illness not only causes individual suffering but has an impact upon social organization, economic independence and political power. These factors, in turn, have an impact on general well-being and health.

For example, illness has a critical impact on educational success. In Australia, childhood illnesses such as chronic ear disease result in between 10 percent and 40 percent of Aboriginal children with hearing loss "significant enough to interfere with education" (Reid and Trompf, 1991:58). Almost three times as many Aboriginal children contract diseases such as meningitis, pneumonia and respiratory tract infections. This rate is also twice as high as that for the Inuit and Navajo in America. Overcrowded living conditions and inadequate diet were seen "to be of importance in the pathogenesis of these diseases" (Reid and Trompf, 1991:60). Childhood in Australia for Aboriginal people is the beginning of a relationship with hospitals that will see them admitted two and a half to three times more often than for children in the total population (Reid and Trompf, 1991:50). As adults they are going to experience such Third World diseases as trachoma (evidenced in 38 percent of Aboriginal population compared to less than two percent of non-Aboriginal), leprosy and tuberculosis. While these diseases are more prevalent in remote regions they serve to highlight that policies of settlement in remote areas without adequate provision of infrastructure have serious consequences for Aboriginal health (Aboriginal Statistics, 1986).

There appears to be a similar pattern in Canada with respect to on-reserve Natives. According to Frideres (1988b:199) "poor health and high mortality on reserves are directly related to poor access to medical facilities, the lack of sewage disposal, the unchecked exposure to disease, and a general lack of health care services." In both countries, Aboriginal people are more likely to suffer from diabetes, heart disease and diseases of the respiratory system. All of these diseases are chronic and affect potential for access in life. The impact upon families is underestimated. Children miss school to tend sick relatives or because of their own illnesses. Parents are deprived of the support of grandparents. In addition, illness and death are occasions for familial and community responsibility. Many trips back to 'their country' are to bury or tend sick relatives - a practice often unacknowledged and referred to in derogatory terms - e.g., 'walkabout' - which refer to the inability of Aboriginal people to integrate or settle down. What is often referred to as 'transience' is an adaptive mechanism to socio-economic inequality and illness as well as cultural maintenance in the face of socio-economic and political repression. Illness therefore reduces the capacity to work and is a drain on already stretched resources. As Table 1 shows, Aboriginal people are disadvantaged in the labour market. Australian Aboriginal employment rates are four times higher than the national average, while Canadian Aboriginal unemployment is three times higher.

Table 2. Leading Causes of Aboriginal Deaths in Australia and Canada.

AUSTRALIA (IN ORDER OF FREQUENCY)	CANADA (IN ORDER OF FREQUENCY)
DISEASES OF CIRCULATORY SYSTEM	DISEASES OF CIRCULATORY SYSTEM
INJURY AND POISONING	INJURY AND POISONING
DISEASES OF RESPIRATORY SYSTEM	NEOPLASMS
NEOPLASMS	DISEASES OF RESPIRATORY SYSTEM
INFECTIOUS AND PARASITIC DISEASES	DISEASES OF DIGESTIVE SYSTEM

Sources: Janice Reid and Peggy Trompf, *The Health of Aboriginal Australia*, (Sydney: Harcourt Brace Jovanovich,1991); James Frideres, "From the Bottom Up:Institutional Structures and the Indian People," in *Social Issues and Contradictions in Canadian Society*, edited by B.S. Bolaria (Toronto: Harcourt Brace Jovanovich, 1991); Mary Jane Norris, "The Demography of Aboriginal People in Canada," in *Ethnic Demography: Canadian Immigrant, Racial and Cultural Variations*, edited by S.S. Halli, F. Trovato and L. Driedger, (Ottawa: Carleton, 1990).

The major causes of death are compared in Table 2. Here we can see the continuation of avoidable 'lifestyle' diseases. For both populations, the incidence of injury and poisoning is extremely high. These reflect a reaction to intolerable situations characterized by poverty reflected in poor housing, unemployment and inadequate incomes. It is interesting to note that, in both countries, death caused by these means is more common on reserves (Frideres, 1988b; Reid and Trompf, 1991) where infrastructure is limited. Alcohol, petrol-sniffing and drug-taking all contribute to health-related problems and directly contribute to violence and abuse in these communities. York found that 70 percent of Manitoba's children and 20 percent of Aboriginal children in the Northern Territory, sniffed gasoline/petrol and that it was under the influence of the inhalant that violent acts occurred (1990:10,17). As York (1990:16) put it, "they are poverty-stricken members of a community that has been overwhelmed by a more powerful outside culture."

The financial stress placed on these communities is exacerbated by the high dependency ratio resulting from unemployment and the number of children of school age. Often it is the most able who leave to seek work in urban areas thus taking potential income with them. Clearly, Aboriginal health is not just an issue of prevention of germ invasion or 'lost culture.' It is related to basic issues concerning income, housing, education and employment and self-determination through land rights. With self-determination, Aboriginal people can change institutionalized racist practices that affect every level of their lives and their physical and mental health. Constitutional reform in Canada promises to insert the right of Aboriginal self-government into the Canadian constitution (*Globe and Mail*, June 15, 1992) but the details have yet to be outlined. In Australia, such developments are not yet even on the political agenda.

Control and Representation

The health of Aboriginal people is therefore determined by a number of factors beyond the individual's immediate control. The treatment of illness is intricately bound up with the understandings that exist within a society. Aboriginal people in Australia and Canada know that the health issues they are facing are a direct result of the conditions in which they live. They also know these conditions result from government policies which have marginalized and excluded their voices.

While western medicine is heavily dependent upon treating the individual body, Aboriginal people have a more holistic approach to the health of their members which recognizes that health is not just the responsibility of the individual but of the whole community. Malloch emphasizes that it "is difficult to talk about Indian medicine and Indian values without relating them to a whole way of life" (1989:105). She goes on to discuss the role of the spirit, body and mind needing to be in balance for good health. Clearly, government policy has undermined Indian lifestyles so that this integrated model of good health has become difficult to maintain. Yet that is what is being fought for at the moment. Self-government is the way to self-determination and therefore potentially a regaining of control over life and a concomitant increase in psychological, physical and mental well-being. However, unless accompanied by improved living conditions and long-term employment opportunities, these gains will be quickly eroded.

The political and economic relations of the Aboriginal communities in Canada to the government have influenced all aspects of native lives, including gender relations (Bourgeault, 1991:130). Traditional relationships between men and women have been eroded and consequent violence and abuse must be understood as part of these changes. However, Indian women, as part of their adaptation to these conditions in which they exist, have set up organizations to deal with these issues (e.g., Native Women's Association of Canada). These responses are initiatives that will deal with concerns at the community level while wider structural issues are also being challenged (Mary Two-Axe Early, *Globe and Mail*, May 29, 1992). Critiques that 'suggest' these women have been invaded by feminists (Lyon, 1992:4) fail to recognize that the women in these communities are also part of a wider society that has seen vast social movements in the last twenty years. How they incorporate or use these processes is for them to determine.

One successful model of autonomous Aboriginal health care in Australia is the Aboriginal Medical Services (A.M.S.). The A.M.S. has developed dual functions of primary health care givers and a political advocacy role. The A.M.S. developed out of a chronic need for health care. In 1971, Aboriginal activists in Redfern, an inner-city Sydney suburb, demanded a health service for their people. At that stage there was no free health care in Australia and Aboriginal people could not afford to pay doctors or join private health funds. Today the A.M.S. has over 60 branches in various communities delivering primary health care and launching health-related campaigns such as immunization, diet and alcohol issues. As Pat Fagan (1991:400) says about the A.M.S.: "[It] sees health not only at the individual disease level but also at the community level, and so adopts a more holistic view, involving itself in the broader concerns of the community that have an impact on health."

Policy issues are thrashed out between the Aboriginal health workers, directors and non-Aboriginal personnel. The A.M.S. is an example of adaptation in an urban context. Criticisms concerning duplication of services do not take into account that Aboriginal people need to visit a medical establishment that takes into account the wider issues involved in health rather than just 'blaming the victim' for their illness.

Although language difficulties vary from place to place, a long-time Aboriginal resident of Redfern commented on "how language was a glass door we walked into BANG all the time and not many white people could see it" (Langford, 1988:231). The rules of interaction and the ways in which information is obtained are all factors that make visits to an Aboriginal Medical Service much more comfortable for Aboriginal people. This does not imply they cannot function in other medical services but rather that historical factors often determine social relationships that may impede health care for Aboriginals in the mainstream health care system.

Increased Aboriginal participation in mainstream institutions is a prerequisite for improved socio-economic and health profiles. However there have been a number of critiques concerning the role of Aboriginal people in state-funded bureaucracies. Daniels (1986) uses the term 'co-optation' to describe what he sees as the involvement of 'Natives' in bureaucracies. He cites abuse of power and the creation of an elite that serve their own needs and do little to change the overall state of 'Native' peoples in general. He eloquently points out these facts, citing a 'few' chiefs while acknowledging the real hard work of the rank and file in these organizations. Daniels has little regard for Aboriginal peoples to be able to effectively bring about change within these structures that will be more democratic and representational. The problem with defining relations between Aboriginal peoples and non-Aboriginal peoples in terms of dominance and co-optation is that it doesn't account for "mutually transformative relations" (Stasiulus, 1990:278). In other words Aboriginal people are not empty vessels which the state dominates. They resist and respond and help shape their own futures.

The same view is expressed in Australia but is labelled 'incorporation.' Once again this has a monolithic view of the state and denies that change is often brought about from within by the meeting of contradictory forces. If we remove the concept of agency from an analysis of Aboriginal affairs, we are merely left with a pessimism that at the least creates inactivity and at the worst continues the paternalistic attitude that 'we know best.' An approach that recognizes "dynamically reproduced and transformed" practices, traditions and world views (Stasiulus, 1990:278) will make sure that no simplistic analyses are made in relation to Aboriginal attempts to deal with the legacy of past policies. The A.M.S. is such an organization and "has played an important role in bringing attention to the political and economic causes of Aboriginal ill health" (Saggers and Gray , 1991:403).

Since Aboriginal people in Australia are not 'contained' within reserves and determine their Aboriginality themselves they have tended in recent years to approach issues such as health, law and education as political and economic issues and call for national strategies. While Aboriginal bureaucracies are definitely burgeoning organizations they are coming to terms with the limitations and strengths of these structures and can utilize them for their peoples' good. Some Canadian Aboriginal groups have been fortunate in that treaties recognized their status and afforded them a legal means through which to negotiate. They are now promised constitutional right to self-government. However, these same ties that bind appear to have been used to contain their lifestyles and to conquer and divide the Aboriginal population in general. So for status Natives it is easier to develop clinics on reserves as long as they can find the workers. However, it is much more difficult for Metis and non-status Natives to determine their lives because they have even less access to political power because they have no formal specified rights.

Conclusion

The importance of analyzing the health of Aboriginal people in Australia and Canada in a political-economy framework is clear. The state of Aboriginal health in both countries is too similar for it to be explained in culturalist terms. This framework also shows how Aboriginal responses have been shaped by historical relationships. Importantly, Aboriginal people have always been part of these relationships and are central to a process of change. Health cannot be separated and compartmentalized and treated in isolation from the conditions in which people live. One Aboriginal concept of well-being is "an absence of trouble" and "active participation in social activities" (Mobbs, 1991:299). That says it all.

Notes

1. In Canada indigenous people include status Natives, non-status Natives, Inuits and Metis. In Australia, the people are the Aboriginals. The term 'Aboriginal' will be used to discuss the indigenous people in both countries.
2. As UNESCO has argued, there is no scientific basis for the concept of race. "Race" is a socially constructed concept, not an objective difference based on phenotype - physical difference - or genotype - genetic difference (Bolaria and Li, 1988:16-17).

References

Australian Bureau of Statistics. 1991. Australia's Aboriginal and Torres Strait Islander People: Census of Population and Housing. June, 1986. Commonwealth of Australia.

Bolaria, B. Singh and Peter S. Li. (eds.). 1988. *Racial Oppression in Canada.* Toronto: Garamond Press.

Bourgeault, Ron. 1991. "Race, Class and Gender: Colonial Domination of Indian Women." Pp. 129-150 in *Racism in Canada.* Edited by O. McKague. Saskatoon: Fifth House.

Brady, Paul. 1983. "The Underdevelopment of the Health Status of Treaty Indians." Pp. 39-55 in *Racial Minorities in Multicultural Canada.* Edited by P.S. Li and B.S. Bolaria. Toronto: Garamond.

Daniels, Douglas. 1986. "The Coming Crisis in the Aboriginal Rights Movement: From Colonialism to Neo-Colonialism to Renaissance." In *Native Studies Review* 2(2): 97-115.

Department of Aboriginal Affairs. 1987. Aboriginal Statistics, 1986. Canberra: Australian Government Publishing Service.

Fagan, Patricia. 1991. "Self-Determination in Action." Pp. 400-401 in *The Health of Aboriginal Australia.* Edited by J. Reid, P. Trompf. Sydney: Harcourt Brace Jovanovich.

Fleras, Augie and Jean L. Elliott. 1992. *The Nations Within.* Toronto: Oxford University Press.

Frideres, James S. 1985. "Native Land Claims." In *Ethnicity and Ethnic Relations in Canada.* 2nd edition. Edited by R.M. Bienvenue, J.E. Goldstein. Toronto: Butterworths.

Frideres, James S. 1988a. "Racism and Health:The Case of Native People." Pp. 135-147 in *Sociology of Health Care in Canada.* Edited by B.S. Bolaria, H.D. Dickinson. Toronto: Harcourt Brace Jovanovich.

Frideres, James S. 1988b. *Native Peoples in Canada: Contemporary Conflicts.* 3rd edition. Ontario: Prentice-Hall.

Frideres, James S. 1991. "From the Bottom Up:Institutional Structures and the Indian People." Pp. 108-132 in *Social Issues and Contradications in Canadian Society.* Edited by B.S. Bolaria. Toronto: Harcourt Brace Jovanovich.

Globe and Mail. "Native Women Cling to Charter." May 29, 1992

Globe and Mail. "For Self-Government, in a Canadian Context." June 3, 1992.

Globe and Mail. June 15, 1992. "Canada: Degrees of Agreement." June 15, 1992.

Gray, Alan and Peggy Trompf, Shane Houston. 1991. "The Decline and Rise of Aboriginal Families." Pp. 80-122 in *The Health of Aboriginal Australia.* Edited by J. Reid, P. Trompf. Sydney: Harcourt Brace Jovanovich.

Haig-Brown, Celia. 1988. *Resistance and Renewal: Surviving the Indian Residential School.* Vancouver: Tillacum Library.

Human Rights Commission. 1991. *Racist Violence: Report of the National Inquiry into Racist Violence.* Canberra: Australian Government Publishing Service.

Langford, Ruby. 1988. *Don't Take Your Love To Town.* Victoria, Australia: Penguin.

Langton, Marcia. 1981. "Urbanizing Aborigines: The Social Scientists' Great Deception." *Social Alternatives* 4(2). Brisbane, Australia: Diamond Press.

Lyon, Noel. 1992. "First Nations and the Canadian Charter of Rights and Freedoms." *The Network.* 2(4). Ontario.

Malloch, Lesley. 1989. "Indian Medicine, Indian Health: Study Between Red and White Medicine." *Canadian Women's Studies* 10(2,3): 105-113.

Mobbs, Robyn. 1991. "In Sickness and Health: The Sociocultural Context of Aboriginal Well-Being, Illness and Healing." Pp. 292-325 in *The Health of Aboriginal Australia.* Edited by J. Reid and P. Trompf. Sydney: Harcourt Brace Jovanovich.

Morrow, Lin. Unpublished. "Colonisation - Alive and Well in Australia Today." Paper delivered at an early Land Rights conference. Sydney, Australia.

Muirhead, Justice J.H. 1988. Interim Report, Royal Commission into Aboriginal Deaths in Custody. Canberra: Australian Government Publishing Service.

Norris, Mary Jane. 1990. "The Demography of Aboriginal People in Canada." Pp. 33-59 in *Ethnic Demography: Canadian Immigrant, Racial and Cultural Variations*. Edited by S.S. Halli, F. Trovato and L. Driedger. Ottawa: Carleton.

O'Neil, John D and James B. Waldram. 1989. "Native Health Research in Canada: Anthropological and Related Approaches" *Native Studies Review* 5(1): 15.

Patterson, E. Palmer. 1988. "Native-White Relations." Pp. 230-234 in *Social Inequality in Canada: Patterns, Problems, Policies*. Edited by J. Curtis, E. Grabb, N. Guppy and S. Gilbert. Ontario: Prentice-Hall.

Read, Peter and Coral Edwards. 1989. *The Lost Children*. New South Wales, Australia: Doubleday.

Reid, Carol. 1991. "Girls on the Block: Aboriginality, Schooling and the Lives of Teenage Girls in Redfern." B.A.Hons. Thesis. Macquarie University (unpublished).

Reid, Janice and Peggy Trompf. 1991. *The Health of Aboriginal Australia*. Sydney: Harcourt Brace Jovanovich.

Reynolds, Henry. 1981. *The Other Side of the Frontier*. Queensland, Australia: James Cook University.

Saggers, Sherry and Dennis Gray. 1991. "Policy and Practice in Aboriginal Health." Pp. 381-420 in *The Health of Aboriginal Australia*. Edited by J. Reid and P. Trompf. Sydney: Harcourt Brace Jovanovich.

Stasiulis, Daiva K. 1990. "Theorizing Connections: Gender, Race, Ethnicity and Class." Pp. 269-305 in *Race and Ethnic Relations in Canada*. Edited by P.S. Li. Toronto: Oxford University Press.

Waldram, James B. 1989. "Native People and Health Care in Saskatoon." *Native Studies Review* 1(5): 97-113.

York, Geoffrey. 1990. *The Dispossessed: Life and Death in Native Canada*. London: Vintage U.K.

16

The Health of Aboriginal People in Saskatchewan: Recent Trends and Policy Implications

Alan B. Anderson

Introduction

While disparities in health status continue to persist among different socio-economic groups, these disparities are even more pronounced between the Native and non-Native populations. Despite recent relative improvements in Aboriginal health status, they continue to have higher morbidity and mortality rates. Diseases of poverty, overcrowding, poor housing and unsanitary living conditions continue to take a heavy toll among Aboriginal peoples. This chapter focuses on recent trends in the health status of Aboriginal people, followed by a discussion of policy alternatives to eliminate health status inequalities. It is argued that to achieve equality of health status it is necessary to address questions of social, economic and political inequality faced by Aboriginal people and a "culturally sensitive" approach to health care.

Aboriginal Health: Recent Trends

It is informative to first look at Indian health and living conditions in Saskatchewan a quarter of a century ago. Back in 1967, the majority of Saskatchewan Indians lived on reserve, and almost all reserves were extremely poor. On at least thirteen reserves, more than 90 percent of families earned under $1,000 a year, while the proportion was 75-89 percent on another sixteen reserves. Three-fifths of 4,380 family units, averaging six people, had annual incomes under $1,000, four-fifths under

$2,000. Most reserves were incapable of self-sufficiency. Housing conditions were deplorable — every third home was classified as "substandard," every fifth "in need of major repair." One out of every five reserve families lived in single-room houses, another two out of five in two-room. Very few Indian homes had electricity or plumbing. For example, only one in five homes were electrified (in five agencies with 240 homes, the ratio was one in fourteen); one in 530 had exclusive private use of a sewer or septic tank within the house; one in 465 an indoor bath; one in 370 running water; one in 230 a telephone. But some reserves were totally lacking all of these facilities. The disparities in health status were quite pronounced. Almost half (46 percent) of all recorded deaths of Indians in Saskatchewan occurred before their first birthday, compared to less than 7 percent at the time in the general population. In fact, two-thirds of whites died at ages over 65, compared with only one in five Indians who attained such an age at death. A fifth of all Indian deaths was by pneumonia (Raby, 1969: 176). The very survival of Indians would not have been ensured for even a single generation if the Indian birth rate had not been double the provincial average.

There has been in recent years a dramatic decline in mortality rates among registered Indians in Saskatchewan. In just one ten-year period, the crude death rate has fallen from 6.0 in 1979 to 3.5 in 1988. Death rates still tend to be higher among registered Indians, particularly on reserve, than the general population. As Table 1 shows, in 1988 the crude death rate on reserve was 4.3, compared to only 2.9 off reserve. While death rates among Canadian Indians as a whole dropped by more than one-third during the 1980s, they are still one and a half times higher than those of the total Canadian population (Toughill, 1990). Indian and Northern Affairs and Statistics Canada have predicted (a) that life expectancy will continue to increase for "regular" Indians, though remaining consistently behind life expectancy of the total Canadian population; (b) that among "regular" Indians, C-31 population, and general population, males do not live, on average, as long as females; (c) that C-31 population will continue to have higher life expectancy than either "regular" Indians or the general population. Still, life expectancy rates for Native people remain almost an average full decade behind the rates for the general population (reported at a meeting of the Canadian Public Health Association in June 1990); earlier, 1986 data from Health and Welfare Canada calculated the differential at 9.2 years for males and 8.0 for females (Farnsworth, 1991). Thus, a Native man born in 1991 could expect to see his 65th birthday, whereas a non-Native man could expect his 74th, as would a Native female, but non-Native women now live past the age of 81 (Canadian Press, June 27, 1990).

Table 1. Selected Vital Statistics for Registered Indian Population of Saskatchewan, 1988

	1984	1988	5-YEAR TREND	ON-RESERVE (1988)	OFF-RESERVE (1988)
LIVE BIRTH RATE	29.7	33.2	+3.5	27.2	40.8
CRUDE DEATH RATE	4.6	3.7	-0.9	4.3	2.9
NATURAL INCREASE RATE	25.0	29.6	+4.6	22.9	37.9
INFANT MORTALITY RATE	14.9	10.2	-4.7	11.2	9.3
NEONATAL DEATH RATE	5.0	3.7	-1.3	2.0	5.1
STILLBIRTH RATE	12.9	7.8	-5.1	8.1	7.5

Source: Health and Welfare Canada. Vital Statistics for the Registered Indian Population of Saskatchewan (annual report), 1988.

Similarly, the infant mortality rate has been falling quite rapidly, while it too is considerably higher than for the general population, especially for reserve Indians. According to a recent report of the First Nations Health Commission (Oct. 1991), Native infants are dying of many diseases at double to triple the rate of other Canadian infants, primarily due to poor living conditions. Mortality rates among Aboriginals are double those of the general population at birth, but triple shortly after birth. The chance of an Aboriginal child developing pneumonia is currently 17 times that of other Canadian children. Moreover, Native children have more ear infections, meningitis, hepatitis, and Native communities have to contend with diverse health problems compounded by substance abuse, such as fetal alcohol syndrome (Canadian Press, October 11, 1991). Across Canada, the infant mortality rate had declined from 82.0 in 1960 to 12.7 by 1988, yet remained twice as high for reserve Indians as the general Canadian rate (Hagey et. al., 1989:6). While in 1960, almost 80 Native babies out of 1,000 died in their first year of life, today, fewer than 15 die. This is still double the Canadian national average (Toughill, 1990). In Saskatchewan, among registered Indians, in little more than a decade the infant mortality rate has virtually been cut in half: 45.8 in 1975, 12.0 in 1980, 9.4 in 1986, 10.2 in 1988 (Tables 1 and 2). According to a study released by the Canadian Institute of Child Health, the infant mortality rate in the Province of Saskatchewan is well above the Canadian rate; their babies are twice as likely to die in infancy as other Canadian children (Laforest, 1990). Reduction of the neonatal death rate (deaths of infants within 28 days after birth) has been even more extraordinary: 16.6 in 1980, 6.6 in 1986. The under-five death rate has fallen from 8.0 in 1979 to 3.1 in 1988, while the death rate for registered Indians aged 65 and over remained fairly constant: 45.1 in 1979, 43.6 in 1988 (Woodard and Edouard, 1991).

Table 2. Infant Mortality Rate and Neonatal Mortality Rate for Native Population and General Population in Saskatchewan, 1980, 1986, and 1992 (projected estimate)

	Native Mortality	General Population
Infant Mortality		
1980	12.0	7.6
1986	9.4	6.1
1992	6.8	4.6
Neonatal Mortality		
1980	16.6	6.0
1986	6.6	5.5
1992	—	5.0

Source: Woodard, G., and L. Edouard. 1991. "Reaching Out: A Community Initiative for Disadvantaged Pregnant Women." Report of the Saskatoon Community Health Research Unit and Development Committee and Department of Community Health and Epidemiology, College of Medicine, University of Saskatchewan.

Nonetheless, as stated above, most types of death rates are still higher among registered Indians in this province than among the general population. This is particularly evident when age cohorts are taken into consideration. For instance, death by fire, suicide, drug and alcohol abuse, accidental poisoning are common for younger-aged status Indians, but rare among young people in general. Also, the motor vehicle accident death rate is relatively more prevalent among registered Indian youth (Health and Welfare Canada, 1988). According to Statistics Canada data, released in Canadian Social Trends, Native Indians are three times as likely to die before age 35 as Canadians generally (Fine, 1989). The death rate among Native 15-44 year-olds is triple the Canadian average (Toughill, 1990). Native children of all ages are four times more likely to die from all causes (Laforest, 1990).

They are 6 times more likely to die in accidents as teenagers (Struthers, 1990). In Canada the suicide rate among Aboriginal youth (aged 10-24) is five to six times higher than the rate in this age group in the general population, and is increasing (First Nations Health Commission, Oct. 1991; Toughill, 1990). The most recent data indicate an increase in suicides among younger Native females — just since the beginning of 1990, female suicides have gone from being rare to approximately equaling the male rate (Platiel, 1991). Earlier data from Indian and Northern Affairs Canada indicated that while the suicide rate among status Indians was decreasing (e.g., from 43 to 34 per 100,000 between 1981 and 1986), it remained more than twice as high as the rate for the total Canadian population (Hagey et al., 1989:7).

Since 1981, the overall rate of violent deaths for status Indians has fluctuated between three to four times the general Canadian rate (Hagey et al., 1989:8). Accidental and violent deaths still account for at least a third of Indian deaths, according to Health and Welfare Canada (Toughill, 1990; Canadian Press, June 27, 1990).

Specifically, according to 1988 Health and Welfare data, one in every five (20.9 percent) deaths of registered Indians in Saskatchewan is due to circulatory system disease, compared with 14.6 percent due to cancer and malignant neoplasms, 11.3 percent respiratory system problems, 9.2 percent suicide (11.4 percent among males, 5.6 percent females), 8.4 percent motor vehicle accidents, and 4.2 percent accidents involving fire. It is noteworthy that the accidental poisoning death rate for female registered Indians is 4.4 percent in general, and climbs to 5.4 percent off-reserve. The potential years of life lost, on and off reserve, because of poisoning and injury comes to an astonishing 50.9 for males and 42.3 for females. For example, in 1988 in Saskatchewan, ten young registered Indians shot themselves, eight hanged themselves, two died from poisoning, another couple from other self-inflicted causes. A disproportionate number of these suicides were found on reserves. Also, there were thirty-three deaths of registered Indians (22 on reserve, 11 off) from alcohol or drug abuse. Nor are these data for one year atypical. Among registered Indians in Saskatchewan, a disproportionately high number of such deaths is consistently found in younger age cohorts (Health and Welfare Canada, Annual Reports, 1987, 1988, 1989).

The incidence of diabetes in Saskatchewan's Indian population has apparently risen dramatically during the past decade; an estimated 119 percent between 1980 and 1990. In fact, this disease has now emerged as a major Native health problem across Canada: the Native rate is now ten times the general Canadian rate. This dramatic increase has been attributed to changing diet related to urbanization, specifically higher consumption of "junk food" carbohydrates, which increase blood sugar levels, further accentuating what nutritionists report is already a high genetic occurrence among indigenous people (Farnsworth, 1991; Regina *Leader-Post*, December 1, 1990).

In Saskatchewan, registered Indian women are more than six times as likely to develop cervical cancer than the rest of the female population, according to a 1991 Statistics Canada report on Canadian cancer statistics (Greenshields, 1991). Saskatchewan Indians aged 45-64 are dying from diabetes at a rate six times greater than the overall rate in these age cohorts, and dying from cirrhosis of the liver at three times the general rate, while Indians aged 25-44 are 12 times more likely to die from pneumonia and influenza (Canadian Press, May 31, 1989).

Respiratory diseases such as bronchitis and pneumonia cause double the deaths among Native people across Canada, as in the general population, but it should be stressed that even when Native people die of the same causes as the general population, they tend to die from them at much younger ages (Canadian Press, June 27, 1990).

Yet, given the overall faster decline in the crude death rate and infant mortality rate among registered Indians, compared to a slow decline or possibly even a temporal increase in the live birth rate and fertility rate, an imbalance (typical of the demographic transition) is created, resulting in relatively high population growth. Also, in Canada as a whole, differences in life expectancy of registered Indians and the total Canadian population are decreasing, especially among females.

Policy Considerations

It is readily apparent that the health of Native people in Saskatchewan, and all across Canada, is closely tied to poverty and living conditions. Abject poverty contributes to dismal living conditions, which make for extraordinarily poor health and high mortality. Therefore, a policy on Native health care is impossible without a policy on alleviating poverty and improving living conditions. A political economy approach to understanding Native health care is absolutely essential.

As the Canadian Institute of Child Health has pointed out, the health problems of Canada's Native children bear a striking similarity to those found in third world countries: "The state of poverty in which they live makes them particularly vulnerable to health hazards. Their powerlessness and social isolation possibly contribute to higher than average suicide rates." Further, "this country cannot ignore the deplorable conditions of Native people. . . . When you look at the overcrowding, the poor housing conditions, the lack of running water in so many Indian communities , there's no reason [this] should exist in Canada" (Struthers, January 27, 1990).

It is quite clear, according to the First Nations Health Commission, why this is a third world health problem right within our society — 60 percent of Native households still lack running water or sewage, and over 30 percent of Native children still live in overcrowded homes (Canadian Press, October 11, 1991).

Of course, one possible explanation could be inadequate Native use of available health facilities. But far more attention continues to be directed at the inadequacy of facilities, not to mention poor quality of service. It has recently been pointed out, for example: "that the lack of accessible medical services is particularly hard on elderly Native people, especially in northern Saskatchewan — unable to speak English, and frightened by being removed to a strange and lonely southern hospital environment, they are reluctant in the extreme to move for better health care — they'd rather stay up north . . . and die" (Mandryk, 1990).

The infant mortality rate could be lowered with improved pre-natal programs for Native mothers, half of whom reportedly smoke during pregnancy. Improved alcohol treatment — better yet, prevention — programs would help to decrease alcohol-related accidental, violent, and suicide deaths (Canadian Press, June 27, 1990).

Most deaths due to house fires could easily be prevented with better fire fighting service on reserve. Few, if any, reserves in Saskatchewan have adequate equipment on reserve, and off-reserve fire services have often been reluctant to serve nearby reserves (for any number of presumed excuses, such as fees not being paid, or agreement not having been made — as was the case recently on the Cote Reserve near Kamsack, where three children died because of the refusal of the town fire department to respond to a desperate call for help from the reserve (Skrapek, 1990).

Regarding accessibility and availability of health services, recently, the Lac La Ronge Indian band has complained about such things as being referred to several doctors for the same illness, then being prescribed sometimes conflicting medications; misdiagnosis or failure to diagnose properly; refusal to refer patients to better treatment centers; failure to recognize the severity of a patient's illness; etc. Currently three full-time and two part-time physicians serve a local population of 13,500 out of a 30-year old hospital (Hoffman, 1992).

Janice Acoose-Pelletier, Native Affairs reporter of the Saskatoon *StarPhoenix*, has recently written:

> We must concern ourselves with the health conditions of Native people. If nothing is done, they will continue to seriously deteriorate. For proof, one simply has to look around at the increasing number of Native people who suffer from various physical disabilities. Statistics confirm that many of the medical problems associated with Native people are either directly or indirectly brought on by socio-economic conditions. However, many more are simply caused by sheer neglect or ignorance on the part of medical professionals. . . . Do Natives receive the same 'professional' care that non-Natives receive? I would truly like to believe they do. . . . However, I have heard of too many incidents where Native people have been turned away by hospitals or doctors because they were supposedly drunk. So what if they were not exactly in the best of shape? Don't they deserve medical attention if they need it? What right do medical 'professionals' have to impose their moral values on people in need of attention? . . . Sadly, some who have been refused medical attention have died, are crippled for life or are severely brain damaged. . . . In some communities, the medical resources available are simply not adequate. Many Native patients do not receive proper care because of archaic medical facilities or second-rate doctors and nurses. Incidents of shoddy medical practices are commonplace in remote communities. . . . Therefore, it is not surprising to learn of the deteriorating health conditions of Native people. This is inexcusable, for this is the twentieth century. While billions of dollars are being poured into space programs and defence operations, Saskatchewan cannot even offer Native communities proper health facilities and professionals (Acoose-Pelletier, 1989).

In conclusion, two additional points may be addressed. First, a unique cultural approach to Native health care seems essential. As James Waldram has pointed out in a recent study in Saskatoon, traditional Native medicine and spirituality could be featured in health care institutions serving or operated by Native people (Struthers, September 27, 1990). Tom Iron, vice-chief of the Federation of Saskatchewan Indian Nations in charge of health, has added that "cultural disintegration in Native communities is a major cause of health problems. . . . [Therefore] Indians themselves must rediscover their traditional values and cultural pride before dramatic progress will be made on social problems" (Struthers, January 27, 1990).

And Janice Acoose-Pelletier has had this to say:

> Because of cultural differences, many Native people refuse to go to hospital or for routine medical examination. This is not surprising, considering the racist attitudes that prevail in broader society. . . . When a Native person is admitted to a hospital, a number of other problems arise because we have our own ways of dealing with illness and care of the sick. Most hospitals don't recognize this or simply don't care. . . . Non-Native medical

personnel do not understand that healing, to many Native people, concerns whole communities or families. . . . To become well and whole again, the sick person must have faith and confidence in the healing process. For Native people, this is difficult and frustrating because in many cases they can't even communicate with doctors. . . . Doctors are just not aware of the cultural differences between Natives and non-Natives regarding disease and care of the sick (Acoose-Pelletier, 1989).

Second, the development of such "culturally sensitive" health care of Native people could constructively be related to the movement for Indian self-government. As Arlene Pete has observed:

Indian 'self-determination' in Indian health care and services means that Indian people would actively participate in the definition of health services and health policies. With 'self-determination' in the area of health care, many problems could be solved. Indian participation would ensure that the communication barrier can be dismantled. The misunderstanding that has long characterized the 'white' health care system, therefore, could be changed. . . . With the use of their own people, it would ensure that empathy for the ill would exist. Native physicians, nurses and therapists could communicate in their own language, to those who, otherwise, wouldn't understand. The resulting level of health services would be greater and more efficient. . . . The most positive aspect of Indian 'self-determination' in health care and services, is the chance for Indian people . . . to prove that their culture offers a low-cost health system and far more efficient means of maintaining health. The rest of Canadian society can learn from Indians, if 'self-determination' over health care becomes concrete (Pete, 1988:13-14).

References

Acoose-Pelletier, Janice. 1989. "Native Health Concerns Need Urgent Attention." Saskatoon *StarPhoenix*, August 31, 1989.

Canadian Press. 1989. "Health Problems Still Major Concern for Natives: Study." Saskatoon *StarPhoenix*, May 31, 1989: A6.

Canadian Press. 1990. "Native Life Expectancy Lags Behind Other Races." Saskatoon *StarPhoenix*, June 27, 1990.

Canadian Press. 1991. "Native Infants Dying at Double Average Rate." Saskatoon *StarPhoenix*, October 11, 1991.

Farnsworth, Clyde, H. 1991. "Diabetes and Other Ills Hit Indians in Canada." *New York Times*, December 8, 1991: 23.

Fine, Sean. 1989. "Report Says Death Rate for Indians Under 35 Triple that of Population." *Globe and Mail*, December 22, 1989.

First Nations Health Commission. 1991. Report, October 1991.

Greenshields, Vern. 1991. "Cervical Cancer Risk Greater for Indian Women in Saskatchewan." Saskatoon *StarPhoenix*, July 27, 1991: A6.

Hagey, N.J. and G. Larocque, C. McBride. 1989. "Highlights of Aboriginal Conditions, 1981 - 2001: Quantitative Analysis and Socio-demographic Research Working Paper Series 89-2." Ottawa: Indian and Northern Affairs Canada.

Health and Welfare Canada. Vital Statistics for the Registered Indian Population of Saskatchewan (annual reports), 1987, 1988, 1989.

Hoffman, Donella. 1989. "Indian Band's Allegation Against Doctors Under Study." Saskatoon *StarPhoenix*, March 18, 1992.

Laforest, Mary Jo. 1989. "High Infant Mortality Rate Needs Remedy Now: Doctor." Saskatoon *StarPhoenix*, January 26, 1990: A18.

Mandryk, Murray. 1990. "Sandy Bay: Frustration and Fear: An Unhealthy Isolation?" Regina *Leader-Post*, March 3, 1990: A17.

Pete, Arlene. 1988. "The Importance of Indian 'Self-determination' on Health Care." Unpublished paper, December 19, 1988.

Platiel, Rudy. 1991. "Suicide Increase Troubles Natives." *Globe and Mail*, June 3, 1991: A1.

Raby, S. 1969. "Saskatchewan Indian Communities." In J. Howard Richards and K.I. Fung (eds.), *Atlas of Saskatchewan.* Saskatoon: University of Saskatchewan, p. 176.

Skrapek, Lyle. 1990. "Kamsack Fire: A Symptom of Prolonged Ignorance." *The Voice* 1:3.

Struthers, Gord. 1990. "Infant Mortality Rates 'Sicken' Native Leader." Saskatoon *StarPhoenix*, January 27, 1990: A8.

Struthers, Gord. 1990. "Doctors, Indians Must Cooperate on Health Care: Professor." Saskatoon *StarPhoenix*, September 27, 1990.

Toughill, Kelly. 1990. "Natives' Health Still Worse Than Average." *Toronto Star*, June 27, 1990.

Woodard G. and L. Edouard. 1991. "Reaching Out: A Community Initiative for Disadvantaged Pregnant Women." Report of the Saskatoon Community Health Research Unit and Development Committee and Department of Community Health and Epidemiology, College of Medicine, University of Saskatchewan.

17

Cultural and Socio-Economic Factors in the Delivery of Health Care Services to Aboriginal Peoples

James B. Waldram

Introduction

It is often assumed that Aboriginal peoples are culturally different from other Canadians and that these differences explain to a large degree their apparent reluctance or inability to utilize biomedical health care services in an "appropriate" manner. In this paper this assumption is challenged on a variety of fronts. I will argue that Aboriginal peoples have suffered from a lumping effect, in which it has been assumed that they are not only culturally similar but, more importantly, uniformly culturally dissimilar from non-Aboriginal Canadians. Furthermore, I will present evidence that "culture" per se does not present a barrier to the utilization of biomedical services for many Aboriginal people. Finally, I will suggest that Aboriginal utilization of biomedical services might be better understood if a new model, combining cultural with socio-economic factors, were employed.

Cultural Determinist Explanations of Health Care Utilization

Many researchers have argued that Aboriginal peoples utilize the health care system differently, and problematically, because they are culturally "different." I would term the totality of these arguments the "cultural determinist" model. This model supposes that cultural differences explain in great measure Aboriginal utilization patterns, and even their ability to understand the biomedical health care system. Cultural trait lists, purporting to typify Aboriginal behaviour, lead to the development of stereotypes concerning health care utilization, which then lead to the assumption of cultural barriers to such utilization. The culmination of this process are calls for more "culturally appropriate" health care.

Brant (1990), in his article on Native ethics and behaviour, presents a discussion of typical traits psychiatrists and others might encounter. While including a disclaimer that the list of ethics and behaviours is not representative of all Aboriginal peoples, Brant's truncated discussion of this issue nevertheless represents an over-generalization and simplification of the contemporary context. Brant (1990:536) presents us with a variety of ethics and behaviours, including an "intuitive, personal and flexible concept of time," and the ethics of non-interference, non-competitiveness and emotional restraint, all of which he suggests have implications for Native mental health and treatment. But these really apply only to a small segment of the Canadian Aboriginal population.

Discussions such as Brant's unfortunately serve to reinforce stereotypes of Native behaviour, rather than demystifying them, as he suggests. Some of the stereotypes commonly associated with Aboriginal health care utilization, and which exist within the medical folklore for this population, include:

Aboriginal peoples are less likely to have regular physicians;

Aboriginal peoples are less likely to know when they are sick, and more likely to report in later stages of illness.[1] Aboriginal peoples prefer intimate contacts with physicians, as they do with traditional healers, and therefore find depersonalized biomedical services to be unacceptable;

Aboriginal peoples are more likely to utilize hospital emergency departments for non-emergency treatment, because they do not understand the purpose of emergency departments;

Aboriginal peoples are less likely to make appointments, and to show up for appointments, because they are past- and present-oriented, and not future-oriented; and

In general, Aboriginal peoples tend to avoid the health care system.

Such stereotypes are, in turn, reflected in explanations of the barriers Aboriginal people face when attempting to utilize the health care system. This is especially true of research pertaining to the urban context. Shah and Farkas (1985), for instance, described the following barriers: different social patterns, including the sharing of money; linguistic and cultural communication problems between Aboriginal patients and Euro-Canadian health care staff (such as different ways of asking and responding to questions); lack of familiarity with urban health care services; and lack of "culturally sensitive" health care. Mears and colleagues (1981), in their study of skid row Indians in Vancouver, argued that they simply did not know where to get the services they required. Both Shah and Farkas and Mears and colleagues allude to the possibility that socio-economic factors play a role in health care seeking behaviour, yet these factors have only a minor role in the overall explanations offered. In effect, the literature emphasizes two broad types of factors to explain Native behaviour: cultural factors (i.e., a discordance between Aboriginal and Euro-Canadian cultures); and knowledge factors (i.e., that Aboriginal peoples have difficulties figuring out the biomedical health care system). The result, no doubt inadvertently, is to present Aboriginal peoples as culturally and socially retarded (Grondin, 1989): they are simply unable to understand what the biomedical system is all about.

This view is problematic for two reasons. First, there have been relatively few actual studies of Aboriginal health care utilization behaviour, and those that have been done, while in some instances superficial, suggest that utilization problems are considerably rarer than the folklore would suggest (Alberta, 1985; Calgary, 1984; Maidman, 1981; Senior Citizens Provincial Council, 1988). Furthermore, studies comparing Aboriginal and non-Aboriginal utilization, which would allow us to see more clearly the consequences of cultural differences, are even rarer, and one such recent study gave considerable weight to the argument that socio-economic factors played a considerably more important role (Waldram and Layman, 1989). Second, proponents of cultural deficiency explanations often seem to confuse behaviour with knowledge. What Aboriginal people, or any people for that matter, actually do with respect to health care utilization cannot be construed as a direct measure of what they know. The real question is not do they know about the biomedical health care system, but rather, how do they act on the knowledge they have and, to a lesser extent, under what circumstances do they seek health care knowledge. This still does not preclude the possibility that they may choose to utilize the health care system differently than the "norm," for either cultural or socio-economic reasons.

Differentiating Cultural and Socio-Economic Factors

Cultural Factors

In order to properly understand the contribution that cultural and socio-economic factors make to Aboriginal health care utilization, it is essential to turn to the available literature. Extensive use of the author's own work in this regard will be supplemented with references to other works where appropriate.

Kaufert (1990) has lamented the propensity to draw boundaries around cultures to make them easier to understand by outsiders. This process of "box-ification" has been applied over the years to Aboriginal Canadians. Indeed, while paying lip service to the fact that these cultures vary greatly, there has been a general tendency among researchers and the public alike to lump them together. Researchers have done so to create a manageable "Native" variable (Edwards, 1992); the public, including medical practitioners, have done so as part of their process of stereotyping. In both instances, the process allows for easier labelling and assessment, just as it allows for differential treatment and discrimination.

Receiving even less attention is the fact that many Aboriginal Canadians actually have no understanding of their Aboriginal cultures, and many others are bicultural, able to survive adequately in both Aboriginal and Euro-Canadian cultural milieux. The author's recent study of Aboriginal offenders at the Regional Psychiatric Centre in Saskatoon (Waldram, 1992) graphically demonstrated what most researchers have known, but ignored: that in terms of cultural adherence, Aboriginal Canadians can be figuratively placed somewhere on a scale ranging from essentially unicultural (Aboriginal) through bicultural to unicultural again (Euro-Canadian). Hence, when one suggests that Aboriginal peoples are culturally different, the real question is not how as a totality they are different from Euro-Canadians, but rather in what ways, if any, are they different at all?

One of the key problematic areas is, no doubt, language. There are many Aboriginal people whose ability to speak and read English or French is poor; this is particularly true of the elderly. Furthermore, there are Aboriginal people who have poorly developed abilities to understand either a Euro-Canadian or an Aboriginal language. The legacy of the residential school system, and an overall inferior education system, are clearly to blame. While written versions of oral Aboriginal languages do exist, relatively few Aboriginal language speakers can also be considered literate in that language. Hence, communication barriers are extremely important. Aboriginal peoples may have difficulty explaining their problems to physicians or other health care personnel, and may have problems understanding instructions. Some will have difficulty reading the labels of prescription and over-the-counter drugs. Obtaining meaningful consent for medical tests and surgical procedures is also a problem. While the successful use of interpreters in hospital settings has been documented, such programs remain relatively rare (Kaufert et al., 1985).

Other cultural problems which may exist have been alluded to earlier. Particularly important are clinical difficulties in questioning and responding; in some instances it is improper to ask direct questions, and Euro-Canadian researchers have long been aware of the propensity of Aboriginal people to provide accommodating answers to questions regardless of their true feelings. There may also be difficulties discussing certain aspects of anatomy, especially in cross-gender clinical encounters, or where the patient is elderly. While it has been demonstrated that some Aboriginal people retain "traditional" beliefs about the etiology, symptomology and treatment of certain problems, it has not been adequately demonstrated that such beliefs significantly impair utilization of the health care system. For instance, it is not uncommon for some Aboriginal patients to consult with both a traditional healer and a physician in a serial or simultaneous manner (Waldram, 1990a,1990b). Furthermore, it has also not been demonstrated that the existence of a traditional belief precludes a parallel, biomedical explanation as well.

While cultural problems certainly do exist, it is not the case that these are exclusive to Aboriginal peoples. Immigrants are also likely to express such beliefs, and all Canadians have recourse to "folk" and "popular" sectors of the health care system, with corresponding folk or non-specialist beliefs about health and illness (Kleinman, 1980). There are a substantial number of Canadians who have literacy problems as well, or who have difficulty discussing anatomy with physicians. Interestingly, there seems to be considerably less medical folklore or stereotyping about the cultural behaviours of Euro-Canadians.[2]

Many of the cultural problems so far described are most likely appropriate for those Aboriginal peoples with the strongest ties to their culture, that is, those who are most traditional. In general, in terms of health care utilization, this would be primarily the older generations, since the younger people are experiencing ever-increasing levels of formal education and hence are considerably more bicultural. Given the current increasing rates of education, it is likely that future generations of elderly Aboriginals will be fully bicultural, able to operate in both the Euro-Canadian and Aboriginal worlds. Cultural problems would then largely disappear: people would clearly understand the Euro-Canadian context of biomedical health care delivery and the clinical encounter, and speak English or French, so if they continued to utilize the system differently it would be for other reasons.

Socio-Economic Factors

As a category, it can be easily argued that Aboriginal peoples in Canada generally represent the most socially and economically disadvantaged group. Despite improving health, social and economic conditions, Aboriginal peoples still tend to experience a disproportionate degree of poverty, both on reserve or in small communities and in urban areas. This poverty is manifested in very high rates of suicide and violent death, alcohol abuse, and domestic violence, areas in which biomedical health care services have had little effect. Poverty is also reflected in poor living conditions; fewer Aboriginal than non-Aboriginal homes are equipped with running water and central heating in Canada. The result is high incidences of infectious diseases, such as scabies and tuberculosis. Low incomes also affect diet and Aboriginal peoples have in recent years developed very high rates of nutritional disorders, such as diabetes and other poverty lifestyle health problems, such as lung cancer and cardiovascular disease (see Feather, 1991; Mao et al., 1986; and Young, 1988 for a discussion of recent health trends). Inevitably, these impoverished conditions would also affect health care utilization patterns. Indeed, it seems logical that if Aboriginal people suffer disproportionately from diseases of poverty that their patterns of health care utilization would also be reflective of their poverty. Surprisingly, there have been relatively few analyses of the socio-economic factors affecting Aboriginal utilization.

In a seminal article, Jarvis and Boldt (1982) graphically described the relationship between poverty and death among Aboriginal people in Alberta. Their analysis determined the paramount role that alcohol played in the sudden death of Aboriginal people, noting that death was often a social event, with individuals dying in the company of others, most frequently on weekends. Although noting that the geographical isolation of many Aboriginals is partly to blame, they stated emphatically that "physical circumstances seem less to blame for short life expectancies and for high rates of Native mortality than are the social conditions under which they live" (1982:1349). These conditions include relatively low levels of education and employment.

Feather (1991) describes some of the barriers to "social health" in northern Saskatchewan; most are applicable to Aboriginal peoples in general. She notes that many families tend to be large and that without adequate income or proper housing, nutritional problems and family stress can result. The higher rate of single parent families and teen pregnancies renders the situation even more problematic. Educational standards are lower in the north and children living in poverty with parents who likely have little formal schooling themselves are at a disadvantage. Unemployment rates are higher in northern Saskatchewan, which means lower incomes and a greater dependence on social assistance. This poverty is "associated with higher than average degrees of family instability, stress, violence, low self-esteem, alcoholism and criminality" (Feather, 1991:35).

How then does widespread poverty affect health care utilization among Aboriginal peoples in Canada? This is a complex question which requires a comparative analysis of Aboriginal and non-Aboriginal Canadians from all socio-economic levels. To date, no such study has been undertaken. However, the author's own study (Waldram and Layman, 1989) attempted to compare Aboriginal and Euro-Canadian health care utilization patterns and barriers among those with the lowest socio-economic status in Saskatoon, and the results were revealing.

The study was undertaken at two locales in the inner city area of Saskatoon: the Westside Clinic, a medical facility, and the Friendship Inn, a social service agency. In this study of 142 Aboriginal people and 84 Euro-Canadians, undertaken in 1987 and 1988, it became apparent that there were relatively few differences between the two populations in terms of utilization patterns and behaviour. This was somewhat surprising, given the medical folklore cited above and the author's own predilection for a "culture matters" hypothesis. Some selected results from this study follow.

Slightly more Aboriginals (79.4 percent) than Euro-Canadians (75.6 percent) indiated that they had a regular physician and were able to provide that person's name. Logically, for many of the respondents, the Westside Clinic physicians were named as their regular physicians. This was particularly true for the Aboriginal respondents, compared to the Euro-Canadians who tended more toward other physicians working in private practice.

Making contact with physicians seemed less problematic than originally hypothesized. For instance, 78 percent of the Aboriginals and 68 percent of the Euro-Canadians reported having consulted their regular physician at least once in the previous three months, and 57 percent of the Aboriginals and 50 percent of the Euro-Canadians reported having had a physical examination within the last year. These differences were not statistically significant, yet the prevailing folklore would have suggested that Aboriginal people in the city would be avoiding physicians. Furthermore, it was even more surprising to learn that the Aboriginal respondents were slightly more likely to agree that having a regular physician was important (see also Waldram, 1990c).

The analysis of data demonstrated that significant factors affecting the utilization of physician services included the length of time a person had lived in the city (those having lived in Saskatoon the longest were more likely to have a regular physician), the existence of dependent children (those with children were more likely to have a regular physician), gender (more females than males were likely to have had contacts with physicians), and marital status (married people were more likely than singles to have a regular physician and have had a recent contact with that individual).

One of the myths extant within the biomedical system, as noted above, is that Aboriginal people prefer "walk-in" type facilities because of an aversion to making appointments, which itself is seen as a manifestation of a cultural trait most colloquially known as "Indian time." The Westside Clinic - Friendship Inn study demonstrated the fallacy of this myth by placing the issue of appointment-making behaviour more squarley within the realm of socio-economic factors. At the Westside Clinic, only 33 percent of the Aboriginal patients had arrived with an appointment on the day of their interview, compared to 59 percent of the Euro-Canadians; such an observation is of the type that leads to the generation of medical myths. A closer look, however, demonstrated that only 29 percent of the Aboriginal patients had telephones, compared to 82 percent of the Euro-Canadians, and that most patients with telephones had made appointments. The reasons why fewer Aboriginal peoples had telephones are not clear, but may be due to the fact that they are, in general, even poorer than the Euro-Canadians living in the same area. Furthermore, having a telephone does not seem to be related to an Aboriginal individual's Euro-Canadian cultural orientation, for, in fact, more people who spoke an Indian language actually had telephones (Waldram, 1990c).

In the urban context, then, socio-economic factors, particularly those related to poverty, seem to explain considerably more of the health-seeking behaviour than cultural factors. In the Saskatoon study, Aboriginal peoples and Euro-Canadians behaved in a similar manner, a strong argument for the uniform effects of poverty. But what about in the rural, remote and/or reserve communities, where there is much greater cultural integrity among the people?

Unlike the city, the small Aboriginal community tends to have few health care options. Most health facilities are staffed by registered nurses, with the support of an array of lay and para-professionals derived from the community who offer various educational and preventive services. In general, access to physicians and other medical specialists occurs in one of two ways. First, these specialists may visit the community on a scheduled basis, often one day a week for physicians. Or second, the patients may be removed, or may go themselves, to another, usually urban community to obtain treatment. Thus, in their home communities, Aboriginal peoples often have access to only one biomedical facility, usually a nursing station, which coordinates the delivery of all types of medical services.[3]

The utilization of biomedical services in these smaller communities has been problematic. A frequently heard complaint offered by the nursing staff is that utilization is "inappropriate" from their perspective, meaning that patients tend to visit the nursing station after regular clinic hours for complaints which, in the mind of the nurses, were of a non-emergency nature. In general, these observations have been borne out by research and by the personal observations of the author; they are not simply medical folklore. However, as O'Neil (1981) notes, what constitutes an "emergency" may be differentially defined in an Aboriginal community, and futhermore, "inappropriate" utilization and other conflict within the health care realm may well be a reaction to the colonial nature of the delivery of biomedical services (O'Neil, 1986). Certainly the Montreal Lake case bears this out.

The William Charles Band, located at Montreal Lake in Saskatchewan, was the first band in Canada to obtain control over health care delivery under the Health Transfer Agreement of the Department of National Health and Welfare.[4] Prior to transfer, the community was experiencing a wide array of social and health problems, including alcoholism. More importantly for this paper, the people of Montreal Lake appeared to have given control for their health care totally to the local clinic and the physicians living about one hundred kilometers away in Prince Albert. They practiced little home management of illness, especially for children. Immunization rates were low. Some people, especially elderly, avoided contact with the nursing station and others made a habit of calling on the nurses after hours. Some Band members recognized that a change was needed, and initiated the long process of planning that ultimately leads to transfer. In a way, the key issue at the community level had to do with ownership and responsibility; the nursing station was seen as a foreign agent, and was exploited as were other government programs and resources. But when the Band gained control in 1988, there was a dramatic change in attitude. Immunization rates increased. Home management improved. Elders began to see the nurses on a regular basis, and after-hours visits to the nursing station decreased. While control over the delivery of health care services was accompanied by new educational and outreach initiatives, there is still no denying that the services themselves came to be viewed as the property of the residents, and the nurses "their" employees. The colonial tie of which O'Neil (1986) spoke was broken, and health care behaviour changed accordingly (Moore et al., 1990). Hence, it is suggested here that Aboriginal health utilization behaviour must be seen in an historical, as well as socio-economic, context.

There is no question that racism exists in Canada, and that Aboriginal peoples have been subjected to all levels of racism, individual, institutional and structural (Hull, 1982). With respect to health care delivery, the role of racism in understanding the clinical encounter, and general health care utilization behaviour, has not been fully investigated. Two studies, however, shed much light on the issue from the perspective of the Aboriginal patients themselves. The first, by Waldram (1992), involved the study of Aboriginal offenders at the Regional Psychiatric Centre (RPC) in Saskatoon. The RPC undertakes the treatment of offenders primarily from the federal correctional system. In this study, thirty Aboriginal offenders were intensively interviewed on a range of topics, including their perceptions of racism within the prison and, more importantly, the treatment program at RPC. The results demonstrated not only perceptions that the predominantly Euro-Canadian staff were racist, treating the Euro-Canadian patients considerably better than the Aboriginals, but also that these perceptions conditioned the responses of the Aboriginal offenders to the overall program. Simply put, some tended to reject the messages because of their perceptions of the treatment staff's perceptions of them.

The other study was done by Sherley-Spiers (1989), who documented perceptions of racism in clinical encounters among the Dakota of southwestern Manitoba. In her study, Sherley-Spiers (1989) presented the views of many Dakota individuals regarding the physicians in particular, and the health care system in general, and noted that those who delivered health care tended to hold common stereotypes of the Dakota. Thus, seriously ill patients were often assumed to be drunk by the attending physicians. Physicians often scolded mothers for not taking proper care of their children and for bringing them to the clinic either when they were not seriously ill, or else when they had reached an advanced state of illness (the inherent contradiction in this, and other myths and stereotypes, is rarely recognized by the medical community). The result ultimately was that some people avoided contact with the clinic.

It is important to note that in the above two cases we are dealing only with the perceptions of certain Aboriginal people and not necessarily the clinical "reality." Furthermore, the perspectives of the clinicians themselves have not been solicited. Nevertheless, the implication of these studies is clear: perceptions of racism, especially in the absence of formal means to discuss them with the others involved, condition the response of Aboriginal people to the health care system. But does this mean that biomedically-based health services, delivered by Euro-Canadians, are too inflexible to meet the needs of Aboriginal Canadians?

Culturally Appropriate Health Care Services

Much has been said in recent years about the need for "culturally appropriate" health care for Aboriginal peoples. While this concept is rarely defined, it usually entails the provision of services in Aboriginal languages, and sensitivity to elements of traditional culture (especially health beliefs and patterns of interpersonal interaction) and the unique life circumstances and living conditions of Aboriginal peoples. The language issue is, of course, fundamental to our understanding of a successful clinical encounter, as I have noted above. With respect to the other aspects of culturally appropriate care, the Montreal Lake case, and other cases of health transfer, demonstrate that local control can be seen as one manner of achieving cultural appropriateness. But when Aboriginal people do obtain such control, they do not discard the biomedical approach to health care delivery; they supplement it with traditional philosophies and the use of the local language. The best examples of this fact are the many Aboriginally controlled alcohol and drug abuse centres in Canada. In general, these centres have adopted biomedical approaches to treatment, including the disease model and Alcoholics/Narcotics Anonymous. But they have also added a component of cultural education and traditional spirituality. Frequently, the spirituality sessions launch each new day, with participants sitting in a circle, smudging with sweet grass and smoking the sacred pipe. Sweat lodges may also be used. Later in the day, however, they will undertake various group therapy exercises which look very much like those used among non-Aboriginals.

Although relatively rare, it is evident that some non-Aboriginal health care institutions have made efforts, often successful, to be "culturally sensitive" to Aboriginal patients. Such care is distinguishable from "culturally appropriate care" in that the latter can really only be offered within the proper cultural context by members of the same culture, whereas "culturally sensitive" care can be offered by non-culture members. As noted earlier, some hospitals have medical interpreters available. There are a few cases in Canada in which traditional healers are actually on the staff of hospitals or clinics, and many more instances in which traditional healing activities are carried on within biomedical institutions. The author is also aware of at least two urban clinics, the Westside in Saskatoon and the Boyle-McAuley in Edmonton, which provide culturally sensitive care to Aboriginal patients. At the Westside, for instance, patients encounter a low-key atmosphere in which the waiting room looks more like a living room, and the clinical staff dress in casual clothing and avoid the ubiquitous medical symbolism found in other clinical settings. Furthermore, they are sensitive to the issue of traditional medicine, and many have had direct experience in third world countries and/or other situations of poverty; they are acutely aware of the barriers poverty erects with respect to health care. As a result, the Westside Clinic has inculcated a very loyal patient load and a city-wide reputation as a good place for Aboriginal peoples to come for their health care needs.

An Integrated Cultural and Socio-Economic Model

The purpose of this chapter has been to examine some of the cultural and socio-economic factors which explain Aboriginal health care utilization. It is suggested here that, in general, socio-economic factors, including broader historical questions, explain to a greater degree the current situation than do cultural factors. This is not to belittle in any way the importance of culture, for as I have suggested there are some areas in which cultural factors are clearly at work, and one of the most serious obstacles to good health care for Aboriginal peoples can be found in the language barrier. But the fact is that many Aboriginal peoples in Canada today are either bicultural or unicultural in the Euro-Canadian sense and future generations will continue to be raised in such a manner. Only the elderly and those in some of the more remote areas of the country (such as the high arctic) still demonstrate a traditional, unicultural persona, and these will decline in numbers in the future. Furthermore, health care services have been available in these areas for many years and the people are now fully acquainted with at least the northern rural or remote delivery mode. Hence, we will see increasingly larger numbers of Aboriginal peoples with an ability to move in both the Aboriginal and Euro-Canadian worlds (as evidenced by increasing urban migration); they will have recourse to both biomedical and traditional services; they will understand the biomedical system, and the English/French languages. Their primary orientation may well be toward their Aboriginal cultural roots, but they will not be crippled by that culture such that they fail to understand what the biomedical system is all about. In such a situation, socio-economic factors and, more broadly, historical and political factors, become more important in understanding health care behaviour. Hence, it is suggested here that a new model needs to be developed, one which adequately addresses cultural as well as socio-economic factors (including class position) and which does not portray Aboriginal peoples as ignorant, passive victims of colonial oppression in the health care realm.

Such an integrated model would propose that there may be a direct relationship between culture and health care behaviour in situations of cultural contact where the culture in question is different from that which underlies the new health care system. In the case of Aboriginal peoples, continued Aboriginal language retention and traditional etiologies will likely affect health care behaviour. But the model would also suggest that relevant cultural traits may be filtered through socio-economic variables in their ability to affect health care behaviour, with the consequence that most behaviour is explainable in terms of such variables as income and employment status, family and marital status, class status, racism and so on. Culture per se would not disappear in such a model, but its effects on health care behaviour would be muted and, I suggest, minimalized in relation to these socio-economic factors. Furthermore, for many Aboriginal peoples with little or no knowledge of their ancestral cultures, the primary explanatory factors would be those of Euro-Canadians in general, explained by socio-economic status (and racism). Finally, the historical relations between the Aboriginal peoples and Euro-Canadian society must be seen as a comprehensive, somewhat diffuse factor which affects both culture and socio-economic status as they pertain to health care utilization.

Conclusion

In attempting to understand Aboriginal health care utilization, it is essential to first eliminate the many stereotypes that characterize the medical folklore regarding these peoples, and then to appreciate the true cultural heterogeneity that exists. It is argued here that the future will likely see socio-economic status and class position become even more significant in explaining health care utilization, as current trends toward increasing urbanization and developing biculturality continue.

Three general trends are required if the health care situation for Aboriginal peoples is to improve: first, there must be a greater cultural sensitivity on the part of non-Aboriginal biomedical practitioners, especially to the linguistic barrier and problems engendered by the life circumstances of Aboriginal peoples; second, there must be a continuing process of acquisition of control over health care services at the community level, so that local customs and initiatives can be taken into account; and third, there must be an overall general improvement in the socio-economic status of Aboriginal Canadians. The first two are relatively easily attainable, and represent current trends. The latter, unfortunately, requires more structural changes in the broader Canadian economic and political milieu, but the continuing progress that is being made toward Aboriginal self-government indicates that even here the future may be better.

Notes

1. For instance, the 1969 Booz-Allen report stated that, "Many Indians have little understanding of the meaning of good health because of cultural differences and education deficiencies. Indians exhibit little awareness of what is meant by good health and because of this lack of awareness there is a tendency to both over and under-utilize health services. . . . Indians frequently fail to recognize significant symptoms and delay seeking treatment until they are acutely ill" (Booz-Allen, 1969:13).
2. The Saskatoon study, for instance, demonstrated that Euro-Canadians were more likely to utilize the emergency department of a city hospital in an inappropriate manner than were the Aboriginals, yet it was the latter who were subjected to stereotyping regarding emergency department utilization.
3. It is this fact that has led people to conclude that Aboriginal migrants to the city become confused by the myriad of health care services available.
4. See Speck (1989) for a description and critique of the health transfer process.

References

Alberta. Native Counselling Services of Alberta and Native Affairs Secretariat. 1985. *Demographic Characteristics of Natives in Edmonton*. Edmonton: Native Affairs Secretariat.

Booz-Allen and Hamilton. 1969. *Study of Health Services for Canadian Indians. Summary Report*. Ottawa: Dept. of National Health and Welfare.

Brant, Clare C. 1990. "Native Ethics and Rules of Behaviour." *Canadian Journal of Psychiatry* 35: 534-539. Calgary. Department of Social Services.

Brant, Clare C. 1984. *Native Needs Assessment*. Calgary: City of Calgary, Department of Social Services.

Edwards, Nancy C. 1992. "Important Considerations in the Use of Ethnicity as a Study Variable." *Canadian Journal of Public Health* 83(1):31-33.

Feather, Joan. 1991. *Social Health in Northern Saskatchewan.* Saskatoon: Northern Medical Services.

Grondin, Jacques. 1989. "Social Support and Decision-Making: The Inuit in the Biomedical System." *Native Studies Review* 5(1): 17-40.

Hull, Jeremy. 1982. *Natives In a Class Society.* Saskatoon: One Sky.

Jarvis, George and Menno Boldt. 1982. "Death Styles Among Canada's Indians." *Social Science and Medicine* 16:1345-1352.

Kaufert, Patricia. 1990. "The 'Boxification' of Culture: The Role of the Social Scientist." *Santé/Culture/Health* 7(2-3): 139-148.

Kaufert, J., J. O'Neil, and W. Koolage. 1985. "Culture Brokerage and Advocacy in Urban Hospitals: The Impact of Native Language Interpreters." *Santé,/Culture/Health* 3(2):2-9.

Kleinman, Arthur. 1980. *Patients and Healers in the Context of Culture.* Berkeley: University of California Press.

Maidman, Frank. 1981. *Native People in Urban Settings: Problems, Needs and Services.* Report of the Ontario Task Force on Native People in the Urban Setting: Toronto.

Mears, B., K. Pals, K. Kuczerpa, M. Tallio and E. Morinis. 1981. *Illness and Treatment Strategies of Native Indians in Downtown Vancouver: A Study of the Skid Row Population.* Vancouver: Health and Welfare Canada.

Mao, Y., H. Morrison, R. Semenciw, and D. Wigle. 1986. "Mortality on Canadian Indian Reserves 1977-1982." *Canadian Journal of Public Health* 77: 263-268.

Moore, Meredith, Heather Forbes and Lorraine Henderson. 1990. "The Provision of Primary Health Care Services Under Band Control: The Montreal Lake Case." *Native Studies Review* 6(1):153-164.

O'Neil, John. 1981. "Health Care in a Canadian Arctic Village: Continuities and Change." In *Health and Canadian Society*, D. Coburn et al. (eds.), pp.123-142. Toronto: Fitzhenry and Whiteside.

O'Neil, John. 1986. "The Politics of Health in the Fourth World: A Northern Canadian Example." *Human Organization* 45(2):119-128.

Saskatchewan Senior Citizens Provincial Council. 1988. *A Study of the Unmet Needs of Off-Reserve Indian and Metis Elderly in Saskatchewan.* Regina.

Shah, C. and C. Farkas. 1985. "The Health of Indians in Canadian Cities: A Challenge to the Health Care System." *Canadian Medical Association Journal* 133 (1): 859-863.

Sherley-Spiers, Sandra K. 1989. "Dakota Perceptions of Clinical Encounters with Western Health Care Providers." *Native Studies Review* 5(1): 41-51.

Speck, Dara Culhane. 1989. "The Indian Health Transfer Policy: A Step in the Right Direction, or Revenge of the Hidden Agenda." *Native Studies Review* 5(1): 187-213.

Waldram, James B. 1990a. "Access to Traditional Indian Medicine in a Western Canadian City." *Medical Anthropology* 12: 325-348.

Waldram, James B. 1990b. "The Persistence of Traditional Medicine in Urban Areas: The Case of Canada's Indians." *American Indian and Alaska Native Mental Health Research* 4(1): 9-29.

Waldram, James B. 1990c. "Physician Utilization and Urban Native People in Saskatoon, Canada." *Social Science and Medicine* 30(5): 579-589.

Waldram, James B. 1992. *Aboriginal Offenders at the Regional Psychiatric Centre.* Unpublished report. Saskatoon.

Waldram, James B. and Melissa Layman. 1989. *Health Care in Saskatoon's Inner City.* Winnipeg: Institute of Urban Studies, University of Winnipeg.

Young, T. Kue. 1988. *Health Care and Cultural Change: The Indian Experience in the Central Subarctic.* University of Toronto Press.

PART 4:

Research Issues and Ethics

18

Problems and Limitations in the Study of Immigrant Mortality

Frank Trovato

Introduction

Migrant studies have been conducted in a variety of disciplines. For epidemiologists, immigrant populations present a unique opportunity to discern patterns in the etiology of disease (Evans, 1987; Hull, 1979; Kruger and Moriyama, 1967; Marmot et al., 1984a, 1984b, 1983; Rosenweike and Shai, 1986; McMichael et al., 1980; Stenhause and McCall, 1970; Haenszel, 1961, 1975; Kasl and Berkman, 1985; Kmet, 1970; Lilienfeld, Levin and Kessler, 1972; Stawszeski et al., 1970). If immigrants differ in their rate from disease X in relation to the host society, but do not differ from their country of origin, inference can be made that the etiology of disease for the migrants is the same as for their nation of origin. When both the immigrants and host population have the same level of risk for disease X, while immigrants and country of origin differ, it can be posited that the foreigners may have assimilated the mortality experience of the host society (see Trovato, 1990 for a more complete discussion of this).

In demography, the emphasis is less on etiology of disease and more on the documentation of differentials (e.g., Jacobson, 1963; Kestenbaum, 1986; Kitagawa and Hauser, 1973; Sharma, Michalowski and Verma, 1989; Vallin, 1985; Michalowski, 1990; Young, 1987, 1991). Few of these works attempt to test competing hypotheses about the nature of mortality differences (see Trovato, 1992, 1985; Trovato and Clogg, 1992; Brahimi, 1980 for exceptions to this).

In sociological research, mortality differentials are usually interpreted as a reflection of socioeconomic inequality between groups

(Tumin, 1967; Simpson and Yinger, 1985; Kitagawa and Hauser, 1973; Kitagawa, 1977). An important theoretical perspective from such research is the social stratification thesis of mortality inequality, which posits an inverse association between socioeconomic position and death rates (Antonosky, 1967; Kitagawa, 1977).

Problems and Limitations

Notwithstanding the many important contributions of the epidemiologic, demographic and sociological literature, there are many problems and limitations inherent in the study of immigrant mortality. In this overview, I discuss both substantive and data quality problems. The discussion is limited to research based on official Vital Statistics and exclude aspects pertaining to prospective surveys of mortality, which is a separate area of discussion, encompassing its own set of problems and limitations (see Kasl and Berkman, 1985).

Data Concerns

In Canada, deaths are recorded on a continuous basis by the national Vital Registration System. The Mortality Data Base (MDB) at Statistics Canada is a file which contains all individual death records by province, age, sex, marital status, country (province) of birth, cause of death, and other pertinent medical information. This comprehensive data source is extremely valuable in the analysis of immigrant mortality, but has some limitations.

A major difficulty arises from the incompleteness of information on the decedents' country of birth (Trovato, 1985). This variable may not get coded regularly by all the provinces, and/or Statistics Canada, therefore, the degree of reporting varies from period to period. During the early eighties over 20 percent of all death records were missing the decedent's country of birth. In 1986, fortunately, this proportion went down to about three percent. A provincial analysis of this situation reveals that some provinces account for a disproportionate share of "unknown," depending on the time period under consideration.

When the numbers of "unknown" nationalities are many (above 10 percent), the statistical results will be affected, particularly if one is interested in analyzing a large number of immigrant groups. The degree of error probably varies in inverse proportion to the number of groups in the analysis due to small numbers on the one hand, and missing information on the other.

When the percentage of "unknowns" is low (less than 10 percent), one may ignore such cases on the assumption that exclusion plays no significant role in the *pattern* of results. Of course, the *magnitude* of rates would be affected (deflation).

Another approach is to apportion the "unknown" deaths on the basis of the known distribution of deaths, the assumption being that both have the same underlying probability of occurrence. This solution may "correct" for the magnitude problem in the derivation of death rates, but may introduce bias in the pattern of differences across groups if the "missing" are not distributed at random. However, when the "unknowns" are relatively few, the overall degree of error is likely to be inconsequential.

A large number of "unknown" country of birth cases poses serious statistical limitations. The distribution of such cases is unlikely to be random, and more likely due to some systematic source of error or bias (e.g., a given province or provinces consistently fail to code country of birth on the death certificate). Therefore, the assumptions outlined above cannot hold in this instance.

Knowledge of the source(s) of this problem would facilitate the application of adjustments. For example, if Province Z consistently fails to report country of birth on the death certificate, it can simply be deleted from the analysis. This procedure, however, introduces the problem that if the province is large, and therefore contains a significant number of immigrants, statistical results may be severely limited in terms of generalizability. Alternative techniques can be applied, but all have their strengths and weaknesses, they overcome certain aspects of the problem, but fail in other respects (see Trovato, 1985; Trovato and Clogg, 1992).

Another limitation of official records pertains to the number of variables coded on the death certificate. Beyond age, sex, marital status, place of birth (province, country), province of death and cause of death, there are no other variables useful for social epidemiological or sociological analysis. Direct information on the decedent's education, occupation, religion, and other background characteristics is not available.

Some analysts have relied on a procedure called record linkage to overcome this limitation, which involves the matching of a decedent's death record with his/her other personal files such as the census return (see Kitagawa and Hauser, 1973). The advantages of this method are obvious: the analyst will have a more complete data file, enabling a more comprehensive and detailed analysis of mortality.

Unfortunately, record linkages suffer from a number of drawbacks. The excessive costs involved in matching records makes this methodology prohibitive. Moreover, in practice not all records can be matched. For example, one may have the death certificate for a decedent, but fail to find the corresponding census return for the same individual. On other occasions, the census file is located, but the death record is not found. Consequently, the number of usable records for analysis is typically fewer than one's anticipated target. Depending on the proportion not matched, statistical results could be severely affected.

An alternative method to the linkage of records is to rely on a quasi-ecological procedure to data set construction and analysis. This approach has promise because while it is less expensive and less time consuming than record linkage, it also allows for an extensive analysis of causes beyond the usual variables often employed in the literature. In ecological investigation, the unit of analysis is typically the census block, the city, the province, the country or the social group. For a given unit one may correlate death rates with corresponding aggregate socioeconomic variables. An analogous approach useful to studying immigrant mortality is to consider the group-age-sex-marital status-province specific cell in a multiway tabulation as the unit of analysis. Aggregated age-sex-marital status-province-nationality group specific variables (e.g., average income) from the Census can be appended to the corresponding death rates for this same cross-classification (e.g., Trovato and Clogg, 1992). If the appropriate data tables are not available in published form, one may compile the desired cross-tabulation from the Public Use Sample Tapes or from the Master Census Files (complete counts) at Statistics Canada. This type of aggregation is midway to the micro and the macro levels. The larger the number of cross-classifiable variables in the death certificate, the more micro the data set — a desirable property from the point of view of statistical inference. Unfortunately, as indicated earlier, the number of cross-classifiable variables on the death certificate are few, limiting the degree of expansion of the data set.

A limitation of this methodology is that in drawing from two (or possibly more) data sources, the compiled data set will probably reflect some degree of error. The deaths cross-classification may not in actuality match the census cross-tabulation (the alive population) in terms of socioeconomic characteristics. For example, the assumption in this procedure is that the socioeconomic characteristics such as average income, education, etc., of the decedents cross-classified by say, age, sex, marital status and province are identical to the corresponding alive population in the census, which serves as the basis for extracting such covariates. In some cases this may not be a true reflection of reality, since it is well established in the literature that mortality varies by socioeconomic characteristics both within and between social groups (e.g., immigrants) (Antonovsky, 1967; Duleep, 1989; Kitagawa, 1977; Stockwell, 1963). However, if the objective of the investigation is to study between-group variation, as in the case of comparing immigrants to the Canadian born, this limitation will be of minor consequence for the statistical results, as long as one assumes homogeneity within categories of cross-classified variables for each social group in the analysis.

A third source of difficulty in the use of official statistics is that it is not possible to investigate the mortality experience of the descendants of immigrants. Incompleteness of information on the death record concerning country of birth of the decedent's parents obviates such investigation. The degree of completeness in the MDB for this variable fluctuates radically from period to period, making it virtually useless in the context of migrant mortality studies. It would be important to discern the level of mortality among first generation immigrants as compared to their descendants in Canada, and to see how mortality probabilities by cause of death change from one generation to the next. Such data would provide more direct clues on whether there may be a convergence process involved in the cause-specific mortality pattern of immigrants, their descendants and the host population.

This point leads to the introduction of a related problem. The MDB (i.e., death records) does not contain any information concerning duration of residency in Canada for foreign born decedents. This is a serious limitation because it restricts one's ability to monitor change in mortality risk over time for the immigrants.

Figures 1 and 2 demonstrate this problem in graphic form. The first diagram represents an ideal case where six individuals enter the host nation in the same year (but at different times in the year). Of these cases, four die before reaching their 51st birthday. Therefore, on average, these four decedents had been residents in their host nation for six months.

However, Figure 2 is a more representative picture of reality. It shows four hypothetical life lines of four immigrants who arrive at different time points and pass through time and age until death at the age of 50. Thus, they all arrive at different times, but die at the same age (between 50 and 51). In this scenario, using age at death as a proxy of duration of residence in the host nation would give a distorted estimate of duration. This difficulty is inherent in official statistics corresponding to immigrant mortality because duration of residence is not coded on the death records.

Age at death is therefore an imperfect proxy for duration of stay in Canada. While it is virtually axiomatic that a foreign born infant death must correspond to a very brief duration of residency in Canada, this

Figure 1. Immigrant Mortality by Duration of Residence

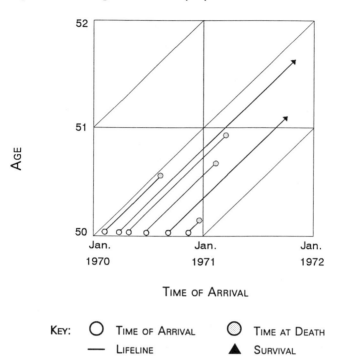

Figure 2. Immigrant Mortality by Duration of Residence

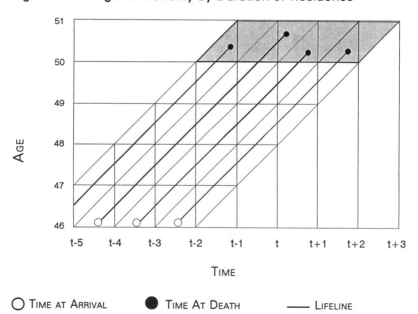

conclusion would be highly dubious in the case of, say, an immigrant who dies within the age group 50-54. Unless direct information about duration is available, we are never certain as to how long the decedent had been a resident of Canada. Within any age class (especially in the adult years), some decedents are of recent duration while others are not. Inability to classify deaths by duration of residency hampers a more complete analysis of disease development over time for immigrants. Because of this limitation, we cannot answer with certainty whether immigrants adopt the disease pattern of the host population the longer they reside in the host country.

Substantive Concerns

It is often assumed that immigrants constitute a select population in terms of their social, economic, psychological and general health characteristics (Brahimi, 1980; Trovato and Clogg, 1992; Trovato, 1992; Kasl and Berkman, 1985). Of particular relevance to the analysis of immigrant mortality is health selection. According to the selectivity explanation, immigrants possess lower death rates than their host society because they are positively selected in their countries of origin and then are screened for medical problems by the immigration process. Immigrants are required to pass a medical test before admittance to the new society. Thus, the question arises: is the lower mortality level of immigrants a function of selection or is it due to other factors?

Information on duration of residency would facilitate an answer to this question, as it would allow the researcher to hypothesize in advance that, in the initial years following immigration, the gap in death rates between the foreign born and the native born would be at its maximum in favour of foreigners, presumably as a function of the health selectivity process, but that this advantage should erode with length of residence in Canada. Unfortunately, we cannot test this thesis in the context of Canada (as far as I know, Australia is the only country that codes duration of residence on the death certificate).

Health selection at the time of entry into Canada may be an important factor accounting for immigrants' apparent superiority in survival probability relative to the Canadian born. But selection may also operate in a different way. Not all immigrants to this land will remain in Canada on a permanent basis. A certain proportion of newcomers return to their home country. Such individuals may form a select group comprised of persons who may be less capable in coping with the adjustment process to the new society, and/or are "weaker" elements healthwise among the foreign born. Return migration, therefore, may be a contributing factor in the apparent advantage in survivorship probabilities for immigrants in relation to the Canadian born. To the extent that the "weaker" and less healthy elements are predisposed to return migration, the death rate of permanent immigrants will be lower than what it would be had such elements remained in the new land. No data exist to allow for a direct test of this hypothesis.

An interesting fact is that a comparison of death rates in infancy between immigrants and the native born will reveal that the former will always display a significantly lower rate. This is an important basis for immigrants' higher life expectancy at age zero in comparison to persons born in Canada. Since very few babies immigrate in any given year, it follows that the number of foreign born babies dying will be small. Immigration involves a great deal of planning and preparation. It is doubtful, therefore, that parents contemplating a migration will time the birth of their babies to coincide with the time of relocation to the new land. In fact, few parents move to Canada with newborn babies. For the most part, foreign born children at the time of entry into Canada are beyond the age of infancy. For example, in 1986 there were only 1,850 foreign born infants in Canada. Of these, it is more than likely that the overwhelming majority will be in the postneonatal period (i.e., older than one month) where death probabilities are significantly reduced in comparison to the neonatal period (first month). Therefore, the higher life expectancy of immigrants at age zero is to a large extent a function of these facts, corresponding to the inherent nature of the immigration process itself.

Researchers typically classify deaths into relatively few nationality groups for the purpose of analysis. For the most part, this is a necessary strategy since many immigrant groups are numerically small and will therefore "produce" few deaths in any given period of observation. Unfortunately, there is considerable loss of precision and generalizability when inferences about death rates are based on few broad regional classes of nationality (e.g., South European, African, South American, etc.). With such classification strategies, it is virtually impossible to conclude anything meaningful about the cultural bases of mortality differentials. The most desirable situation would be to group deaths by specific nationality (e.g., Greek, Italian, English, etc.) so that more meaningful inferences can be made about the nature of disease and the possible role of culture in this process. Unfortunately, as indicated above, this strategy is not always possible due to the smallness (demographically) of many immigrant groups. This fact also hampers our ability to investigate the mortality experience of refugees and recent immigrant groups that are numerically small.

A disappointing feature of most studies in this area of investigation is the apparent disregard for theory development and synthesis. Few analysts have attempted to go beyond the mere description of their data and to formulate theory about immigrant mortality in host nations (see Trovato, 1992; Trovato and Clogg, 1992; Kliewer, 1979). Thus, we are still faced with the task of answering the fundamental question: under what conditions do immigrants experience different mortality levels and patterns than their countries of origin and destination? This question cannot be answered adequately without the formulation of a theory of immigrant mortality.

Some fundamental weaknesses and problems prevail not only in immigrant studies but also in more general analyses of mortality trends, levels and patterns. For example, a common assumption in the literature is that causes of death are independent of each other. In a strict sense, this is fundamentally incorrect, as in many cases death is a function of the interplay of more than one cause or ailment. The main reason behind the independence assumption is to facilitate the statistical analysis, as the most widely used tests and procedures assume independence. A more realistic picture would emerge if causes of death were treated as dependent, rather than independent, competing risks. No attempts have been made at analyzing causes of death simultaneously under the mathematical model of competing risks. Separate analyses for causes of death fail to capture the reality that death often occurs as a function of two or more causes acting simultaneously. More work and development is needed in order to rectify this aspect of mortality analysis.

Our knowledge of what causes the death of individuals is limited. While it can be established with certainty that a death has occurred, specification of the process leading to death is difficult. From the available statistics we cannot discern how the life style, health behaviours, attitudes about safety, risk taking and other pertinent behavioural aspects of a decedent's background may have contributed to his/her death. Thus, the end result is a certainty, but the chain of causation leading to death is uncertain.

This final point suggests that a promising avenue for future research lies in the execution of prospective studies over long periods of time. Such designs would facilitate the collection of behavioural and attitudinal data for individuals and the correlation of such information with mortality risk (see for example, Berkman and Syme, 1979; Marmot and Syme, 1976; Reed et al., 1972).

Conclusion

Vital Statistics data pertaining to immigrant mortality have serious weaknesses and limitations. Notwithstanding their drawbacks, mortality data collected by the official accounting system are the best available source of information on immigrant mortality. Prospective surveys would overcome many of the data limitations indicated in this review, but would introduce problems and limitations of their own. For example, sample sizes may not be adequately large to do in-depth detailed analyses of a large number of immigrant groups. Generalizability from sample to population may be problematic when results are based on small samples. Cost and time would also introduce additional sources of concern, as prospective panel surveys are costly, take a long time to complete, and often suffer from sample attrition due to some respondents failing to continue with follow-up.

Therefore, it maybe concluded that official data are quite valuable for the analysis of immigrant mortality and when used judiciously, can be an important source of information. Familiarity with data problems and their limitations is an essential requisite before pursuing this area of investigation. In the opinion of this writer, of the issues discussed in this review, the most serious limitation of official statistics is the lack of information on the death certificate concerning decedent's duration of residency in Canada. Unfortunately, it is doubtful that much can be done about this deficiency unless recording practices are changed and this variable is introduced as a required piece of information on the death certificate.

This research was supported by a Research Grant from the Social Sciences and Humanities Research Council (Grant No. 5567408).

References

Antonovsky, A. 1967. "Social Class, Life Expectancy and Overall Mortality." *Milbank Memorial Fund Quarterly* 45:31-73.

Berkman, L.F. and S.L. Syme. 1979. "Social Networks, Host Resistance and Mortality: A Nine-Year Follow-up Study of Alameda County Residents." *American Journal of Epidemiology* 109(2):186-204.

Brahimi, M. 1980. "La Mortalite des Etrangers en France." *Population* 35:603-622.

Duleep, H.O. 1989. "Measuring Socioeconomic Mortality Differentials." *Demography* 26(2):345-351.

Evans, J. 1987. "Introduction: Migration and Health." *International Migration Review* 3(21):5-14.

Haenszel, William. 1961. "Cancer Mortality Among the Foreign-Born in the United States." *Journal of the National Cancer Institute* 26(1):37-132.

Haenszel, William. 1975. "Migrant studies." Pp. 361-370 in *Persons at High Risk of Cancer: An Approach to Cancer Etiology and Control*, edited by J.F. Fraumeni Jr. New York: Academic Press.

Hull, D. 1979. "Migration, Adaptation and Illness." *Social Science and Medicine* 13A:25-36.

Jacobson, P.H. 1963. "Mortality of the Native and Foreign-Born Population in the United States." Proceedings, International Population Conference, IUSSP, New York, 1961; Volume 1:667-674.

Kasl, S.V. and L. Berkman. 1985. "Health Consequences of the Experience of Migration." *Annual Review of Public Health* 4:69-80.

Kestenbaum, Bert. 1986. "Mortality by Nativity." *Demography* 23(1):87-90.

Kitagawa, E. 1977. "On Mortality." *Demography* 14(4):381-389.

Kitagawa, E. and P.M. Hauser. 1973. *Differential Mortality in the United States*. Cambridge: Harvard University Press.

Kliewer, Erich. 1979. *Factors Influencing the Life Expectancy of Immigrants in Canada and Australia*. Ph.D. Dissertation, The University of British Columbia.

Kmet, Janet. 1970. "The Role of Migrant Population in Studies of Selected Cancer Sites: A Review." *Journal of Chronic Diseases* 23:305-324.

Kruger, D.E. and I.M. Moriyama. 1967. "Mortality of the Foreign Born." *American Journal of Public Health* 57(3):496-503.

Lilienfeld, A.M., M.L. Levin, D. Irving and I. Kessler. 1972. *Cancer in the United States*. Cambridge, MA: Harvard University Press.

Marmot, M.G., A.M. Adelstein and L. Bulusu. 1984a. Immigrant Mortality in England and Wales 1970-78. Cause of Death by Country of Birth. Studies on Medical and Population Subjects No. 47 (HMSO, London, England).

Marmot, M.G., A.M. Adelstein and L. Bulusu. 1984b. "Lessons From the Study of Immigrant Mortality." *Lancet* 1:1455-1457.

Marmot, M.G., A.M. Adelstein and L. Bulusu. 1983. "Immigrant Mortality in England and Wales." *Population Trends* 33:14-17.

Marmot, M.G. and S.L. Syme. 1976. "Acculturation and Coronary Heart Disease in Japanese-Americans." *American Journal of Epidemiology* 104(3):225-247.

McMichael, A.J., M.G. McCall, J.M. Hartshorne, and T.L Woodings. 1980. "Patterns of Gastrointestinal Cancer in European Migrants to Australia: The Role of Dietary Change." *International Journal of Cancer* 25:431-437.

Michalowski, M. 1990. "Mortality Patterns of Immigrants: Can They Measure the Adaptation?" Paper presented at the XIIth Congress of Sociology. Madrid, Spain, July 9-13, 1990.

Reed, D., D. McGee, J. Cohen, K. Yano, S.L. Syme, and M. Feinleib. 1982. "Acculturation and Coronary Heart Disease Among Japanese Men in Hawaii." *American Journal of Epidemiology* 115:894-905.

Rosenweike, I. and D. Shai. 1986. "Trends in Cancer Mortality Among Puerto Rican-Born Migrants to New York City." *International Journal of Epidemiology* 15(1):30-35.

Sharma, R.D., M. Michalowski and R.B.P. Verma. 1989. "Mortality Differentials among Immigrant Populations in Canada." Paper presented at the 21st IUSSP meetings in New Delhi, India, September 20-27.

Simpson, G.E. and J.M. Yinger. 1985. *Racial and Cultural Minorities: An Analysis of Prejudice and Discrimination.* New York: Harper and Rowe.

Stawszeski, J., J.S. Lomska, C.S. Muir, and D.K. Jain. 1970. "Sources of Demographic Data on Migrant Groups for Epidemiological Studies of Chronic Diseases." *Journal of Chronic Diseases* 23:351-373.

Stenhause, N.S. and M.G. McCall. 1970. "Differential Mortality from Cardiovascular Disease in Migrants from England and Wales, Scotland and Italy, and Native-Born Australians." *Journal of Chronic Diseases* 23:423-431.

Stockwell, E.G. 1963. "Socioeconomic Status and Mortality." *American Journal of Public Health* 6:956-969.

Trovato, F. 1990. "Immigrant Mortality Trends and Differentials." Pp. 91-109 in *Ethnic Demography: Ethnic and Cultural Variations*, edited by S.S. Halli, F. Trovato and L. Driedger. Ottawa: Carleton University Press.

Trovato, F. 1992. "Violent and Accidental Mortality Among Four Immigrant Groups in Canada, 1970-72." *Social Biology* 39(1-2).

Trovato, F. and C.C. Clogg. 1992. "General and Cause-Specific Adult Mortality Among Immigrants in Canada, 1971 and 1981." *Canadian Studies in Population* 19(1): 47-80.

Trovato, F. 1985. "Mortality Differences Among Canada's Indigenous and Foreign-Born Populations, 1951-1971." *Canadian Studies in Population* 12(1):49-80.

Trovato, F. and J.K. Jarvis. 1986. "Immigrant Suicide in Canada, 1971 and 1981." *Social Forces* 65(2):433-457.

Tumin, M.M. 1967. *Social Stratification: The Forms and Functions of Inequality.* Englewood Cliffs: Prentice Hall.

Vallin, J. 1985. "La Mortalite des Immigres en Engleterre et Galles." *Population* 1:156-161.

Young, C.M. 1987. "Migration and Mortality: The Experience of Birthplace Groups in Australia." *International Migration Review* 21(3):531-554.

Young, C.M. 1991. "Changes in the Demographic Behaviour of Migrants in Australia and the Transition Between Generations." *Population Studies* 45:67-89.

19

Cultural Diversity, Dual-Roles and Well-Being: A Research Note

Manfusa Shams

Introduction

The majority of women in Western societies today simultaneously occupy demanding work and family roles. In 1980, 60 percent of women between 16 and 64 years of age were employed (Sorensen and Verbrugge, 1987). Yet women continue to shoulder the main responsibility for household tasks and child care. Research is now accumulating on the issue of women's multiple responsibilities and attendant role conflicts. Research evidence so far is inconsistent. Thus, some studies showed that performing dual-roles is a difficult task and women in this situation experience a great deal of stress (Rapaport and Rapaport, 1978; Bebbington, 1973); other studies showed that both spouses in dual-earner marriages reported high self-esteem, high career commitment and high life satisfaction (Holahan and Gillbert, 1979). Several theoretical models have been proposed to explain the psychosocial costs associated with dual-roles.

Theorizing dual-roles, the "multiple-role hypothesis" proposes that multiple-roles are beneficial to health. It is argued that the positive gains from each role accumulate to produce increments in well-being and defense against depression (Thoits, 1986; Brenett and Baruch, 1985; Kendel, Davies and Ravies, 1985; Froberg, Gjerdingen and Preston, 1986). In contrast to this hypothesis, the "role-overload" hypothesis focuses more on the negative aspects of multiple role demands and the associated stress.

Research on employment and mental health of married women (Brown and Harris, 1978; Cochrane and Stopes-Roe, 1981; Radloff, 1975;

Rosenfield, 1980, Warr and Parly, 1982), impact of work and non-work variables on job satisfaction and life satisfaction of dual-earner families (Beutell and Greenhaus, 1981; Greenhaus and Kopelman, 1981; Sekaran,1983) and the impact of certain life-stages, organizational, extra-organizational and individual difference variables on stress-manifestations (Lewis and Cooper, 1987) are evident among the British population. However, these issues amongst Asian dual-earner families are so far under-researched. The psycho-social costs relating to multiple roles and the experiences of dual-earner families will vary from culture to culture due to different levels of cultural expectations, fixed sets of norms for men and women and overall social and organizational framework.

Empirical evidence in the Indian subcontinent showed that employed married women with high job pressure describe their lives more favourably than those with low job pressure. Job pressure was also found to be significantly related to dyadic adjustment. The higher the job pressure, the poorer is the dyadic adjustment (Sorcar and Rahman, 1985). A significant difference between working married women and full-time housewives on marital satisfaction has also been observed (Rahman and Sorcar, 1981). Better mental health was also reported amongst working women in comparison to housewives (Shams, 1985). It is argued that monetary security obtained through paid jobs moderates the feelings of stress associated with their dual role in the family. Moreover, performing dual roles per se may be beneficial for this group and a defense against illness.

These findings need to be re-examined amongst married employed Asian women in Britain. A search for empirical research on dual-earner Asian households shows few descriptive accounts of the lives of Asian women. Bhachu's (1981) account of the lives of Sikh women in Britain argues strongly for the way in which waged work empowers Sikh women and has definite effects within the domestic sphere, giving Sikh women more resources with which to negotiate changes in the division of labour within the home and also in the patterns of expenditure. Women's experience of paid work outside the home enables them to obtain autonomy as managers exercising power and control. The importance of paid work and the way in which women's roles are socially constructed through familial ideologies is crucial. Bhachu argues that gender roles have been redefined in the nuclear households as they are more conducive to egalitarian relationships. There is not necessarily a radical shift in perceptions of what is 'masculine' and 'feminine' but there is a revision of male and female roles which has resulted in men being more involved in the household due to women's involvement in the labour market.

It is believed that the primary reasons given for Asian women seeking work outside the home are economic. Asian women work primarily to supplement the incomes earned by their husbands and in most cases they enter the workforce at a stage in the family life cycle when domestic responsibilities and expenses are at their heaviest, and the psycho-social costs associated with this role are enormous. Due to the so-called 'homemaker' role for Asian women, few married Asian women regard paid work as a liberating experience.

This chapter aims to give a theoretical and experiential account of Asian dual-earner households in Britain.

Asians in Britain: Cultural Diversity and Gender Roles

The Asians in Britain are a distinctive cultural group, characterized by strong family ties, shared values and norms within different sub-groups. Despite the traditional trend observed among Asian women as housewives, a growing number of this group has entered into the job market in recent years. A social survey (Brown, 1984) has highlighted that among Asian women in Britain, 42 percent of those 19 years old, 20 percent of those 20-24 years old, 17 percent and 14 percent of those 25-34 and 35-44 years old, respectively, are active in the labour market. The marital status of these groups is not shown in this survey, nevertheless, in line with the tradition of these cultural groups (marriage at an early age is a common feature for women), it can be assumed that the majority of these women are married. The family and societal demands for this group are different, as their roles, expectations, norms, values, economic necessity, career salience and aspiration levels are different. Moreover, the extended family system among Asians in Britain is still in practice. Thus, economically active women have to bear the major extended domestic responsibilities irrespective of their employment status, and are expected to perform the homemaker role. The socio-cultural constraints in association with role overloads (joint responsibilities of household and career) is believed to raise the level of stress and hence, illness.

Gender-role socialization for this cultural group is strongly determined by the traditional male/female typology. The assignment of a set of traits (e.g., submissiveness, compliance, passivity, helplessness, weakness) for Asian women is so strong as to be mistaken as innate or inevitable characteristics, the absence of which is termed as 'deviant' or 'abnormal.' The degree of assigning these traits vary across different cultures.

In discussing the ethnic and cultural issues of dual-earner families, therefore, we have to focus our attention on some of the ethnic and cultural factors, which may enable us to understand the similarity or differences in dual-role experiences among men and women in a diverse socio-cultural context. Some of the important issues are outlined below:

1. **Culturally embedded female traits.** Cultural variations in assigning traits to women, degree and extent, as discussed earlier.

2. **Social expectations and the role model.** Society expects women, especially Asian women, to take up the role of homemaker only. This stereotyped belief is supported by the observation of some women in this category. In the Asian community, it is often thought that men have "instrumental" (task-oriented) roles and women have "socio-emotional" roles which can only be fulfilled through the homemaker role. When women enter into the labour market they are challenging these existing roles and as a result, they begin to experience high levels of stress. It is unlikely that a woman's career is viewed as primary in dual-career marriages among British Asians. A wife's employment in a traditional position can also strongly affect her husband's self-concept by violating his role expectations with regard to his wife, threatening him, and causing him to feel more competitive.

3. **The male work ethic and role overload.** The male model of work assumes continuous employment from education to retirement, making no allowance for breaks for childbirth and child care, and is inappropriate for most women. In addition, the assumption of a full-time helpmate to provide domestic and child care support means that long and demanding work schedules incompatible with the dual earner lifestyles are often the norm. Hence many dual earner spouses suffer from overload, due to excessive demands at home and at work. The male model of work assumes a separation between the domains of work and family, but in reality they are interdependent

4. **Translation of biological differences among men and women.** In a traditional culture, such as Asian, the role of women is explained in terms of their physical features and is used to portray expected female behaviour such as child-bearing and care-giving. Women's working outside the home exceeds this biological deterministic theory and may cause conflicts and contradictions in their adjustment to the immediate environment.

5. **Role of religion and cultural beliefs.** The social definition of religion sometimes contradicts women's dual roles. Thus, some of the dominant orthodox religious groups discourage women from taking paid jobs, a practice congruent with the wider societal beliefs about

Asian women. This is more common among lower income groups, where both orthodox religious beliefs and stereotyped gender roles may have stronger influence. Employment among Asian women from this social group is rarely observed.

6. Ethnic hierarchy in the society. The position of women within their ethnic boundaries is an important determinant of the levels of stress or conflicts experienced in performing dual roles. Immigration to a new country further imposes a structure where men came to work and women came to care for the home. This arrangement is disrupted when women enter into the labour market, creating an imbalance in marital harmony and causing family discord.

7. The distribution of multiple roles. Cultural and familial ways of sharing roles vary from culture to culture. For example, in a traditional family system, domestic labour can be shared among the female members of the family, but in a nuclear family it has to be shared between husband and wife. In the latter case, tension can be increased if the labour is not distributed equally. Extended households with several dual-career couples are rare in Britain but dual-earner families in an extended family setting are not uncommon amongst Asians living in Britain. The most frequently cited example is the self-employed Asian household. It is not known to the author whether performing housework is stressful for self-employed partners. The nature of the distribution of multiple roles within this type of household has not been well-documented. This issue deserves research attention.

Conclusion

In summary, despite strong interest in Asian culture, marriage and family system in Britain, little attention has been given to the gendered division of labour, the extent to which Asian women are influenced by the Western work ethic, and the feminist movement among diverse socio-cultural groups. These issues need to be empirically examined. In this chapter an attempt is made to identify some of the salient socio-cultural factors which may enable us to better understand the similarities or differences in dual-role experiences of men and women and the relationship of these experiences to well-being.

This paper was developed while the author was at the Social and Applied Psychology Research Unit, Sheffield, England. Part of this paper was presented at the International Conference on Dual-Earner Families in London, 23 April, 1992.

References

Barnett, R.C. and G.K. Baruch. 1985. "Women's Involvement in Multiple Roles and Psychological Distress." *Journal of Personality and Social Psychology* 49:135-145.

Beutell, N.J. and J.H. Greenhaus. 1981. "Inter-Role Conflict Among Married Women: The Influence of Husband and Wife Characteristics on Conflict and Coping Behaviour." Working Paper, Seton Hall University and Drexel University.

Bebbington, A.C. 1973. "The Function of Stress in the Establishment of the Dual-Career Family." *Journal of Marriage and the Family* 35.

Bhachu, P. 1981. *Marriage and Dowry Among Selected East African Sikh Families in the UK.* Unpublished Ph.D. thesis, University of London.

Brown, G.W. and T. Harris. 1978. *Social Origins of Depression: A Study of Psychiatric Disorder in Women.* London: Tavistock.

Brown, C. 1984. *Black and White Britain. The Third PSI Survey.* London: Heinemann.

Cochrane, R. and M. Stopes-Roe. 1981. "Women, Marriage, Employment and Mental Health." *British Journal of Psychiatry* 139:373-381.

Froberg, D., D. Gjerdingen and M. Preston. 1986. "Multiple Roles and Women's Mental and Physical Health: What We Have Learned." *Women and Health* 11:79-96.

Greenhaus, J.H. and R.E. Kopelman. 1981. "Conflict Between Work and Non-Work Roles: Implications for the Career Planning Progress." *Human Resource Planning* 4:1-10.

Holahen, C.K. and L.A. Gillbert. 1979. "Inter-Role Conflict for Working Women: Career vs Jobs." *Journal of Applied Psychology* 64:80-90.

Kendel, D.B., M. Davies and V.H. Ravies. 1985. "The Stressfulness of Daily Social Roles for Women: Marital, Occupational and Household Roles." *Journal of Health and Social Behavior* 26:64-66.

Lewis, S., and L.C. Cooper. 1987. "Stress in Two-Earner Couples and Stage in the Life-Cycle." *Journal of Occupational Psychology* 60:289-303.

Radloff, L.S. 1975. "Sex Differences in Depression: The Effects of Occupation and Marital Status." *Sex Roles* 1:249-265.

Rahman, M. and N. Sorcar. 1981. "Working Women, Job Pressure and Marital Satisfaction." *The Dhaka University Studies* XV:112-124.

Rapaport, R. and R.N. Rapaport. 1978. *Working Couples.* New York: Harper and Row.

Rosenfield, S. 1980. "Sex Differences in Depression: Do Women Always Have Higher Rates?" *Journal of Health and Social Behavior* 21:33-42.

Sekaran, U. 1983. "Factors Influencing the Quality of Life in Dual-Career Families." *Journal of Occupational Psychology* 56:161-174.

Sorensen, G. and M.L. Verbrugge. 1987. "Women, Work and Health." *Annual Review of Public Health* 8: 235-251.

Sorcar, N. and M. Rahman. 1985. "Job Pressure, Life Description and Dyadic Adjustment of Career Women." *The Journal of Social Development* 2:1-12.

Shams, M. 1985. "Mental Health and Dual Career Women." *Dhaka University Journal of Psychology* I5:59-67.

Thoits, P.A. 1986. "Multiple Identities: Examining Gender and Marital Status Differences in Distress." *American Sociological Review* 51:259-272.

Warr, P. and G. Parry. 1982. "Paid Employment and Women's Psychological Well-Being." *Psychological Bulletin* 91:498-516.

20

Challenges of Research with Seniors

M. Peggy MacLeod

Although we tend to categorize them, seniors are a very diverse group. Even divisions such as young old, 65- 75 years; old, 75-85 years; and old old, 85 years and over, are not enough to allay the problems with attempts to view those over 65 as a group. It is recognized that people become more disparate as they age, not only because of physical differences but because of life experiences, which includes immersion in a cultural climate. However there are some general problems encountered in research with those 65 years of age and over. The challenges pertain to the aging process, sampling bias, and ethical considerations. Recommendations for dealing with these challenges will follow.

There are many sensory changes to deal with at varying levels; those applicable to research mainly involve auditory and visual senses. Auditory changes can be expected, especially when one considers that 30 percent of the older population have significant hearing loss (Matteson and McConnell, 1988). The visual constraints vary, often dependent on the current correction. The current corrections for vision will more and more depend on ability to pay in our province. However, all the techniques to aid communication must be tried - including altering background noise, employing the best lighting, attention to size of print and colour of stationery.

The most noticeable difference in dealing with seniors and a younger group is the *pace*. Seniors are slow when answering a questionnaire. They ponder. The conclusion that this is due to a slowing of mental function is premature - it can be more likely attributed to weighing the answer they wish to give. They have a lot more to consider. The other reason they are slower is they may not be as familiar with forms as we of the younger cohort have become. This is a generality, there will be those who are quite familiar with paperwork. The most efficient gentleman I encountered was one who had been in the insurance business.

There are other differences in this population as well. Jobe and Mingay (1990) reported that respondents found difficulty translating frequency information asked for in questionnaires into the categories specified. Often the answer they gave was more specific than the one asked for. Surveys, because of the potential wide number of people reached, are frequently used in research design. Kaye, Lawton and Kaye (1990) demonstrated a decline in willingness to participate associated with increasing age. Thus the representativeness of the sample becomes questionable.

If a convenience sample is used, senior buildings are a prime source of subjects. It makes good use of time and is cost effective when a high density concentration of seniors are found in one place. Unfortunately, they may not be representative of the total population. Different buildings tend to attract distinct populations. The populations in the buildings can be differentiated by religious affiliation, ethnic background, or area of settlement, i.e., home town area. This can be a benefit if a specific population is sought but caution must be used to extrapolate to the total population.

Telephone surveys do not have a good representation of older adults, personal interviews are preferred (Carter et al., 1991). Seniors who do agree to participate in research are more positive about being used as a subject, giving samples or being examined, feeling pleasant after answering questions, not considering it an intrusion, feeling that the research will help others, enjoying answering questions, telling their real feelings, not feeling upset after answering the questions and participating in a study of new medicines (Kaye et al., 1990). These authors concluded that if the benefits of the research are explained and the interviewer is a pleasant and non-threatening person, the response rate would be higher.

Research is difficult. A co-operative, able subject is a boon to enable data collection. Communication in some form or another is mandatory. If we as researchers have decided to use a written questionnaire that must be completed by the respondent, the language in which the questionnaire is printed is an important consideration. For instance if the language is English, we may exclude a certain proportion of the cohort who are over 65 now because of Saskatchewan immigration patterns. According to Freisen (1987), almost half of all prairie residents at the start of the First World War had been born in another country. The proportion was still one in three as late as 1931. Recent immigration patterns point to an increasing cultural and linguistic diversity in Canada. If the subject speaks another language, a translator can be employed, yet this too can be fraught with difficulties. We can also insure that we choose questionnaires that are administered verbally if the subjects can understand English, which addresses the problem of literacy or visual impairment.

In a sample I used, the response rate for an interview format was very different in two buildings. In a building which had a distinct cultural background, the response rate was 35.7 percent; while in the building which had representation of an English-speaking culture, the response rate was 74.6 percent. As researchers it is important to be aware of sampling biases - from language barriers, complications of aging which include auditory and visual changes, and also from requiring too much from the subjects. If we exclude the subjects who cannot read our questionnaires, who either cannot understand or read English, who are not comfortable, then our samples tend to be representative of the most able, English speaking seniors. If we fall prey to convenience sampling and rely on seniors' buildings, those samples are representative of the most able of a particular community.

Difficulty in reading can also limit the selection of subjects because of the ethical requirement of a consent form. To address this requisite, the researcher may read the consent form with or to the subject, have it in large dark print on a white or yellow background and leave a copy of the consent with the subject.

The limitations of employing only one type of research in this population can lead to an inadequately researched issue. Qualitative data can be exceedingly rich with this group. Qualitative methods allow time for reflection and exploration of an issue in order to investigate the question thoroughly. Although quantitative methods are still funded more readily and in some circles given more credence, qualitative methodology is gaining momentum. The advantages for using it in this group are that it can be presented orally, the interview is usually relaxed and the subjects are not faced with unfamiliar paperwork.

My recommendations for doing research with people age 65 and over are:

- If possible use personal interview for data collection.
- Employ a personable interviewer who is able to explain the benefits of the research.

- Use a large print consent form but read it with them.

- If a tool in the form of a questionnaire is to be administered use one that can be administered orally.

- Take into consideration the setting for the interview. Comfort of the subject is important; a well lit, quiet environment is ideal.

- Qualitative research methods are particularly appropriate for this age group. The use of triangulation would be wise to employ in the research design so that an accurate portrayal of the issue is reached.

Seniors, disparate as they are, offer unique challenges in research. If we want to generalize to the senior population, a representative sample will include seniors of other cultures and those who speak and read languages other than the two official languages in Canada. Careful consideration of their potential limitations and innovative designs can mediate most problems encountered.

References

Carter, W.B., R. Elward, J. Malmgren, M. Martin and E. Larson. 1991. "Participation of Older Adults in Health Programs and Research: A Critical Review of the Literature." *The Gerontologist* 31: 584-592.

Friesen, G. 1987. *The Canadian Prairies: A History.* Toronto: University of Toronto Press.

Jobe, J.B. and D.J. Mingay. 1990. "Cognitive Laboratory Approach to Designing Questionnaires for Surveys of the Elderly." *Public Health Reports* 105: 518-524.

Kaye, J., P. Lawton, and D. Kaye. 1990. "Attitudes of Elderly People About Clinical Research on Aging." *The Gerontologist* 30: 100-106.

Matteson, M.A. and E.S. McConnell. 1988. *Gerontological Nursing: Concepts and Practice.* Toronto: W.B. Saunders Co.

21

Arranged Marriages and Mental Health Among Immigrant Women

Lou Heber

Introduction

The increasing cultural diversity of the Canadian population offers new opportunities for research in the health care field. One such area is the health consequences of migration and cultural adjustment and adaptation to a new country. Anderson (1985), Stern (1985), and Taft (1985) focus on immigrant women's psychosocial health, occupation and cultural differences, and adjustment problems in the host country. They provide some awareness of how minority women adjust, work, and maintain self-esteem as a wife, a worker, and as a client in the health care system. As Canada continues to welcome new immigrants, it is becoming clear that the resettlement experience can have profound impacts on the social and psychological well-being of some of these immigrants, especially those involved in intercultural and interracial marriages.

This chapter examines the issue of arranged marriages and mental health among immigrant women from the Philippines in Canada. Arranged marriages here refers to marriage through "pen pal" courtship and "mail order" brides. Arranged marriages were once a phenomenon of World War II "war brides." There were many successes in these marriages, but there were also some adjustment problems. The findings are based on observations and psychiatric assessments of 21 cases of immigrant women, 12 of whom were involved in arranged marriages.

Adjustment Process

The process of adjustment follows several stages. These are: a honeymoon stage, a period of culture shock, a surface (superficial) adjustment stage, a period of unresolved problems, and full adjustment (Range, 1984). The first four stages are the most relevant to this research and are discussed below.

Honeymoon Stage

The Filipina and her family in the Philippines have expectations for immigration abroad that encourage marriages. These expectations include economic and social mobility in that financial support for the bride's family is enhanced, and social elevation in a stratified society becomes possible. Family pressures for the immigrant to meet these expectations are often extreme and long-lasting. Ongoing expectations create initial euphoria for the immigrant's family, but create stress for the immigrant woman.

The Canadian Government is also involved in the Honeymoon Stage through immigration requirements as a set of expectations based on a point system for Landed Immigrant Status (Bonavia, 1974). The Canadian Government ends its involvement with the immigrant woman once these requirements are met, and it does not intervene or follow-up on the adjustment process.

Culture Shock Period

Culture shock is a condition of disorientation when an individual is suddenly exposed to a foreign social and cultural environment. Culture shock is described by Range (1984: 60) in the following manner: "The excitement is gone; things are not like 'back home'; social cues and relationships are difficult; there are feelings of alienation and homesickness, temporary dislike of the host culture." The Culture Shock Stage for the immigrant bride exacerbates the adjustment to marriage and increases the individual immigrant's level of stress, often beyond the point of emotional or psychological tolerance.

Surface Adjustment Stage

The immigrant bride experiences a period of initial adjustment to marriage. This adjustment may be part of the Honeymoon Stage; appearance of adjustment may be minimal in concrete changes due to increased familiarity with the social and cultural conditions, and not to the adjustment to an arranged marriage. This false adjustment may be a permanent condition causing underlying unresolved problems.

Period of Unresolved Problems

For some immigrant women, unresolved adjustment problems due to the social and cultural environment and to marriage may become manifest early in the individual's experience. For others, these problems may be expressed later in married life, depending upon the severity of the problems and the individual's ability to cope. Unfamiliarity with the values, institutional systems, and lifestyle of the host environment poses some difficulties in the adjustment process that may produce increased individual stress. However, emotional stress may also come out of feelings of guilt, loss of self-esteem, or from isolation. Immigrant women who are party to arranged marriages are faced with a unique set of adjustment problems that are often personal in nature and for which outside support or recognition is lacking.

Unresolved problems of adjustment to an arranged marriage can become manifest through psychological breakdown with psychiatric symptoms of depression (underactive behavior), withdrawn behavior, or disorientation. The following two case studies are provided to indicate the degree of affect that can occur for immigrant brides facing unresolved problems in adapting or failing to adapt to their new condition.

Case Studies

As illustrations, two case studies are presented here.

Case Study I

Client History

A psychiatric client diagnosed as having "chronic schizophrenia," an 18-year-old Filipina from the City of Cebu, married after a brief courtship in the Philippines to a Canadian of Scottish ethnic background. The parents felt their daughter's marriage to a Canadian would be secure and happy since Canada is more stable economically and politically than the Philippines. They also felt that a Canadian husband could provide financial security for their daughter and financial support to her family. The client was passive, limited in English, and had little education and working experience. She was left for long periods with her husband's family, while he was away working in the Canadian North. The attending psychiatrist requested my opinion, and formal consultation was done in my office.

Initial Client Interview

The client was smiling and pleasant on approach and was "pleased" to see me as an acquaintance and countrywoman. She immediately spoke in "Visayan" and discussed openly her problems. She cried and felt "shame" for her marriage troubles. She appeared "fearful" of her husband, and some of her responses were vague. During subsequent visits, the client was heavily medicated and often "hysterical." I asked her if she would like to go home to the Philippines. She stated, "My mother won't let me, and she does not know what's happening to me now." She expressed that she wanted to go home, but she cannot because her husband won't let her go. The following findings were recorded during the series of interviews and counselling sessions:

Findings

1. **Isolation** - client was linguistically, socially, and physically isolated.
2. **Lack of Support** - client's husband was absent for long periods. Client was kept from visiting her only friend.
3. **Abuse** - client's in-laws had a history of drug abuse, and drew the client into drug and sexual abuse.
4. **Helplessness** - client felt pressures of obligation to meet her parents' and family's expectations in the Philippines. These obligations produced feelings of guilt and helplessness, which increased as her emotional condition deteriorated. Psychiatric care was not effective in resolving the client's problems. Follow-up care and intervention was hampered by the intransigent attitude of the husband.

Case Study II

Client History

Mrs. Y., a 45-year-old female, former school teacher from the Visayan region, Philippines, married after a pen pal courtship to a farmer in Central Saskatchewan. They took up residence on the farm in a remote rural area of the province.

Arranged Marriages and Mental Health

A year after the birth of their son, Mrs. Y. started to cry and act bizarre, as observed by neighbors. During the winter, she attempted to run away with her baby and was found several miles from home without shoes or warm clothing. I was requested by a friend of the family to visit her.

Findings

1. **Isolation.** Mrs. Y. lives in physical isolation on a rural farm in Central Saskatchewan. She has no driving skills and minimal working skills.
2. **Lack of Support.** Mrs. Y. has cultivated no friends in the community and has no relatives in Canada. Her husband is socially retarded, meaning poor interpersonal relations, and has few friends.
3. **Helplessness.** Mrs. Y. felt she had no way out of her situation and finally became resigned to her condition.

Case Profile Summaries

This section summarizes the characteristics of those women interviewed who had arranged marriages, in terms of age, length of stay in Canada, courtship process, circumstances of marriage, behavior pattern and nursing diagnosis.

    A. **Age Range**
Brides:
41% - (N-5) - 17 years to 34 years old
58% - (N-7) - 35 years to 58 years old
Husbands:
66% - (N-8) - 25 to 54 years old
33% - (N-4) - 55 to 72 years old

    B. **Length of Stay in Canada (Filipino Women)**
33% - (N-4) - 3 months to one year
25% - (N-3) - 2 years to 3 years
41% - (N-5) - 4 years to 7 years

    C. **Courtship Process**
66% - (N-8) - pen pal
16% - (N-2) - mail order bride
16% - (N-2) - introduced by friends and married after a brief courtship

D. **Circumstances of Marriage**
    - pen pal communication was superficial
    - lack of knowledge of the life skills and 'values' of fiance
    - husband is conservative with poor interpersonal relations
    - couple live in relative isolation
    - lack of friends and support
    - breakdown in communication between wife and spouse
    - lack of client's understanding of spouse's family background
    - expressed prejudices to the client by members of the spouse's family

E. **Behavior Pattern (Immigrant - Married Filipino Women)**
    - passive and nonassertive
    - underactive, crying episode, and low self-esteem
    - anxious, indecisiveness
    - resigned to her duty as housewife
    - maintained a "master-servant" relationship
    - culture shock still apparent

F. **Nursing Diagnosis** - when referral was sought by a friend or psychiatric referral for further cultural and mental health assessment.
    50% - (N-6) - withdrawal with some psychotic features
    33% - (N-4) - severe depression
                    (underactive with low self-esteem)
    16% - (N-2) - anxious - indecisiveness

Summary of Identified Problems of Arranged Marriages

This section provides a summary of many of the problems of arranged marriages.

1. **No friends or support system.**
    - no socialization and interaction outside of the home
2. **No relatives in host country.**
    - no blood relative nor extended family member in Canada
3. **English language skills at minimum.**
    - spoke 'Piglish" as practised in rural Philippines ("Piglish" is a mixture of Filipino and English)
    - educational background ranges from grade 7 to college education in the Philippines
    - English language spoken at minimum in home country

4. **Non-assertive personality.**
   - no eye contact
   - incongruency of verbal and nonverbal
   - will not openly confront husband regarding own feelings
5. **No driving skills.**
   - unable to drive
   - no license
   - discouraged by husband.
6. **No employment opportunity.**
   - credentials from the Philippines not acceptable by Canadian standards
   - distance of home also a factor (some live in rural farm communities)
7. **Minimal working skills.**
   - no background of Canadian work ethic
   - lack of competitiveness
   - only domestic or service work related areas identified

Conclusions

This study focussed on health consequences of arranged marriage for a small sample of immigrant women from the Philippines. Many of these women experienced depression and withdrawn behavior and displayed some degree of social and psychological trauma that could be attributed to their adjustment to marriage and to the new environment. Studies involving larger populations and different ethnocultural immigrant groups will provide valuable data on health status and health behavior of immigrants which could also be useful for health policy and delivery of health care to these groups.

References

Anderson, J. 1985. "Perspective on the Health of Immigrant Women: A Feminist Analysis." *Advances in Nursing Science* October.

Andrews, M. and P. Ludwig (eds.). 1984. "Nursing Practice in a Kaleidoscope of Culture." Conference Proceedings. Salt Lake City: University of Utah.

Heber, L. 1986. "Ethnic Women and Self-Esteem." Paper presented at the International Health Conference for Women's Issues, Halifax, Nova Scotia.

Heber, W. 1979. *Filipino Ritual Kinship: A Study of Filipino Social Integration in Nova Scotia.* Unpublished thesis. Halifax, Nova Scotia: St. Mary's University.

Range, M. 1984. "Preparation for International Nursing: Ivory Tower vs. Trial and Error." In M. Andrews and P. Ludwig (Eds.), *Nursing Practise in a Kaleidoscope of Culture.* Salt Lake City: University of Utah.

Stern, P. (ed.). 1985. *Women, Health and Culture.* Washington, D.C.: Hemisphere Publishing Co.

Taft, L. 1985. "Self-Esteem in Later Life: A Nursing Perspective." *Advances in Nursing Science* October.

22

Ethics and Research

Michael Owen

Introduction

It is not unusual for researchers in Canadian universities to encounter ethical dilemmas in the conduct of their research, especially when that research crosses cultural boundaries and disciplinary boundaries, and impacts on gender or gender relations. While researchers inevitably rely on the ethical guidelines developed by professional societies (e.g., the American Psychological Association or the Canadian Sociological Association) research councils (e.g., the Medical Research Council or the Social Sciences and Humanities Research Council), or international protocols (e.g., The Declaration of Helsinki), inevitably these guidelines do not provide the researcher with all the necessary information, advice and direction for the conduct of research related to health, medicine, racial minorities and women. These are some of the issues that I wish to address.

As with many individuals in universities, I wear three hats: university teacher, researcher and administrator. Each is distinct but not isolated from the other. As a teacher, one is careful to present to students the collective wisdom of scholars in one's field, within the context and boundaries of a course. As I teach in the history of education, research from social historians, feminist historians, sociologists, psychologists and education, influence the way in which I present to students issues in educational history - women as teachers, students and mothers; schools and ethnic minorities; concepts of childhood; and the relations between state policy and educational practice. Each of these sub-categories requires one to be sensitive to the needs and backgrounds of the students in the particular class, including their gender, ethnicity and social origins; both in the way in which one approaches a particular subject and the way in which different individuals may react to one's presentation. While university teachers need to be true to their disciplinary focus, the presentation of a particular subject matter needs to be contextualised to reflect the way in which social institutions impact on women, children, ethnic and racial minorities, and social classes.

As a researcher who conducts research on the role of women and the interaction between mainline institutions and ethnic minorities, often in the provision of social and medical services, I am particularly concerned that the research I conduct, primarily in institutional and public archives, meets with the standards imposed on me by my profession and by the archives as custodians of personal papers, government documents, and other materials. As a historian, I am confronted with the need to read beyond the official reports of church societies and missionaries, even women missionaries, to determine how their activities were accepted or deflected by their clients. The need exists within my field to reflect faithfully the intentions of the women and men missionaries and, perhaps more importantly, the way in which these services had an impact on the Aboriginal or new Canadian clients. Ethical dilemmas arise on a regular basis in this research, in what to research and how to interpret the historical record. Ethical dilemmas also arise in how one handles sensitive documents, especially personal letters and confidential assessments of colleagues or clients, that make their way into archival records.

As a university administrator, coordinating requests for ethical reviews of research in the social sciences and health sciences, my task is as much educational as it is monitorial. Much of the debate that occurs within universities, here and elsewhere, is why it is necessary for researchers from all disciplines and at all stages in their careers to have their research protocols reviewed by Institutional Review Boards (IRBs).

Role of Institutional Review Boards (Ethics Committees)

From my perspective, IRBs serve four major roles: (1) to protect human subjects who are expected to participate in the research, by ensuring that the research protocol is ethically sound and, particularly, that the subjects are fully aware of the objectives of the research and any risks and/or benefits that may accrue to them as a result of their participation; (2) to protect researchers by providing them with arms-length reviews of their protocols and assurances that their rights will be protected (e.g., protection under an institution's liability insurance for clinical or behavioural procedures that may present risks to the subjects, or for suits brought against the researcher by subjects); (3) to provide the institutional ethical review for research proposals submitted to outside agencies (e.g., Social Sciences and Humanities Research Council, the National Cancer Institute of Canada, Health and Welfare Canada NHRDP, National Institutes of Health (US)); and (4) to assist researchers (faculty and students) in their research endeavours. Institutional Review Boards are not roadblocks to the conduct of research. Institutional Review Boards do not unnecessarily delay approval of protocols, although they may from time to time request that researchers justify the use of particular procedures, the use of deception, the lack of use of consent forms when conducting interviews, and the disposition of data, especially audio- and video-tapes. By reviewing protocols and seeking clarification on particular aspects of the protocol, IRBs should be seen as facilitators, as yet another set of eyes to review the research protocol to protect the rights of the subjects, the community, the researchers, and the institution. Thus the questions that should be asked are: (1) how can IRBs assist researchers; (2) what are the researcher's responsibilities; and (3) what are the institution's (IRBs) responsibilities?

General Guidelines on Research Ethics

IRBs work on the assumption that the researcher (either the faculty member or the student under the supervision of the faculty member) is a professional and an ethical person.

Each professional association (e.g., psychologists, sociologists, clinicians) subscribe to specific ethical practices, all of which have some common bases (advancement of knowledge/science, advancement of social behaviour, to assist populations, to cause as little discomfort to subjects, etc.) Moreover, researchers at universities are expected to adhere to the ethical guidelines of granting agencies (e.g., SSHRC and NRC) and to international conventions (e.g., The Declaration of Helsinki). Combined professional standards and agency guidelines provide the researcher and the IRS with sufficient information on how best to develop research protocols from an ethical perspective and the basis on which to evaluate these protocols.

An underlying assumption contained in all guidelines and the work of SRBs is that the proposed research is ethical and is scientifically/

academically valid. In an educational institution we cannot proceed from any other basis. The IRBs, then, rarely review proposals to provide a stamp of academic or scientific validity. That is the responsibility of the researcher, the graduate supervisor/committee, the department head and dean, and/or the external peer review process. Institutional Review Boards review proposals for ethical concerns that from time to time are underestimated, ignored or slip by researchers in the development of the research methodology.

Issues that Confront IRBS that Relate to the Themes of this Conference -- Women, Racial Minorities, Medicine & Health

Issues that confront IRBs when presented with protocols that impact on any one or more of the sub-themes, e.g., racial or ethnic minorities and medicine, are many. Institutional Review Boards require that the researcher inform subjects of the nature of the research, why it is being conducted, what the subjects' roles are and why, what the risks and benefits (if any) are, that the services received by the subjects are not dependent on participation in the research project, that they may withdraw at any time or not respond to the questions or procedures, the right to confidentiality, and how the subjects will be informed of the results of the research or debriefed if deception has been employed. In short, IRBs need to be assured that the subject's participation in any research activity is voluntary and informed and that the subject's rights/person are protected.

Now these may appear, on the surface, to be common-sense types of things that any researcher would do. It is surprising, however, how many proposals, both in the health sciences and behavioural sciences, do not do so. There are many questions of an ethical nature (some raised at this conference) that need consideration.

(A) One difficult area that IRBs deal with is research with dependent/captive populations (e.g., prisoners, the homeless, those requiring services in hospitals, clinics and/or social agencies). When one incorporates into this equation issues of culture and gender, then additional responsibilities are placed on the researcher, whether they are an academic or a medical practitioner. How does one ensure that dependent and captive populations are informed of their rights? How does one ensure that they understand their rights to participate? How do subjects' dependencies on drugs, or subjects who are not literate in the language in which the researcher is operating, or whose age and mental abilities do not allow them to understand the research description and instructions, especially if related to their health, and which impact on their ability to consent to participate in a research study, provide assent to become involved in the study? What is the role of surrogates in providing consent for these individuals? These are concerns confronted by researchers and IRBs on a regular basis.

In some instances, particularly with native populations, it is essential that the researcher obtain the permission of, and in some cases involve, the governing authority of a band before a research study can be undertaken with the members of the band or tribal council. While this is important, especially in the area of providing adequate information in culturally appropriate ways to study participants, is the permission of the authorities enough or must the researcher also have individual consent forms signed by the subjects, as a protection for the subject and the researcher?

(B) When conducting research that crosses cultural boundaries, either recent immigrant populations or groups that have amalgamated into the larger society (e.g., the Scots), the researcher needs to be careful to understand, as much as possible, the cultural milieu in which she/he will be operating. This is important not only for access to the cultural group, but also for ensuring the validity of the data, i.e., the subjects have understood the purposes of the research and have responded to the questions or other modes of inquiry accurately. One method used successfully by many researchers is to employ an individual from that cultural group to help formulate the questions, to assist in the conduct of the research, and to interpret that data. Again when one introduces gender into the equation, depending on the nature of the research and the cultural and religious population, the researchers are placed under additional constraints.

(C) A major problem arises when the research population is small, from an isolated region or a peculiar institution, or from dependent populations. Researchers, subjects and IRBs are interested in how best to protect the identity of the subjects and their rights to privacy. It is not unusual in the information provided to subjects, either in written form or orally, that the identity of the subjects will remain confidential and that the responses provided cannot be traced to an individual. But are these assurances realistic when the number (N) is very small? In addition, when dealing with gender, racial or ethnic minorities and health issues, it is not unusual to have research studies focussed on small populations with identifiable characteristics, e.g., diabetes mellitus among Aboriginal populations. When researchers work among populations that are small, it may not always be possible to ensure the anonymity of participants and the confidentiality of an individual's responses. This becomes especially problematic when the researcher provides a debriefing to participants in a small community.

(D) What happens to the data after they are collected, analyzed, manipulated? How are the data stored? It is always a concern that confidential research data will be used for purposes for which they were not intended. Researchers need to state clearly the purpose for which the data, especially audio- and video-tape data are being used, how and where they are to be stored, and how they will be disposed of at the end of the project. Unless such assurances of secure storage and disposition are provided, then it is not unreasonable for potential subjects to refuse to participate in a study. The SSHRC recommends that data collected from large surveys are preserved and stored with an organization (e.g., archives, university survey centre or data bank) "which can ensure preservation and distribution and that they are used in an ethical way." The usual protection of anonymity of respondents is provided.

The SSHRC guidelines for researchers who conduct survey research has provided excellent advice for researchers on the storage of data collected with public funding. This advice, I feel, is appropriate for all data collected through research studies that utilize the public as subjects or public funds. In its guidelines, SSHRC states that "data collected in a survey supported by the Council are public property and not the property of the principal investigator. They must eventually be made available to other scholars." Such storage and accessibility of data ensure that the data become sources for other scholarly works and for replication and re-analysis. It is possible that these data banks, identified by the SSHRC, could become fruitful sources for graduate students who need survey materials for their research but for whom resources to conduct large scale surveys are scarce.

(E) How do we inform the people with whom we have conducted research on the results of that research? Why should we do so? One of the most interesting aspects of the ethics review process is that of debriefing. I use the term "debriefing" not in its formal sense related specifically to studies that involve deception but in the way that the public would use the term, that is, to inform the study participants of the results of the research. Many researchers ignore the need to provide some mechanism for debriefing subjects. At the University of Saskatchewan, debriefing, or informing subjects of the results of the research, has become an important part of the review process. One reason for a mechanism to debrief participants is good public relations, especially if one's research is being conducted in an inter-cultural setting. The main reason, however, is that subjects should know what the results of the research study were. If we as researchers are interested in maintaining good relations with ethnic or racial groups with whom we wish to work, it is essential that we inform them about the results of the research that we conducted with them. If we do not keep them informed of the results of our research, these individuals become the objects of research and it is unlikely that they would be willing to participate in follow-up or future studies. As health prevention and health care research, including attitudes toward health care and medicine among ethnic or racial groups and between genders, attain a higher priority among national granting agencies and provincial health departments, longitudinal and short term studies that are follow-up studies of previous research become important. If we as researchers consider only publication of the results of our research in academic journals as the primary goal, then we do a disservice to the people on whom we rely for details of their individual lives and cultural insights.

Moreover, debriefing is not an onerous responsibility. Depending on the nature of the study, debriefing could be an article in a professional journal, a short story in a local newspaper, or a brief note in a newsletter that is distributed widely in a community. Debriefing could be more intensive and include a presentation to a band council and then one to the wider community in which principal researchers and their co-researchers outline the results of the research and respond to questions from the community on the implications of the findings for that community.

(F) With the funding agencies' current emphasis on inter- and multi-disciplinary research and with research conducted by teams who come from different universities and jurisdictions, researchers confront the problem of multiple approvals. Each institution requires its own review of the research protocol. Although this does not usually pose a problem, it is not unusual for different IRBs to request different additions or changes to a protocol. Ideally an approval from one committee should be enough. As one recent national study on relations between male and female students demonstrated, not all IRBs had similar concerns. The researchers and the collaborators at each institution needed to address sensitive issues including those of confidentiality of the questionnaires, the administration of the questionnaires in large lecture theatres in ways that permitted confidentiality and privacy, and adequate information on the purposes of the study prior to the administration of the questionnaire and debriefing of the respondents, both immediately after the administration of the questionnaire and, later, once the results of the larger study become known.

Conclusion

There are, of course, many other issues which could be considered. There are, from some perspectives, good reasons for "deception" in the conduct of research with human subjects, for example in the study of "glass ceilings" with respect to gender or ethnicity in certain organizations or occupations. The use of deception in any study requires, from the perspective of an IRB, good justification and not be seen from simply a political perspective. We know, for example, of studies conducted in the past that would be considered unethical by any standards. Institutional Review Boards and researchers need to be cautious that studies conducted for narrowly political reasons, however laudatory now, are not similarly condemned in the future.

The role of ethics committees at universities in the review of protocols - either behavioural or health sciences - must be seen as a necessary step in any research study, as necessary as the development of clear hypotheses and methods. Indeed, in most cases, the development of a good research study that involves human subjects would necessarily address all the questions required or concerns raised by an ethics committee. Moreover, the review of any study by an ethics committee should be seen as an asset to the researcher and not as a barrier. Such reviews are usually completed promptly and conditions or advice for revisions of questionnaires, consent forms or other instruments enhance the clarity of the study and should ensure that the researcher obtains as good if not more precise data. Moreover, such reviews provide the subject, researcher, and the institution with a measure of protection and confidence.